Arrhythmias in Adult Congenital Heart Disease

Arrhythmias in Adult Congenital Heart Disease

A Case-Based Approach

SESHADRI BALAJI, MBBS, MRCP(UK), PhD
Professor
Department of Pediatrics
Division of Cardiology
Oregon Health & Science University
Portland, OR, United States

RAVI MANDAPATI, MD, FHRS, FACC
Professor of Medicine & Pediatrics
Director, Loma Linda University International Heart Institute
Director, Cardiac Electrophysiology
Loma Linda University Health
Loma Linda, CA, United States

GARY D. WEBB, MD, FRCP(C)
Editor of the CHiP Network and the ACHD Learning Center
Editor of the Congenital Heart Disease Center of Excellence
Consultant to the Pediatric Learning Center
Consultant to the Cincinnati Adult Congenital Heart Program
Cincinnati, OH, United States
Consulting Cardiologist for the Toronto Congenital Cardiac Centre for Adults
Toronto, ON, Canada

ELSEVIER

ELSEVIER

3251 Riverport Lane
St. Louis, Missouri 63043

ARRHYTHMIAS IN ADULT CONGENITAL HEART DISEASE

Content Strategist: Robin Carter
Content Development Manager: Kathy Padilla
Content Development Specialist: Megan Ashdown
Publishing Services Manager: Shereen Jameel
Project Manager: Nadhiya Sekar
Designer: Gopalakrishnan Venkatraman

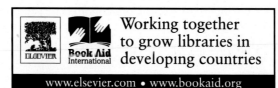

Working together to grow libraries in developing countries

www.elsevier.com • www.bookaid.org

List of Contributors

Victor A. Abrich, MD
2nd Year Electrophysiology Fellow
Mayo Clinic
Phoenix, AZ, United States

Rafael Alonso-Gonzalez, MD, MSc, FESC
Adult Congenital Heart Centre and National
    Centre of Pulmonary Hypertension
Royal Brompton Hospital
Imperial College London
London, United Kindgom

Reza Ashrafi, MBBS, BSc, MD, MRCP
North West Congenital Heart Disease Partnership
Liverpool Heart and Chest Hospital
Thomas Drive
Liverpool, United Kingdom

Peter F. Aziz, MD
Division of Pediatric Cardiology
Cleveland Clinic Children's Hospital
Cleveland, OH, United States

J.P. Bokma, MD, PhD
Department of Cardiology
Academic Medical Center
Amsterdam, The Netherlands

David J. Bradley, MD
Professor of Pediatric Cardiology
Section of Electrophysiology
CS Mott Children's Hospital
University of Michigan
Ann Arbor, MI, United States

Anica Bulic, MD
4th Year Fellow
Pediatric Cardiology
Stanford University
Stanford, CA, United States

Bryan Cannon, MD
Department of Pediatrics
Vice-Chair of Education
Division of Pediatric Cardiology
Director
Pediatric Arrhythmia and Pacing Service
Mayo Clinic
Rochester, MN, United States

Frank Cecchin, MD
Professor
Department of Pediatrics
Director
Division of Pediatric Cardiology
NYU Langone Medical Center
New York, NY, United States

**Santabhanu Chakrabarti, MBBS, MD, FRCPC,
    FRCP (Edin), FRCPCH, FACC, FHRS**
University of British Columbia
Department of Medicine
Division of Cardiology
Heart Rhythm Services
Vancouver, BC, Canada

Henry Chubb, MBBS, PhD
Postdoctoral Fellow
Pediatric Cardiac Electrophysiology
Stanford University
Palo Alto, CA, United States

Marc G. Cribbs, MD, FACC
Director
Alabama Adult Congenital Heart Program

Director
UAB Comprehensive Pregnancy & Heart Program

Assistant Professor
Medicine and Pediatrics
University of Alabama at Birmingham
Children's of Alabama
Birmingham, AL, United States

Damien Cullington, MBChB (Hons), MD, MRCP, FESC
Consultant
Adult Congenital Cardiologist
Leeds General Infirmary
Leeds, United Kingdom

Lara Curran, MBBS, BSc
Adult Congenital Heart Centre and National
    Centre of Pulmonary Hypertension
Royal Brompton Hospital
Imperial College London
London, United Kindgom

Joris R. de Groot, MD, PhD
Professor of Cardiac Electrophysiology
Department of Cardiology, Heart Center
Amsterdam University Medical Centers
University of Amsterdam
Amsterdam, The Netherlands

Natasja M.S. de Groot, MD, PhD
Department of Cardiology
Erasmus Medical Center
Rotterdam
The Netherlands

Konstantinos Dimopoulos, MD, MSc, PhD, FESC
Adult Congenital Heart Centre and National
    Centre of Pulmonary Hypertension
Royal Brompton Hospital
Imperial College London
London, United Kindgom

Anne M. Dubin, MD
Professor of Pediatrics
Pediatric Cardiology
Stanford University
Stanford, CA, United States

Vivienne Ezzat, MBChB
Consultant Electrophysiologist
Special Interest—Congenital Heart Disease
Barts Heart Centre
St. Bartholomew's Hospital
West Smithfield, London, United Kingdom

Frank Fish, MD
Professor of Pediatrics and Medicine
Director
Pediatric Electrophysiology
Vanderbilt University
Nashville, TN, United States

Kaveshree Govender, MD
University of British Columbia
Department of Medicine
Division of Cardiology
Vancouver, BC, Canada

Matthias Greutmann, MD, FESC
Congenital Heart Disease Unit
University Heart Center, Cardiology
Zurich, Switzerland

Louise Harris, MBChB, FRCP(C)
Staff Cardiologist
Peter Munk Cardiac Centre
University Health Network
Toronto Congenital Cardiac Centre for Adults
Professor
University of Toronto
Toronto, ON, Canada

Gabriele Hessling, MD
Professor
Pediatric Cardiology
Department of Electrophysiology
German Heart Center
Technical University of Munich
Munich, Germany

Charlotte A. Houck, MD
Department of Cardiology
Erasmus University Medical Center
Rotterdam, The Netherlands

Anna Kamp, MD, MPH
Electrophysiology and Pacing
Associate Fellowship Director
Nationwide Children's Hospital
Assistant Professor
Ohio State University
Columbus, OH, United States

Ronald Kanter, MD
Director of Electrophysiology
Nicklaus Children's Hospital
Miami, FL, United States

Peter P. Karpawich, MsC, MD, FAAP, FACC, FAHA, FHRS
Director
Cardiac Arrhythmia Services, Children's Hospital of Michigan
Professor
Wayne State University School of Medicine
Detroit, MI, United States

Naomi J. Kertesz, MD
Director of Electrophysiology and Pacing
Associate Medical Director of Cardiology
Nationwide Children's Hospital
Professor of Pediatrics
Ohio State University
Columbus, OH, United States

Jeffrey J. Kim, MD
Section of Pediatric Cardiology
Department of Pediatrics
Baylor College of Medicine
Texas Children's Hospital
Houston, TX, United States

Madhukar S. Kollengode, MD
ACHD/Cardiovascular Fellow
University of Colorado Denver
Division of Cardiology
Aurora, CO, United States

Wilson W. Lam, MD
Sections of Pediatric Cardiology & Cardiology
Departments of Pediatric and Internal Medicine
Baylor College of Medicine
Texas Children's Hospital
Houston, TX, United States

Andrea Lee, MD, FRCPC
University of British Columbia
Department of Medicine
Division of Cardiology
Vancouver, BC, Canada

Christopher J. McLeod, MBChB, PhD
Director of the Adult Congenital Arrhythmia Clinic
Division of Heart Rhythm Services
Department of Cardiovascular Disease
Mayo Clinic
Rochester, MN, United States

Tabitha G. Moe, MD
Adult Congenital Cardiology
Phoenix Children's Hospital
Phoenix, AZ, United States

Jeremy Moore, MD
Associate Clinical Professor & Program Director
Department of Pediatrics
Division of Cardiology
David Geffen School of Medicine
University of California Los Angeles
Los Angeles, CA, United States

Elisabeth M.J.P. Mouws, MD
Department of Cardiology
Erasmus Medical Center
Rotterdam
The Netherlands
Department of Cardiothoracic Surgery
Erasmus Medical Center
Rotterdam
The Netherlands

Barbara J.M. Mulder, MD, PhD
Professor of Cardiology
Department of Cardiology, Heart Center
Amsterdam University Medical Centers
University of Amsterdam
Amsterdam, The Netherlands
Netherlands Heart Institute
Utrecht, The Netherlands

Krishnakumar Nair, MBBS, CCDS, CCEP
Staff Cardiologist
Peter Munk Cardiac Centre
University Health Network
Toronto Congenital Cardiac Centre for Adults
Assistant Professor
University of Toronto
Toronto, ON, Canada

Duy T. Nguyen, MD
Associate Professor of Medicine
Section of Cardiac Electrophysiology
University of Colorado
Aurora, CO, United States

James Oliver, MBChB, PhD, MRCP
Consultant in Adult Congenital Heart Disease
Leeds Teaching Hospitals NHS Trust
Leeds, United Kingdom

Akash R. Patel, MD
Department of Pediatrics
UCSF School of Medicine
Division of Pediatric Cardiology
UCSF Benioff Children's Hospital
San Francisco, CA, United States

Department of Pediatrics
Director
Pediatric and Congenital Arrhythmia Service
UCSF Benioff Children's Hospital
San Francisco, CA, United States

Sruti Rao, MD
Division of Pediatric Cardiology
Cleveland Clinic Children's Hospital
Cleveland, OH, United States

Edward K. Rhee, MD
Director
Electrophysiology
Phoenix Children's Hospital
Clinical Associate Professor Child Health
University of Arizona College of Medicine
Phoenix, AZ, United States

Eric Rosenthal, MD FRCP
Consultant Paediatric and Adult Congenital
    Cardiologist
Evelina London Children's Hospital
St Thomas' Hospital
London, United Kingdom

Berardo Sarubbi, MD, PhD
Director
Adult Congenital Heart Disease Unit
Monaldi Hospital
Naples, Italy

Honorary Professor
Cardiovascular Disease
Parthnope University of Naples
Naples, Italy

Maully Shah, MBBS
Director of Electrophysiology
Division of Cardiology
The Children's Hospital of Philadelphia
University of Pennsylvania School of Medicine
Philadelphia, PA, United States

Kevin Shannon, MD
Clinical Professor
Ahmanson/UCLA Adult Congenital Heart Disease
    Center
UCLA Health Sciences
Los Angeles, CA, United States

Adam J. Small, MD
Adult Congenital Cardiology Fellow
Ahmanson/UCLA Adult Congenital Heart Disease
    Center
UCLA Health Sciences
Los Angeles, CA, United States

Narayanswami Sreeram, MD
Department of Cardiology
Heart Center
University Hospital of Cologne
Cologne, Germany

Daniel Steven, MD
Department of Cardiology
Heart Center
University Hospital of Cologne
Cologne, Germany

**A.G. Stuart, MBChB, PgCert (Genomics), MSc,
    FRCP, FRCPCH, FESC**
Consultant Cardiologist and Electrophysiologist
Bristol Royal Hospital for Children/Bristol Heart
    Institute
Bristol, United Kingdom

Reina Bianca Tan, MD
Pediatric Electrophysiology Fellow
Division of Cardiology
The Children's Hospital of Philadelphia
Philadelphia, PA, United States

Ronn E. Tanel, MD
Department of Pediatrics
UCSF School of Medicine

Director
Pediatric and Congenital Arrhythmia Service
UCSF Benioff Children's Hospital
San Francisco, CA, United States

Oktay Tutarel, MD, FESC
Co-Head
Adult Congenital Heart Disease Unit
Consultant Cardiologist
Department of Paediatric Cardiology and Congenital
    Heart Disease
German Heart Centre Munich
Technical University of Munich
Munich, Germany

Jim T. Vehmeijer, MD
Research Fellow
Department of Cardiology, Heart Center
Amsterdam University Medical Centers
University of Amsterdam
Amsterdam, The Netherlands

Edward P. Walsh, MD
Professor
Harvard Medical School
Associate Chief of Clinical Affairs
Director of Electrophysiology
Children's Hospital
Boston, MA, United States

Darryl Wan, MD
University of British Columbia
Department of Medicine
Vancouver, BC, Canada

Frank Zimmermann, MD
Director of Electrophysiology
Advocate Children's Heart Center
Oak Lawn, IL, United States

Preface

This book is the result of the realization that didactic textbooks and monographs on arrhythmias in adults with congenital heart disease (ACHD) fail to capture the complexity and uniqueness of most such patients.

We routinely see cases with unique features and for whom there are few guidelines on what to do.

A case-based textbook is, we realize, by its very nature, somewhat subjective.

However, it is also less pedantic and more revealing of the complex gray areas that need to be dealt with while managing such patients.

We contacted a large group of ACHD specialists and asked them to send us actual case scenarios of tough and unique cases of ACHD patients with arrhythmias.

We were fortunate that so many of them volunteered to send us such cases. For all their work in preparing and summarizing these cases, we are immensely grateful to these authors.

We then approached electrophysiology specialists through personal contact and by reputation and asked them to provide a commentary for these cases.

Again, we are profoundly grateful to these experts, who volunteered their time and effort to provide the commentaries in this book.

This book may be considered not as another textbook but more like a collection of short stories.

It is not meant to be read from end to end or to provide any didactic teaching on a specific topic.

Rather, we encourage the readers to dip into the book as they see fit and read the scenarios and the commentaries to get a "feel" of the thinking that goes into making management decisions in these unique and complex patients.

We hope you enjoy reading this book as much as we have enjoyed working on it.

Seshadri Balaji, MBBS, MRCP(UK), PhD
Ravi Mandapati, MD, FHRS, FACC
Gary D. Webb, MD, FRCP(C)

Contents

CHAPTER 1

Sudden Death Risk in Congenitally Corrected Transposition With Ventricular Dysfunction

Patient case submitted by Matthias Greutmann, MD, FESC

CASE SYNOPSIS

We report the case of a patient diagnosed with congenitally corrected transposition of the great arteries (ccTGA) at the age of 1 year. He developed severe systemic tricuspid valve regurgitation at the age of 6 years when it was decided to perform a double switch operation to prevent systemic right ventricular (RV) failure. As preparation for the double switch procedure, to "train" the subpulmonic left ventricle (LV), progressive pulmonary artery banding (PAB) was performed in two stages over a 3-month period. At this point, systolic pressures in the subpulmonic LV had risen to about 90% of systemic pressures, and due to the shift of the interventricular septum and improved tricuspid valve geometry, the degree

of tricuspid regurgitation (TR) had improved from severe to mild.

Although LV ejection fraction (EF) was noted to be mildly impaired (45%–50%), a double switch operation was performed. The postoperative course was complicated by rapid, progressive systemic LV failure, requiring escalation of medical therapy. For persistent LV dysfunction despite a narrow QRS width of 96 ms, the patient underwent implantation of biventricular epicardial pacemaker (CRT-P) in 2005 at the age of 9 years (Fig. 1.1). No improvement of LVEF or exercise capacity was noted after pacemaker implantation.

At the age of 16 years, a new pacemaker system was implanted due to electrode dysfunction. Between the age of 10 and 18 years he had recurrent episodes of

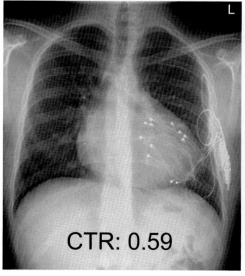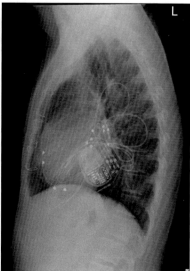

CTR: 0.59

FIG. 1.1

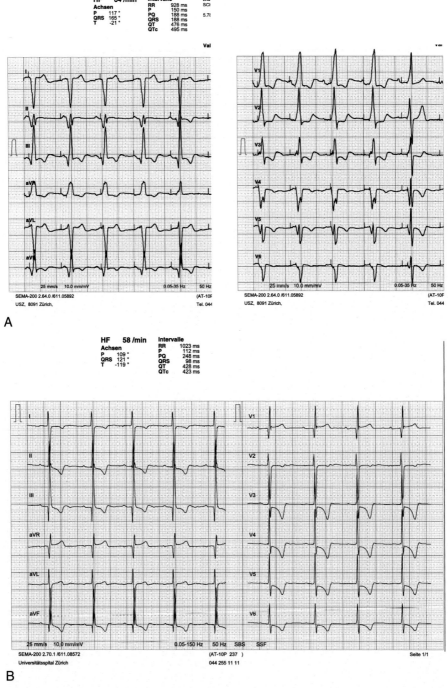

FIG. 1.2

intraatrial reentrant tachycardia, requiring multiple direct current cardioversions and ablation procedures. When the patient was transitioned to adult care at the age of 18 years he remained in heart failure with NYHA functional class III and had undergone his last electrical cardioversion 3 weeks prior to transition.

Transthoracic echocardiography showed a grossly dilated LV with severely impaired EF below 20%. Resting ECG showed broad QRS complexes with QRS duration of 188 ms, and on pacemaker interrogation, he was noted to be 43% atrial and 100% biventricular paced. As there had been growing evidence of lack of effectiveness of biventricular pacing in patients with narrow QRS complexes since the implantation of the device, it was decided to discontinue pacing and the pacemaker was reprogrammed to VVI 30-mode. ECGs on biventricular pacing and without pacing are displayed in Fig. 1.2. The QRS duration of native QRS complexes was 98 ms. After reprogramming of the pacemaker and intensification of medical heart failure therapy, symptoms of exercise intolerance improved (increase in peak VO$_2$ from 13.1 to 20.4 mL/kg/m^2), NT-ProBNP levels decreased (from 1544 to 356 ng/L),

and LVEF mildly improved (from <20% to around 30%).

Despite persistent severely impaired LV function, it was decided not to implant an AICD for primary prevention at this time due to stenosis of the superior vena cava baffle and uncertain risk-benefit ratio. Because modification of pacemaker programming and modification of medical heart failure therapy, the patient had remained clinically stable in NYHA functional class II without recurrence of sustained arrhythmias during a follow-up of 27 months.

Questions

1. Does the patient now need a defibrillator?
2. Was it a mistake to place a biventricular pacemaker for LV dysfunction with a narrow QRS complex?

Consultant Opinion #1

ANICA BULIC, MD • ANNE M. DUBIN, MD

This is an interesting case that highlights several important arrhythmia and device management issues in a patient with ccTGA (l-TGA). *The first issue to discuss, and one that perhaps dictated this patient's outcome, is the timing of the double switch procedure.* These patients are vulnerable to LV deconditioning and are at a high risk of RV failure and TR over time. LV "retraining" is performed by PAB in an attempt to confer a pressure load on the LV and stimulate LV hypertrophy to be able to contract against systemic vascular resistance. Our institution has published data to support an LV retraining program in patients with l-TGA with excellent midterm results. The criteria used to assess LV readiness following PAB for a double switch procedure include LV pressure 90% of systemic pressure; normal LV systolic function with an LVEF greater than 55%; LV end diastolic pressure less than 12 mmHg; mild or less mitral valve insufficiency; and LV mass by MRI greater than 50 g/m^2 in children and greater than 65 g/m^2 in adults.[1] Careful monitoring of LV size and systolic function both intraoperatively and postoperatively is crucial as there is some evidence to suggest that excessive tightening can cause subendocardial ischemia and potentially myocardial fibrosis in the long term. Five-year follow-up showed that all

patients demonstrated that their LVs could retrain in response to PAB and that the majority of those patients who had undergone a double switch procedure had normal LV systolic function. The influence of age on the success of LV retraining is controversial, but some evidence suggests that the older the patient, the less the likelihood of success.[2] One could argue that this patient was not a good candidate for a double switch procedure as LV systolic dysfunction after banding is a risk factor for death following a double switch procedure.[3]

The second issue that warrants discussion is the appropriateness of biventricular pacing, or cardiac resynchronization therapy (CRT), in a patient with repaired two-ventricle congenital heart disease. There are no randomized controlled trials in the pediatric or adult congenital heart disease (ACHD) populations, and the criteria for CRT are extrapolated from the adult literature. In adult heart failure patients with an NYHA class II−IV despite optimal medical management, LV systolic dysfunction (LVEF 35% or less), and a left bundle branch block (LBBB) with QRS 150 ms or wider, CRT has been shown to improve cardiac output, heart failure symptoms, exercise tolerance, and survival. Pediatric and ACHD CRT studies are limited but do support the hemodynamic and functional benefits seen in the adult population. In the largest multicenter pediatric study of 103 patients who underwent CRT, Dubin and colleagues showed that CRT decreased QRS duration by approximately 38 ms from a baseline of 166 ms, and improved EF from approximately a mean of 26% to a mean of 40%.[4] Subsequent studies have suggested that the benefits of CRT in congenital heart disease may depend on the underlying anatomy of the systemic ventricle, the presence and degree of systemic atrioventricular valvar regurgitation, ventricular myocardial scarring, and the type of electrical dyssynchrony. Janousek and colleagues have reported that patients with a systemic RV, systemic atrioventricular valvar regurgitation, and a poor initial NYHA class responded less favorably to CRT.[5,6] With regards to the efficacy of CRT in heart failure patients with a narrow QRS, there are studies to suggest its harmful effects. The LESSER-EARTH trial showed that in symptomatic adult heart failure patients with an LVEF of 35% or less and a QRS of 120 ms or less, CRT did not improve exercise tolerance, LV dimensions, or EF. In fact, CRT patients had a reduction in the 6-min walk test, an increase in QRS duration, and showed a trend toward heart failure–related hospitalizations.[7] *According to a published PACES/HRS expert consensus statement on the management of arrhythmias in ACHD patients, this patient with LV systolic failure, but a narrow QRS, would not meet criteria for CRT implantation.*[8]

Little is known about the risk factors for sudden cardiac death (SCD) in patients with l-TGA. The few published studies to date suggest that unrepaired l-TGA with a failing systemic RV and associated cardiac lesions are associated with a higher risk of SCD.[9] Koyak and colleagues in their multicenter case-control study investigating the risk factors for SCD in ACHD reported that out of 12 l-TGA patients with SCD, 9 had associated defects such as a ventricular septal defect (VSD), pulmonary stenosis, and Ebstein malformation of the tricuspid valve.[10] Heart failure symptoms, a history of atrial flutter or fibrillation, and impaired systemic ventricular function conferred a higher risk of SCD. Of the combined l-TGA and d-TGA cohort following surgical repair, 90% of those who had SCD had a systemic RV. One plausible explanation for this is impaired myocardial perfusion to a hypertrophied RV, particularly the anterior and inferior walls, as well as the interventricular septum.[11] It remains to be seen whether the timing and type of surgical repair, a history of ventricular arrhythmias, or results from programmed ventricular stimulation can further stratify SCD risk. *According to the PACES/HRS guidelines, ACHD patients with biventricular physiology, NYHA class II or III symptoms, and a systemic ventricular EF 35% or less represent a class I indication for implantable cardioverter-defibrillator (ICD) implantation, such as in this patient.*[8]

ICD implantation in l-TGA patients involves certain technical aspects that are unique to this patient population. Transvenous access through the atrial baffles can prove to be challenging, especially in the setting of superior vena cava (SVC) baffle stenosis, as in the case of this patient. Thoracotomy or hybrid procedures are used in as many as 2/3 of the cases.[6] Subcutaneous ICDs have recently been shown to be a safe and viable alternative in ACHD patients and would be a possibility in this patient. Moore and colleagues published their retrospective multicenter studies of subcutaneous ICD implantation in ACHD patients, involving 21 patients over a 5-year period, half of whom had single ventricle physiology and only one of whom had l-TGA. Ventricular arrhythmia was induced in approximately 80% and all were rescued with 80 J or less. There was one case of device infection, which did not result in device removal. The benefits of avoiding transvenous access come at the expense of a high rate of inappropriate discharges (21%), which are from SVT, T wave oversensing, and in one case, low amplitude artifact from subcutaneous air.[12] As in most clinical cases where there is a paucity of evidence-based literature, the decision to implant an ICD should be made on a case-by-case basis, with careful consideration of the risks and benefits for each particular patient.

REFERENCES

1. Ibrahimiye AN, Mainwaring RD, Patrick WL, Downey L, Yarlagadda V, Hanley FL. Left ventricular retraining and double switch in patients with congenitally corrected transposition of the great arteries. *World J Pediatr Congenit Heart Surg*. 2017;8:203–209.
2. Myers PO, del Nido PJ, Geva T, et al. Impact of age and duration of banding on left ventricular preparation before anatomic repair for congenitally corrected transposition of the great arteries. *Ann Thorac Surg*. 2013;96:603–610.
3. Winlaw DS, McGuirk SP, Balmer C, et al. Intention-to-treat analysis of pulmonary artery banding in conditions with a morphological right ventricle in the systemic circulation with a view to anatomic biventricular repair. *Circulation*. 2005;111:405–411.
4. Dubin AM, Janousek J, Rhee E, et al. Resynchronization therapy in pediatric and congenital heart disease patients: an international multicenter study. *J Am Coll Cardiol*. 2005; 46:2277–2283.
5. Janousek J, Gebauer RA, Abdul-Khaliq H, et al. Cardiac resynchronisation therapy in paediatric and congenital

heart disease: differential effects in various anatomical and functional substrates. *Heart.* 2009;95:1165–1171.

6. Janousek J, Kubus P. Cardiac resynchronization therapy in congenital heart disease. *Herzschrittmacherther Elektrophysiol.* 2016;27:104–109.

7. Thibault B, Harel F, Ducharme A, et al. Cardiac resynchronization therapy in patients with heart failure and a QRS complex <120 milliseconds: the Evaluation of Resynchronization Therapy for Heart Failure (LESSER-EARTH) trial. *Circulation.* 2013;127:873–881.

8. Khairy P, Van Hare GF, Balaji S, et al. PACES/HRS Expert Consensus Statement on the Recognition and Management of Arrhythmias in Adult Congenital Heart Disease: developed in partnership between the Pediatric and Congenital Electrophysiology Society (PACES) and the Heart Rhythm Society (HRS). Endorsed by the governing bodies of PACES, HRS, the American College of Cardiology (ACC), the American Heart Association (AHA), the European Heart Rhythm Association (EHRA), the Canadian Heart Rhythm Society (CHRS), and the International Society for Adult Congenital Heart Disease (ISACHD). *Heart Rhythm.* 2014;11:e102–e165.

9. Walsh EP. Sudden death in adult congenital heart disease: risk stratification in 2014. *Heart Rhythm.* 2014;11:1735–1742.

10. Koyak Z, Harris L, de Groot JR, et al. Sudden cardiac death in adult congenital heart disease. *Circulation.* 2012;126:1944–1954.

11. Myocardial Perfusion Defects ccTGA.pdf.

12. Moore JP, Mondesert B, Lloyd MS, et al. Clinical experience with the subcutaneous implantable cardioverter-defibrillator in adults with congenital heart disease. *Circ Arrhythm Electrophysiol.* 2016;9.

Consultant Opinion #2

FRANK CECCHIN, MD

This is a complex case that evolved over a very long period of time. *The first question I would like to address is What is the rationale for a double switch in ccTGA?*

ccTGA is the term used to define the cardiac malformation associated with atrioventricular and ventriculoarterial discordance. This double discordance results in a physiologically balanced circulation. It can be an isolated anomaly (20%), although it is often associated with other anatomic anomalies; the most common of which is a VSD in 60%–80%, pulmonary stenosis in 50%, and abnormalities of the conduction system in 15%–50% of ccTGA patients. The classic surgical approach has been to repair the associated lesions and is termed a "physiologic repair," which leaves the tricuspid valve and RV as part of the systemic circulation. However, a long-term result of this approach is progressive TR and RV failure. This led to the introduction of a true "anatomic repair" in which the LV and mitral valve support the systemic circulation. The true anatomic repair is accomplished by either a venous and arterial switch operation (double switch) or by a venous switch operation and a Rastelli procedure (RV to pulmonary artery [PA] conduit with an overriding VSD). If pulmonary stenosis or a large VSD are not present, then the LV will become deconditioned soon after birth and will need to be retrained as a ventricle able to handle the systemic circulation. The placement of a PA band will provide a high-resistive load for the LV to regain its ability to be a systemic ventricle.[1–4]

The case under review involved an individual with ccTGA and no associated lesion who was diagnosed at 1 year of age. *My recommendation today would be to start LV retraining prior to the development of RV failure.*

It remains controversial as to whether patients who are born with ccTGA, an absence of a ventricular septal defect, and an absence of pulmonary stenosis should undergo prophylactic PAB. The reason is that patients in this subset with good tricuspid valve function have the most favorable natural history, and there is insufficient data to compare this natural history with an anatomic repair pathway. The impetus to proceed with placement of a PAB is based on the observation that the prognosis for patients undergoing a double switch is more favorable in patients who never experienced detraining compared with patients who require retraining. A group in France reported their experience with an aggressive surgical management protocol for isolated ccTGA. They reported the results of 11 infants in whom primary PAB was performed.[5] There was no hospital mortality and all the children maintained normal RV function; tricuspid valve function was stabilized or improved, and systemic competence of the LV was maintained. They concluded that neonates with isolated ccTGA, "prophylactic PA banding is safe and carries a low morbidity." An additional case series from Boston looked at 25 patients with ccTGA who underwent PAB for LV preparation prior to anatomic repair.[6] For the 18 patients who underwent anatomic repair at a median of 10 months from PAB, LV dysfunction developed in 4 of 7 patients repaired after age 3 years compared with 0 of 11 repaired before 3 years. The caveat is that LV retraining should occur as early in age as possible to preserve long-term LV performance.

The clinicians in this situation chose to band the PA at 6 years of age because severe tricuspid (systemic atrioventricular) regurgitation had developed. This was done in the hope that improvement in TR would occur and the child could undergo a double switch procedure. The absence of pulmonary stenosis meant that the LV would need preparation prior to a double switch. The PA banding procedure in ccTGA can be used for two purposes. One is preparation of the LV for anatomic repair. This concept was initially described by Yacoub in 1977 and Mee in 1986 as a means to retrain the morphologic LV in patients with dTGA to allow a late arterial switch operation for patients who had previously undergone an atrial level switch.[7,8] The second purpose is as a palliative procedure aimed at improving RV function by reducing TR. This reduction in TR occurs by restoring normal geometric relationships between the RV, interventricular septum, tricuspid valve, and subvalvar structures. The PA band achieves this by elevating the LV pressure which in turn reduces septal shift toward the LV. This provides better tricuspid valve coaptation, reducing RV size, systemic heart failure, and preventing further tricuspid annular dilation.

In this patient the PA band procedure was performed in two stages over a 3-month period. At this point, systolic pressures in the subpulmonic LV had risen to about 90% of systemic pressures, and due to the shift of interventricular septum and improved tricuspid valve geometry, the degree of TR had improved from severe to mild. Although LVEF was noted to be mildly impaired (45%–50%) a double switch operation was performed. The postoperative course was complicated by rapid, progressive systemic LV failure, requiring escalation of medical therapy.

That brings up the third question: Why do patients develop LV dysfunction after a true anatomic repair?

The early- and intermediate term results of the double switch operation have been favorable, although, there have been more recent concerns regarding the long-term function of the retrained LV. Brawn and colleagues published their late results in 44 double switch subjects, comparing those who required LV retraining (n = 11) and those who did not (n = 33).[9] The 30-day hospital mortality was (4.5%) and the long-term raw mortality was (11%). The rate of death and transplantation combined was (16%). The actuarial freedom from death, transplantation, or the development of moderate-to-severe LV dysfunction was 85% at 1 year, 80% at 5 years, and 72% at 10 years. The incidence of moderate-to-severe LV dysfunction at 1 year following double switch was 39% in subjects requiring LV retraining, compared with 6% of subjects not requiring retraining. Thus, retraining an LV increases the risk of late LV dysfunction.

Preparing an LV to handle a systemic pressure load requires a delicate balance between providing enough resistance to develop hypertrophy without inducing ischemia and fibrosis. Animal models have demonstrated that retrained ventricles display subendocardial edema, myocardial necrosis, and fibrosis with reduced ventricular work index.[10,11] In some patients who do not tolerate a tight band, it may be necessary to progressively tighten the band over time to avoid damaging the LV. The key to successful retraining is stepwise training and rigorous testing of the retrained ventricle to make sure it develops "clean hypertrophy" without significant fibrosis. The Stanford cardiovascular surgical team has successfully retrained the LV in 24 ccTGA patients, with 18 undergoing a double switch procedure using the following protocol.[12]

Assessment of LV preparedness for a double switch:
1. LV pressure 90% of systemic pressure
2. LV systolic function EF >55%
3. LV end diastolic pressure less than 12 mmHg
4. Mitral valve function mild or less insufficiency
5. LV mass (by MRI) $> 50 \, g/m^2$ (in children); $>65 \, g/m^2$ (in adults)

Using the above criteria, the case study patient would not have met criteria for double switch. Either more time or a third PAB would have been needed prior to moving onto the double switch.

Then because of persistent LV dysfunction despite a narrow QRS width of 96 ms, the patient underwent implantation of biventricular epicardial pacemaker (CRT-P) in 2005 at the age of 9 years.

Was it a mistake to place a biventricular pacemaker for LV dysfunction with a narrow QRS complex? The answer to this question is YES it was a mistake to perform narrow QRS pacing, although this fact was not known at the time of the resynchronization procedure. A consensus conference in 2014 published recommendations for ACHD arrhythmia management and listed the following as a class III CRT indication:

Class III: CRT is not indicated in adults with congenital heart disease (CHD) and a narrow QRS complex (<120 ms).[13]

CRT is a powerful tool to counter mechanical and electrical dyssynchrony associated with worsening ventricular performance. CRT was first developed to relieve electrical dyssynchrony in the setting of LBBB and LV dysfunction. The best results are achieved in those with classic LBBB pattern and widest QRS duration. The technique was expanded to those in heart block and eventually the concept of mechanical dyssynchrony came to be understood. Mechanical dyssynchrony is defined as actual discoordinated contraction of ventricular segments versus pure electrical delay as defined by prolonged QRS duration. Successful CRT occurs when optimal LV lead position is achieved, as defined as the viable myocardial region with the latest contraction onset. Thus, narrow QRS CRT is rarely going to meet these criteria because electrical delay is nearly always coupled with mechanical dyssynchrony. When there is a mismatch between electrical and mechanical dyssynchrony, typically the myocardium associated with mechanical dyssynchrony is fibrotic.

In 2008, investigators from 115 centers attempted to investigate the effect of CRT on morbidity and mortality among patients with symptomatic heart failure, a narrow QRS complex, and echocardiographic evidence of LV dyssynchrony.[14] In 2013, after recruiting and following 809 patients for 19 months, the study called Echocardiography Guided Cardiac Resynchronization Therapy (EchoCRT) was stopped for futility on the recommendation of the data and safety monitoring board. There were 45 deaths in the CRT group and 26 in the control group (11.1% vs. 6.4%; hazard ratio 1.81; 95% CI 1.11−2.93; $P = .02$). The investigators concluded in the NEJM publication "that in patients with systolic heart failure and a QRS duration of less than 130 ms, CRT does not reduce the rate of death or hospitalization for heart failure and may increase mortality."

Then in 2015, Sohaib et al. identified all trials comparing CRT with no CRT, which reported Kaplan-Meier curves in groups defined by QRS duration: narrow, non-LBBB broad, and LBBB broad.[15] For each trial, the change in life span every 3 months was calculated. Four trials (MADIT-CRT [Multicenter Automatic Defibrillator Implantation Trial-Cardiac Resynchronization Therapy], RAFT [Resynchronization-Defibrillation for Ambulatory Heart Failure Trial], REVERSE [Resynchronization reVErses Remodeling in Systolic left vEntricular

dysfunction], and EchoCRT [Echocardiography Guided Cardiac Resynchronization Therapy]), totaling 4717 patients, reported curves for mortality or heart failure–related hospitalization. In patients with LBBB broad QRS duration (within MADIT-CRT), life span gain increased in proportion to time. In contrast, in patients with non-LBBB broad QRS (within MADIT-CRT) and patients with narrow QRS (EchoCRT), life span was lost in proportion to time. The nonlinear growth of life span gained when a CRT device is implanted in patients with LBBB broad QRS is unfortunately mirrored by a similarly progressive loss in life span in narrow QRS heart failure. This suggests the culprit is a progressive physiological effect of pacing rather than implant complications. They suggested that a randomized controlled trial of deactivating CRT in patients with narrow QRS is needed, with a primary endpoint of increasing survival.

The patient in this study never demonstrated any gain in ventricular performance with narrow QRS CRT and ultimately improved when CRT was deactivated. Thus, it is likely that myocardial scar developed during PAB placement for LV retraining and that pacing causes additional electrical delay without adequate offsetting improvement in mechanical synchrony. If narrow QRS CRT was to be reconsidered in this patient, then advanced myocardial imaging techniques to guide LV lead placement position, such as tissue Doppler imaging, 2D and 3D speckle tracking echocardiography, cardiac magnetic resonance imaging, and nuclear imaging could be utilized.[16] Myocardial viability at the optimal LV lead position is a key factor in enhancing CRT response rate. The quantification of scar burden in LV dyssynchrony is essential in the evaluation of CRT candidates because extensive scar burden can negatively impact LV functional outcomes. Recent studies show that preserved viability in the LV lead segment is related to greater LV reverse remodeling and functional benefit.[17−19]

The final question is Does the patient now need a defibrillator? I would argue that this is the exact type of patient that would benefit from ICD therapy.

In the 2014 ACHD consensus statement this patient would qualify as a class I indication "ICD therapy is indicated in adults with CHD and a systemic LVEF <35%, biventricular physiology, and New York Heart Association (NYHA) class II or III symptoms."[13] A 2017 study by Moore et al. looked at the incidence of SCD in ACHD and found that ccTGA was one of the top four anatomic diagnosis with the highest rate of SCD.[20] Eisenmenger syndrome was the leading diagnosis at 4.8 SCD/1000 patient years, and then ccTGA,

Fontan, and dTGA ranged from 2.0 to 2.4. In this study and others, atrial arrhythmias have been found to be associated with SCD in ACHD.[20,21] Based on the failed LV retraining via PAB placement, I would assume that significant fibrosis is present. This would be the substrate for malignant ventricular arrhythmias when the EF is less than 35%.

Implant considerations always play a factor in deciding whether ICD therapy is appropriate for an adult with ACHD. However, there are many options available to overcome the common technical challenges of ACHD ICD therapy, such as poor venous access, high DFT's, valve regurgitation, and cardiac malposition. The implant choices include joint cardiac interventional procedure (SVC stent placement), hybrid procedure (use epicardial pace sense leads and add transvenous and or subcutaneous coils), epicardial system (add a combination of pericardial, pleural, or subcutaneous coils), or a total subcutaneous system.[22,23] My choice in this patient would be a conventional joint interventional procedure via placement of an SVC stent, transvenous ICD lead, and atrial leads. If atrial lead placement was difficult then the atrial epicardial lead could be used. Having atrial pacing and atrial antitachycardia pacing provides a distinct advantage over a total subcutaneous device.

Recommendation: Proceed with ICD implantation in conjunction with cardiac interventional team SVC stent placement, a new transvenous ICD lead, and either a new transvenous atrial lead or reuse of the chronic epicardial atrial lead. I would do atrial and ventricular programmed stimulation at the time of implant to customize antitachycardia pacing.

TAKE-HOME POINTS (EDITORS)

1. ACHD patients with systemic ventricular failure and a narrow QRS are not suitable candidates for biventricular pacing.
2. If biventricular pacing leads to poor response or clinical worsening, it is better to turn off pacing (if possible) and leave the patient with their native QRS complex.
3. Patients with severe forms of CHD and severe systemic ventricular failure need to be considered for ICD implantation.

REFERENCES

1. El-Zein C, Subramanian S, Ilbawi M. Evolution of the surgical approach to congenitally corrected transposition of the great arteries. *Semin Thorac Cardiovasc Surg Pediatr Card Surg Annu.* 2015;18(1):25–33.
2. Ibawi MN, DeLeon SY, Backer CL, et al. An alternative approach to the surgical management of physiologically corrected transposition with ventricular septal defect and pulmonary stenosis or atresia. *J Thorac Cardiovasc Surg.* 1990;100:140–145.
3. Yagihara T, Kishimoto H, Isobe F, et al. Double switch operation in cardiac anomalies with atrioventricular and ventriculoarterial discordance. *J Thorac Cardiovasc Surg.* 1994;107:351–358.
4. Prieto LR, Hordof AJ, Secic M, Rosenbaum MS, Gersony WM. Progressive tricuspid valve disease in patients with congenitally corrected transposition of the great arteries. *Circulation.* 1998;98:997–1005.
5. Metton O, Gaudin R, Ou P. Early prophylactic pulmonary artery banding in isolated congenitally corrected transposition of the great arteries. *Eur J Thorac Cardiovasc Surg.* 2010; 38(6):728–734.
6. Myers PO, del Nido PJ, Geva T, et al. Impact of age and duration of banding on left ventricular preparation before anatomic repair for congenitally corrected transposition of the great arteries. *Ann Thorac Surg.* 2013;96(2):603–610.
7. Yacoub M, Radley-Smith R, Maclaurin R. Two-stage operation for anatomical correction of transposition of the great arteries with intact interventricular septum. *Lancet.* 1977;1: 1275–1278.
8. Mee RB. Severe right ventricular failure after Mustard or Senning operation. Two-stage repair: pulmonary artery banding and switch. *J Thorac Cardiovasc Surg.* 1986; 92(3 Pt 1):385–390.
9. Brawn WJ, Barron DJ, Jones TJ, et al. The fate of the retrained left ventricle after double switch procedure for congenitally corrected transposition of the great arteries. *Semin Thorac Cardiovasc Surg Pediatr Card Surg Annu.* 2008;11:69–73.
10. Davis KL, Laine GA, Geissler HJ, et al. Effects of myocardial edema on the development of myocardial interstitial fibrosis. *Microcirculation.* 2000;7:269–280.
11. Muhlfeld C, Coulibaly M, Dorge H, et al. Ultrastructure of right ventricular myocardium subjected to acute pressure load. *Thorac Cardiovasc Surg.* 2004;52:328–333.
12. Ibrahimiye AN, Mainwaring RD, Patrick WL, Downey L, Yarlagadda V, Hanley FL. Left ventricular retraining and double switch in patients with congenitally corrected transposition of the great arteries. *World J Pediatr Congenit Heart Surg.* 2017;8(2):203–209.
13. Khairy P, Van Hare GF, Balaji S, et al. PACES/HRS expert consensus statement on the recognition and management of arrhythmias in adult congenital heart disease: developed in partnership between the Pediatric and Congenital Electrophysiology Society (PACES) and the Heart Rhythm Society (HRS). Endorsed by the governing bodies of PACES, HRS, the American College of Cardiology (ACC), the American Heart Association (AHA), the European Heart Rhythm Association (EHRA), the Canadian Heart Rhythm Society (CHRS), and the International Society for Adult Congenital Heart Disease (ISACHD). *Can J Cardiol.* 2014;30(10):e1–e63.

14. Ruschitzka F, Abraham WT, Singh JP, et al. EchoCRT Study Group. Cardiac-resynchronization therapy in heart failure with a narrow QRS complex. *N Engl J Med.* 2013;369(15): 1395–1405.

15. Sohaib SM, Finegold JA, Nijjer SS, et al. Opportunity to increase life span in narrow QRS cardiac resynchronization therapy recipients by deactivating ventricular pacing: evidence from randomized controlled trials. *JACC Heart Fail.* 2015;3(4):327–336.

16. Tang H, Tang S, Zhou W. A review of image-guided approaches for cardiac resynchronisation therapy. *Arrhythm Electrophysiol Rev.* 2017;6(2):69–74.

17. Lehner S, Uebleis C, Schubler F, et al. The amount of viable and dyssynchronous myocardium is associated with response to cardiac resynchronization therapy: initial clinical results using multiparametric ECG-gated [18F] FDG PET. *Eur J Nucl Med Mol Imaging.* 2013;40:1876–1883.

18. Bilchick KC, Kuruvilla S, Hamirani YS, et al. Impact of mechanical activation, scar, and electrical timing on cardiac resynchronization therapy response and clinical outcomes. *J Am Coll Cardiol.* 2014;63:1657–1666.

19. Taylor RJ, Umar F, Panting JR, et al. Left ventricular lead position, mechanical activation, and myocardial scar in relation to left ventricular reverse remodeling and clinical outcomes after cardiac resynchronization therapy: a feature tracking and contrast-enhanced cardiovascular magnetic resonance study. *Heart Rhythm.* 2016;13: 481–489.

20. Moore B, Yu C, Kotchetkova I, Cordina R, Celermajer DS. Incidence and clinical characteristics of sudden cardiac death in adult congenital heart disease. *Int J Cardiol.* 2017. pii: S0167-5273(17) 36168-5.

21. Graham TP, Bernard YD, Mellen BG, et al. Long-term outcome in congenitally corrected transposition of the great arteries; a multi-institutional study. *J Am Coll Cardiol.* 2000;36:255–261.

22. Tan RB, Love C, Halpern D, Cecchin F. Rise in defibrillation threshold after postoperative cardiac remodeling in a patient with severe Ebstein's anomaly. *Heart Rhythm Case Rep.* 2017;3(6):302–305.

23. Cecchin F, Halpern DG. Cardiac arrhythmias in adults with congenital Heart disease: pacemakers, Implantable cardiac defibrillators, and cardiac resynchronization therapy devices. *Card Electrophysiol Clin.* 2017;9(2):319–328.

CHAPTER 2

Complex Transposition With the Risk of Sudden Death While Awaiting Transplant

Case Report by Berardo Sarubbi, MD, PhD

CASE SYNOPSIS
Case Description

A 27-year-old male was admitted to our cardiac tertiary center because of increasing dyspnea and progressive exercise intolerance.

He had been followed up by different hospitals during his life.

At birth, he was diagnosed with transposition of great arteries with ventricular septal defect and pulmonary outflow tract obstruction.

At the age of 9 months, he underwent the Blalock-Hanlon atrial septectomy and at 3 years the Rastelli procedure with homograft implant, ventricular septal defect enlargement, and atrial septal defect closure.

At 12 and 15 years, he underwent percutaneous angioplasty of the conduit with the use of balloon expandable stents to relieve conduit stenosis, but with unsatisfactory results.

At 16 years, he underwent an uncomplicated right ventricle–pulmonary artery (RV–PA) conduit replacement.

At 21 years, during routine echocardiographic assessment he was found to have moderate conduit stenosis (peak gradient up to 45 mmHg).

At the age of 25 years, due to an episode of syncope and a 24-h Holter documenting a symptomatic pause related to second-degree atrioventricular block, he underwent a dual chamber pacemaker implant.

At 26 years, he had a hospital admission for congestive heart failure, despite taking high-dose diuretics treatment and intravenous inotropic drugs (dobutamine and later levosimendan).

On admission to our department, he had severe dyspnea on mild to minimal effort and peripheral edema. There was a third heart sound and a systolic murmur (grade 4/6) at the left sternal border. Percutaneous peripheral oxygen saturation was 96% and his blood pressure was 100/60 mmHg.

Electrocardiogram showed sinus rhythm at 80 bpm, QRS axis at −40 degrees on the frontal plane, and incomplete right bundle branch block (QRSd, 110 ms).

Transthoracic echocardiographic examination revealed left ventricle enlargement (left ventricular end-diastolic diameter, 65 mm; left ventricular end-systolic diameter, 60 mm), with severe global dysfunction (ejection fraction, 15%); massive mitral regurgitation; a restrictive transmitral flow pattern (E/E′:18); severe RV enlargement (RV end-diastolic diameter, 52 mm) with severe global dysfunction (tricuspid annular plane systolic excursion, 7 mm); and severe tricuspid regurgitation, with the systolic pulmonary artery pressure estimated to be 50 mmHg.

To confirm the anatomic and hemodynamic findings, the patient underwent cardiac catheterization. During angiography, severe RV–PA conduit stenosis was confirmed.

He was then scheduled for heart transplant assessment.

During hospitalization, telemetric electrocardiography and 24-h electrocardiographic Holter monitoring showed repeated symptomatic nonsustained ventricular tachycardia runs (Fig. 2.1) and so he was started on amiodarone.

Owing to the presence of potentially life-threatening ventricular arrhythmias, despite amiodarone treatment, as a bridge for heart transplant, we decided to implant a subcutaneous implantable cardioverter defibrillator (S-ICD), as an upgrade of the existing pacemaker to a transvenous ICD was considered to be a higher procedural risk (Figs. 2.2–2.4).

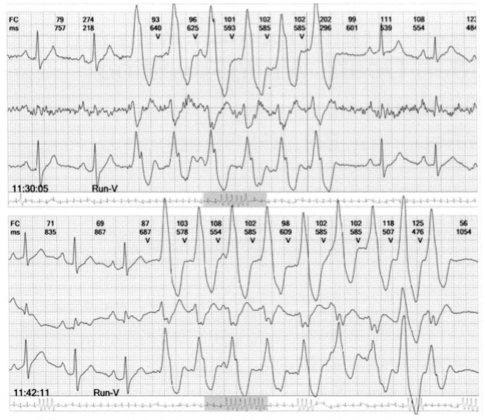

FIG. 2.1 Electrocardiographic Holter monitoring traces showing nonsustained ventricular tachycardia runs.

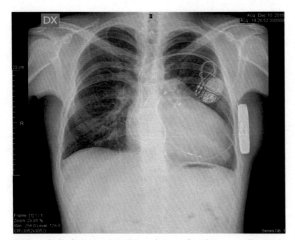

FIG. 2.2 Anteroposterior view of chest radiograph demonstrating the subcutaneous implantable cardioverter defibrillator and the permanent transvenous pacemaker.

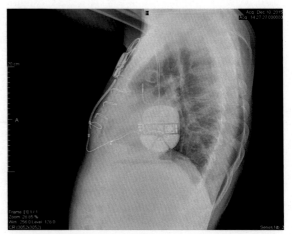

FIG. 2.3 Lateral view of chest radiograph demonstrating the subcutaneous implantable cardioverter defibrillator and the permanent transvenous pacemaker.

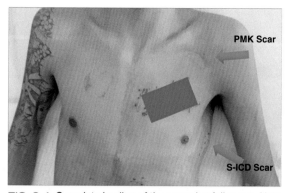

FIG. 2.4 Complete healing of the wound at follow-up. Note the scar of the previous pacemaker (PMK) implant and the subcutaneous implantable cardioverter defibrillator (S-ICD) scar. A tattoo on the chest is masked to protect patient's confidentiality.

QUESTIONS

1. Was amiodarone the right choice for antiarrhythmic treatment in such a patient with severe ventricular dysfunction or should a different antiarrhythmic have been chosen?
2. Could the pacemaker have been the cause of his ventricular dysfunction?
3. Did he definitely need an ICD while on the waiting list for heart transplant?
4. Was S-ICD the correct choice?

Consultant's Opinion #1

KAVESHREE GOVENDER, MD • SANTABHANU CHAKRABARTI, MBBS, MD, FRCPC, FRCP (EDIN), FRCPCH, FACC, FHRS

Was amiodarone the right choice for antiarrhythmic treatment in such a patient with severe ventricular dysfunction or should a different antiarrhythmic have been chosen?

This is a young adult with complex congenital heart disease with a Rastelli repair, significant RV–PA conduit stenosis, severe biventricular enlargement and dysfunction with severe mitral and tricuspid valve regurgitation, a dual chamber transvenous pacemaker, and nonsustained ventricular tachycardia listed for cardiac transplantation.

From the information available, it is unclear if the patient is on a target dosage of β-blocker for heart failure optimization and arrhythmia suppression. Amiodarone is a good choice in this situation in conjunction with a β-blocker to suppress ventricular tachycardia but, if used alone, may not provide a survival benefit. Hence, concomitant use of defibrillator therapy is indicated.[1–4]

Could the pacemaker have been the cause of his ventricular dysfunction?

The patient has a dual chamber transvenous pacemaker. The ventricular lead appears to be in the right ventricular apex (RVA). *There may be multiple mechanisms by which the pacemaker system may contribute to heart failure.* The Mode Selection Trial (MOST) suggests that more than 40% cumulative RVA pacing is associated with an increased incidence of atrial fibrillation, heart failure, hospitalizations, and even death.[5] Interestingly, the risk might be reduced to approximately 2% if RVA pacing is minimized. In contrast, the relative risk of heart failure in the VVIR mode cannot be reduced regardless of minimization of RVA pacing, and this risk is increased to up to 2.5-fold when cumulative RVA pacing exceeds 80%.

In patients with a normal left ventricular ejection fraction and no history of heart failure, the adverse effect of ventricular pacing on heart failure is modest. However, there are data suggesting that RVA pacing with preexistent ventricular dysfunction may result in early symptomatic deterioration of heart failure.[6]

Other causes of heart failure in this scenario may be from pacemaker lead–induced tricuspid valve dysfunction and pacemaker lead endocarditis.

Did he definitely need an ICD while on the waiting list for heart transplant?

Yes, this patient should have an ICD while being listed for cardiac transplant. Evidence suggests amiodarone alone does not prevent mortality in patients with significantly reduced heart function when compared with ICD therapy.[1] The mortality benefit of ICD progresses over time. In a study of 310 consecutive patients on a cardiac transplantation wait list, ICD implantation and β-blocker treatment were the strongest predictors of survival. Furthermore, ICD therapy was associated with improved survival independent of concomitant treatment with a β-blocker or amiodarone. Among patients with ICD and without ICD who were treated with a β-blocker or amiodarone, survival at 1 and 4 years were 93% versus 69% and 57% versus 32%, respectively, proving the significant benefit of having ICD and medication over medical therapy alone.[7]

Was S-ICD the correct choice?

Although ICD therapy is recommended in this patient, the choice between S-ICD and transvenous ICD is open to debate. The S-ICD was implanted, as the patient was very sick. Although S-ICD is feasible in adult congenital heart disease (ACHD), we are still on a learning curve with improvements in S-ICD technology, especially in device size, battery longevity, and discriminatory algorithms, to avoid inappropriate ICD shocks.

Data suggest that S-ICD in ACHD is associated with high incidence of inappropriate shocks (approximately 20%).[8] T wave oversensing and double-counting of atrial or ventricular pacing artifacts can also be a potential problem. The usual indication of S-ICD in ACHD has been the presence of intracardiac shunts and challenging venous access. For this index patient, the addition of a transvenous ICD system is a very viable option, as this would prevent double-counting of pacing artifact and inappropriate ICD therapies.

REFERENCES

1. Bardy GH, Lee KL, Mark DB, et al. Amiodarone or an implantable cardioverter-defibrillator for congestive heart failure. *N Engl J Med.* 2005;352(3):225−237.
2. Boutitie F, Boissel JP, Connolly SJ, et al. Amiodarone interaction with beta-blockers: analysis of the merged EMIAT (European Myocardial Infarct Amiodarone Trial) and CAM-IAT (Canadian Amiodarone Myocardial Infarction Trial) databases. The EMIAT and CAMIAT investigators. *Circulation.* 1999;99(17):2268−2275.
3. The Cardiac Insufficiency Bisoprolol Study II (CIBIS-II): a randomised trial. *Lancet Lond Engl.* 1999;353(9146):9−13.
4. Sim I, McDonald KM, Lavori PW, Norbutas CM, Hlatky MA. Quantitative overview of randomized trials of amiodarone to prevent sudden cardiac death. *Circulation.* 1997;96(9):2823−2829.
5. Sweeney MO, Hellkamp AS, Ellenbogen KA, et al. Adverse effect of ventricular pacing on heart failure and atrial fibrillation among patients with normal baseline QRS duration in a clinical trial of pacemaker therapy for sinus node dysfunction. *Circulation.* 2003;107(23):2932−2937.
6. Saad EB, Marrouche NF, Martin DO, et al. Frequency and associations of symptomatic deterioration after dual-chamber defibrillator implantation in patients with ischemic or idiopathic dilated cardiomyopathy. *Am J Cardiol.* 2002;90(1):79−82.
7. Ermis C, Zadeii G, Zhu AX, et al. Improved survival of cardiac transplantation candidates with implantable cardioverter defibrillator therapy: role of beta-blocker or amiodarone treatment. *J Cardiovasc Electrophysiol.* 2003;14(6):578−583.
8. Moore JP, Mondésert B, Lloyd MS, et al. Clinical experience with the subcutaneous implantable cardioverter-defibrillator in adults with congenital heart disease. *Circ Arrhythm Electrophysiol.* 2016;9(9).

FURTHER READING

1. Steinberg C, Chakrabarti S, Krahn AD, Bashir J. Nothing inside the heart - combining epicardial pacing with the S-ICD. *HeartRhythm Case Rep.* 2015;1(6):419−423.

Consultant's Opinion #2

KEVIN SHANNON, MD • JEREMY MOORE, MD

QUESTIONS

1. Was amiodarone the right choice for antiarrhythmic treatment in such a patient with severe ventricular dysfunction or should a different antiarrhythmic have been chosen?
2. Could the pacemaker have been the cause of his ventricular dysfunction?
3. Did he definitely need an ICD while on the waiting list for heart transplant?
4. Was S-ICD the correct choice?

This case is likely to be a scenario that will be seen with increasing frequency as patients with complex heart disease reach adulthood after multiple interventions at multiple centers. The standard approach to a patient presenting with severe heart failure secondary to congenital heart disease would be to first assess any reversible hemodynamic or electrophysiologic burdens that may be contributing to symptoms and/or ventricular dysfunction. In this example, there are at least three issues to consider. The first is the residual prosthetic pulmonary stenosis, which may be contributing to the heart failure symptoms and the arrhythmia. The presence of severe left ventricular dilatation and dysfunction would suggest that relieving the pulmonary stenosis is unlikely to be of significant benefit. The second consideration is the presence of chronic RV pacing. The chest radiograph (Figs. 2.2 and 2.3) shows an apical and anterior RV pacing lead, which is very likely to result in pacing-induced cardiomyopathy; however, the patient has second-degree heart block and has normal conduction on the only two rhythm strips available. *It would be helpful to know the QRS duration during RV pacing and the pacing burden to help determine the likelihood that pacing is contributing to this patient's cardiomyopathy.* The final consideration is the arrhythmia burden. The rhythm strips provided and the history would not support a diagnosis of tachycardia-induced cardiomyopathy. Thus, based on the information provided, there does not appear to be a reversible component to this patient's cardiomyopathy.

Once the decision has been made to list this patient for transplant, the next consideration would be whether or not an ICD and/or amiodarone treatment would be indicated to bridge this patient to transplant. These decisions would be based in part on the ability to manage this patient's heart failure as an outpatient and in part on his overall risk of sudden cardiac death (SCD) while waiting. If he needs inpatient heart failure management, then an ICD is less likely to be of benefit, but this decision may be subject to multiple institution-specific factors, including the ability to provide constant cardiac monitoring and a rapid response to acute events. *The choice of amiodarone for antiarrhythmic therapy is very reasonable,* in that it is the only antiarrhythmic agent that has been shown not to increase the risk of SCD in patients with a high baseline risk. Although the data on risk reduction is inconsistent, a meta-analysis of studies comparing amiodarone with placebo[1] showed a 29% reduction in SCD and 18% reduction in cardiovascular death. A small decrease in all-cause mortality was not significant in that meta-analysis. Amiodarone may exacerbate pacing-induced cardiomyopathy by increasing the pacing burden and slowing intraventricular conduction. If treatment is indicated because of symptoms, then amiodarone would be the only safe choice. If treatment is being considered for prevention of sudden death, then an ICD is clearly a better choice.[2] The use of amiodarone is concerning in this scenario owing to its very long half-life and its potential effects on the graft after transplant. A study suggests that there may be a survival benefit in avoiding the use of amiodarone.[3]

If the patient is a candidate for outpatient management, then implantation of an ICD is likely indicated.[4] The choice of an S-ICD versus a transvenous device would need to be based first on the surface electrogram screening, which would need to be done with both the native QRS and the paced QRS. Only about one-third of patients with RVA pacing were candidates for S-ICD in at least one study. If both the QRS morphologies pass with the same vector, then an S-ICD would be a consideration. There is data to support the safety and efficacy of an S-ICD in the presence of permanent RV pacing[5] but there is no data available to date on intermittent RV pacing. *It is not clear why this patient was not considered to be a candidate for transvenous ICD,* but elevated RV pressures and severe tricuspid regurgitation are certainly concerning when placing a high-voltage lead across the tricuspid valve. The use of S-ICDs in congenital heart disease appears to be safe and effective in at least one multicenter trial.[6] However, this trial should be viewed with caution, as it did not include any patients with pacemakers.

In summary, this is an increasingly common scenario in the severe ACHD population for whom we have inadequate answers.

TAKE-HOME POINTS (EDITORS)

1. In any patient with intermittent pacing and heart failure examine the pacing burden. Always consider that pacing may be the cause of the heart failure.
2. Amiodarone is a reasonable option to treat patients with ventricular arrhythmia who are on the transplant list. However, amiodarone use needs to be individualized based on the patient's concurrent morbidities.
3. S-ICD is an attractive but relatively untested treatment for suitable patients who are on the transplant list.

REFERENCES

1. Piccini JP, Berger JS, O'Connor CM. Amiodarone for the prevention of sudden cardiac death: a meta-analysis of

randomized controlled trials. *Eur Heart J.* 2009;30(10):
1245−1253.

2. Bardy Gust H, Lee Kerry L, Mark Daniel B, et al. Amiodarone
or an implantable cardioverter−defibrillator for congestive
heart failure. *N Engl J Med.* 2005;352:225−237.

3. Cooper LB, Mentz RJ, Edwards LB, et al. Amiodarone use in
patients listed for heart transplant is associated with
increased 1-year post-transplant mortality. *J Heart Lung
Transpl.* 2017;36(2):202−210.

4. Ghai Akash, Silversides Candice, Harris Louise, Webb Gary
D, Siu Samuel C, Therrien Judith. Left ventricular

dysfunction is a risk factor for sudden cardiac death in
adults late after repair of tetralogy of Fallot. *J Am Coll Cardiol.* 2002;40(9):1675−1680.

5. Ip JE, Wu MS, Kennel PJ, et al. Eligibility of pacemaker patients
for subcutaneous implantable cardioverter defibrillators.
J Cardiovasc Electrophysiol. 2017;28(5):544−548.

6. Moore JP, Mondésert B, Lloyd MS, et al. Alliance for Adult
Research in Congenital Cardiology (AARCC). Clinical experience with the subcutaneous implantable cardioverter-
defibrillator in adults with congenital heart disease. *Circ
Arrhythm Electrophysiol.* 2016;9(9).

CHAPTER 3

Atrial Flutter in a Repaired Tetralogy of Fallot Patient With Unusual Venous Anatomy

Submitted by Reza Ashrafi, MBBS, BSc, MD, MRCP and A.G. Stuart, MBChB, PgCert (Genomics), MSc, FRCP, FRCPCH, FESC

CASE SYNOPSIS
History
A 51-year-old male underwent primary repair of tetralogy of Fallot (ToF) in 1974 at the age of 9 years. The repair included a Dacron patch to close the ventricular septal defect and a pericardial patch in the right ventricular outflow tract. He remained well throughout childhood and early adult life with regular, but infrequent, outpatient follow-up. By the age of 48 he had developed progressive right ventricular dilatation with severe and increasing pulmonary regurgitation on serial echocardiography. He had no exercise-related symptoms and exercise tolerance was good (VO2 max 33 mL/kg/min). Coronary angiography was normal. The right ventricle measured 5.7 cm at the base on echocardiography but there was reasonable long axis function (tricuspid annular plane systolic excursion 18 mm). There was good left ventricular function with no branch pulmonary artery stenosis or other cardiac pathology.

The 12 lead ECG prior to surgery showed sinus rhythm with a broad right bundle branch block pattern with a QRS width of 160 ms and QRS axis of −80 degrees. A preprocedural MRI showed normal biventricular function with severe pulmonary regurgitation and no late gadolinium enhancement. He underwent elective pulmonary valve replacement (26 mm perimount bioprosthesis; Edwards Lifesciences, Irvine, Calif, USA) and a ring annuloplasty was carried out on the tricuspid valve. He made an excellent postoperative recovery (Fig. 3.1).

A year after his procedure he described reduced exercise tolerance with shortness of breath. An echocardiogram showed minimal pulmonary and tricuspid valve regurgitation and normal right ventricular pressures. Left ventricular function was good but his right ventricle had remained dilated with reduced function postoperatively.

ELECTROCARDIOGRAM
A resting 12 lead ECG from the patient in sinus rhythm is shown below with typical features of previously repaired ToF.

Below is a second ECG from the patient with the patient experiencing his typical symptoms of shortness of breath but no palpitations.

He was commenced on Bisoprolol 2.5 mg and given his symptom burden; a decision was made to carry out a diagnostic electrophysiology study (EPS) with a plan to proceed to ablation.

ELECTROPHYSIOLOGY STUDY
When the patient attended for his EPS he was in his tachycardia from a symptomatic viewpoint and his 12 lead ECG shown was identical to his clinic ECG (Fig. 3.2) suggesting one important macroreentrant circuit.

His antiarrhythmic medication had been stopped 5 days prior to the procedure but his oral anticoagulant (warfarin) was not interrupted with his international normalized ratio (INR) on the day of the procedure less than 2.5.

Femoral vein ultrasound confirmed a large left femoral vein and a small but patent right femoral vein.

17

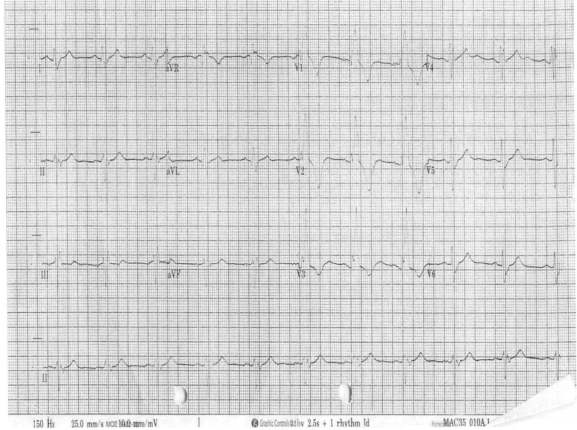

FIG. 3.1 An ECG from the patient 4 months following his operation showing sinus rhythm with positive inferior P waves with a pronounced right bundle branch block pattern, QRS width 166 ms, and QRS axis of −85.

A 7Fr and 8Fr sheath was placed in the right femoral vein percutaneously without complication. A 5Fr quadripolar electrophysiology catheter was advanced through the 8Fr sheath but did not cross the midline on abdominal fluoroscopy. The catheter was withdrawn. A 5Fr sheath was then inserted into the left femoral vein and a 0.035 mm wire advanced toward the heart. This took an unusual course parallel to the left of the spine. The sheath pressure was low suggesting a venous structure as opposed to inadvertent arterial puncture. A 5Fr multipurpose catheter was then advanced toward the heart and a hand angiogram demonstrated a left-sided inferior caval vein with hemi-azygos continuation into left-sided superior caval vein

(SCV) draining to the coronary sinus (CS). A formal venogram was then performed (Figs. 3.3—3.8) which demonstrated a CS measuring 4.8 cm in diameter.

Once the anatomy had been confirmed, a fixed decapolar catheter was placed in a small side branch of the large coronary sinus as a reference catheter and using the CARTO system (Biosense Webster Inc., Diamond Bar, CA, USA) a local activation time map was created using the DecaNav multipolar mapping catheter (Biosense Webster Inc.).

Entrainment maneuvers confirmed a macroreentrant circuit with a cycle length of 270 ms around the cavotricuspid isthmus (CTI) encompassing a large area of the lateral wall of the right atrium (RA).

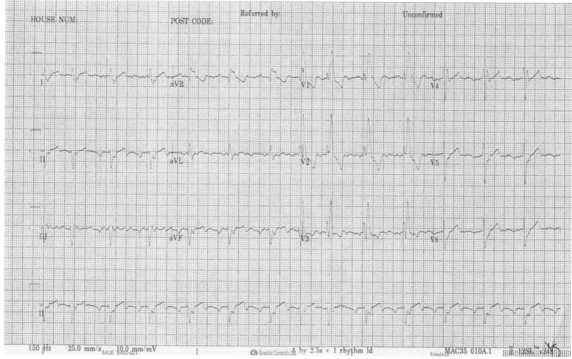

FIG. 3.2 ECG in with evidence of a macroreentrant tachycardia with negative inferior P waves suggestive of a counterclockwise flutter circuit and 3:1 atrioventricular block.

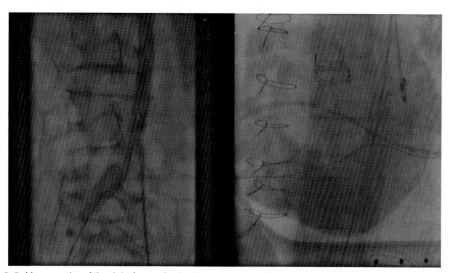

FIG. 3.3 Venography of the right femoral vein demonstrating a left-sided infrarenal inferior vena cava followed by a pump injection into the left hemiazygos to left superior vena cava to coronary sinus.

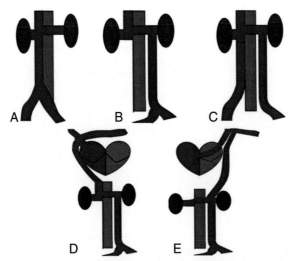

FIG. 3.4 **(A)** Normal inferior vena cava (IVC) arrangement at the prerenal and suprarenal level referenced to the aorta and renal veins; **(B)** Left-sided IVC; **(C)** Double IVC; **(D)** Left-sided IVC with azygous continuation into the superior vena cava (SVC); **(E)** Left-sided IVC with hemiazygos continuation into the left subclavian draining into the right atrium via a left SVC to coronary sinus.

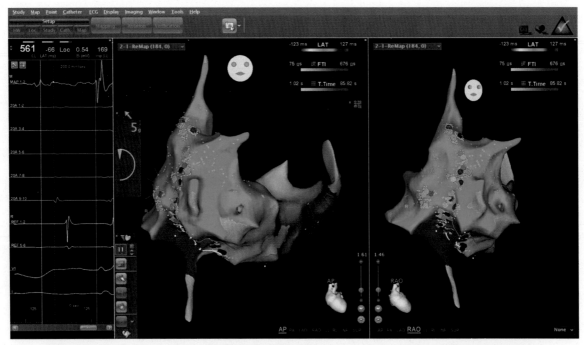

FIG. 3.5 An activation map from the EP study of the patient in the anterior-posterior (AP) and right anterior oblique (RAO) views. In the former, activation begins around the area of CTI and CS os. Ablation lesions are seen marked as pink and red dots with color guidance lines.

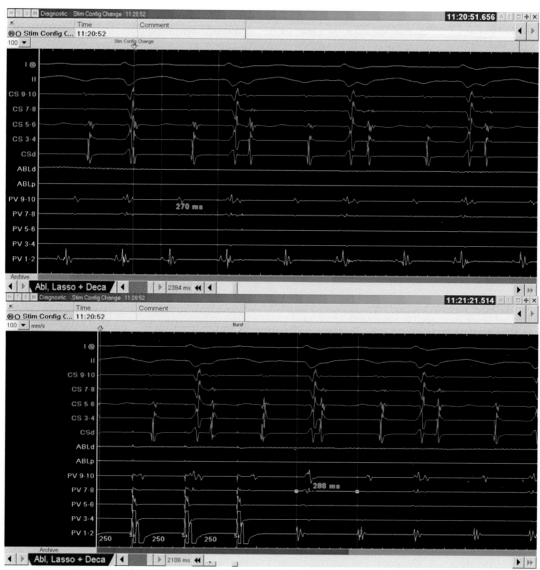

FIG. 3.6 Intracardiac electrograms from the case demonstrating a tachycardia with a cycle length of 270 ms in the upper panel and then entrainment from the from distal poles of the DeacNav catheter at the cavotricuspid isthmus (CTI) with a postpacing interval of 38 ms suggesting a CTI-dependent mechanism.

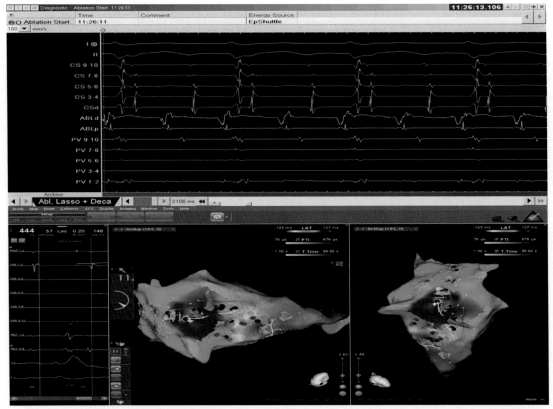

FIG. 3.7 Above, signals from the ablation catheter. Below, rotated local activation time maps from the case showing the extensive lines of ablation drawn from the coronary sinus os and cavotricuspid isthmus to the superior vena cava. Again, ablation lesions marked in pink and red and areas of interesting signals in blue.

Ablation was performed over a wide area the lateral wall down onto the CTI area (there not being an inferior vena cava so defining a true isthmus end was difficult) and CS os using a ThermoCool SmartTouch catheter (Biosense Webster Inc.).

Despite this the tachycardia was not slowed or terminated and subsequently was remapped with identical results. The anomalous venous course hampered stability of the ablation catheter (particularly in reference to doubling back on to the CTI line) and despite further ablation, the tachycardia remained. At this point using extra sedation, the patient was externally electrically cardioverted with a single 200J shock restoring sinus rhythm.

The following day he was discharged home on his antiarrhythmics and warfarin. He was subsequently followed up again after 8 months having suffered a recurrence of his arrhythmia which on the surface ECG appeared identical to the previously identified arrhythmia.

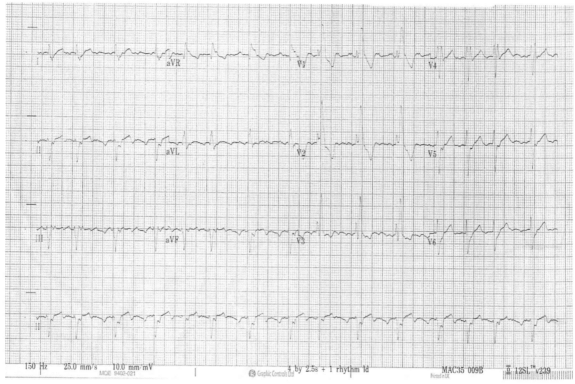

FIG. 3.8 A routine ECG from the patient in clinic confirming a recurrence of his macroreentrant tachycardia.

Questions

1. What are the common atrial arrhythmias encountered in postsurgical correction of ToF?

2. What are the common vascular anomalies encountered?

3. What other options are there for this patient?

Consultant Opinion #1

ELISABETH M.J.P. MOUWS, MD • NATASJA M.S. DE GROOT, MD, PHD

Postoperative atrial arrhythmias and ablation strategies after total tetralogy of Fallot (ToF) correction

This case represents a patient with repaired ToF who developed postoperative atrial tachyarrhythmias approximately 4 decades after the initial repair. Three-dimensional electroanatomical mapping studies prior to ablative therapy revealed that atrial tachyarrhythmias in this patient population **include intraatrial reentrant** tachycardias (macroreentrant circuits around surgical scars, sutures, and so on), **cavotricuspid isthmus–dependent atrial flutter, or focal atrial tachycardias** (electrical activation originating from a small circumscriptive region from where it expands more or less centrifugally to the remainder of the atrium).[1,2] The arrhythmogenic substrate of these atrial tachyarrhythmias is mainly located in the right atrium, near sites related to surgical incisions created at repair. Another frequently occurring tachyar-rhythmia in patients with ToF is atrial fibrillation, which develops on average at the age of 44 years.[3]

The incidence of late postoperative atrial tachyar-rhythmias rises with time after surgical repair and they are the main cause of morbidity due to heart failure, stroke, and even sudden cardiac death. Effective therapy is therefore essential and ablative therapy may be a potentially curative treatment modality.

If ablation is not successful despite targeting the crit-ical isthmus of the reentrant circuit it can be the result of insufficient lesion depth or persisting gaps in the linear lesion. The authors describe difficulty in acquiring a sta-ble position of the ablation catheter due to the complex cardiovascular anatomy. **For such a patient, a redo pro-cedure guided with the magnetic navigation system with a floppy catheter to reach 'the difficult spots' may offer an alternative approach, although it may be complicated by insufficient contact force. Another option may be an ablation procedure using the supe-rior caval vein approach.**

In this case, particularly the venous anomaly in which there is no true inferior vena cava (IVC) isthmus and the inability for stable positioning of the catheter made the procedure challenging.

The authors describe the venous anomaly, which was confirmed by angiography, as the combination of

a left-sided IVC with hemiazygos continuation into a left-sided superior vena cava (SVC) draining to the cor-onary sinus (CS). While this makes ablation difficult, we would recommend another attempt utilizing the ap-proaches given above. **If a second attempt (as described) also fails, we would recommend increasing or altering his medical therapy. Based on the recently published guidelines for management of arrhythmias in the ACHD population[2], we would attempt the use of sotalol (with cardioversion to convert to sinus rhythm after 48 h of sotalol), and, if that fails to maintain sinus rhythm, a trial of Dofe-tilide with appropriate precautions for both drugs as described in the literature.**

REFERENCES

1. de Groot NMS, Lukac P, Schalij MJ, et al. Long-term outcome of ablative therapy of post-operative atrial tachyar-rhythmias in patients with tetralogy of Fallot: a European multi-centre study. *Europace*. 2012;14:522−527.
2. Khairy P, Van Hare GF, Balaji S, et al. PACES/HRS expert consensus statement on the recognition and management of arrhythmias in adult congenital heart disease. *Heart Rhythm*. 2014;11:e102−e165.
3. Teuwen CP, Ramdjan TTTK, Götte M, et al. Time course of atrial fibrillation in patients with congenital heart defects. *Circ Arrhythm Electrophysiol*. 2015;8:1065−1072.

Consultant Opinion #2

REINA BIANCA TAN, MD • MAULLY SHAH, MBBS

Tetralogy of Fallot (ToF) is the most common cyanotic congenital heart defect and accounts for 7%−10% of all congenital cardiac lesions.[1,2] With continuing advance-ments in surgical and medical care, most patients with ToF survive into adulthood; however, a number of he-modynamic and electrophysiologic abnormalities in-crease the morbidity and mortality rate starting in the third decade of life.[3,4] Up to 30%−43% of adults with surgically repaired tetralogy of Fallot (rTOF) develop a clinically sustained arrhythmia.[1,5,6] The prevalence of arrhythmias increases with increasing age. The incidence of sudden cardiac death is 0.2%/year of follow-up and is mostly due to sustained ventricular

arrhythmia; however, a small portion is due to rapidly conducting atrial tachycardia.[1]

Atrial arrhythmias occur in 2%−34% of patients with rTOF with increasing incidence over time.[1,4,5,7-9] Patients are frequently symptomatic and present with palpitations, dizziness, shortness of breath, and exercise intolerance. It is considered a poor prognostic sign and is associated a 50% increase in mortality and twofold increased risk of heart failure or stroke.[3-5,10,11]

Intraatrial reentrant tachycardia (IART) is the most common atrial arrhythmia encountered in the adult CHD population, particularly in patients younger than 45 years of age.[5,12] IART is the general term used to describe macroreentrant circuits localized in the right atrium (RA) in patients with CHD. These include atrial flutter (AFL) through the cavotricuspid isthmus (CTI) and incisional tachycardias, which are atypical circuits through regions of fibrosis from suture lines or patches in combination with natural conduction barriers (crista terminalis, valve orifices, and the superior and inferior caval orifices).[6,11-14] If a tricuspid valve is present, the CTI is a common component of such atypical circuits. Incisional tachycardia is typically slower than typical flutter with atrial rates ranging between 150 and 250 bpm. The slower atrial rate can result in 1:1 atrioventricular conduction with rapid ventricular response and hemodynamic compromise. The mechanism for development of IART is likely multifactorial. Specific risk factors predisposing to IART in rTOF include (1) atrial scarring from prior atriotomy, other surgical manipulation of right atrial tissue, long suture lines, atrial enlargement, and pericardial inflammation; (2) abnormal atrial wall stress secondary to elevated right atrial pressures; (3) other hemodynamic factors such as significant pulmonary regurgitation with resulting right ventricular dilation and left ventricular systolic dysfunction; and (4) older age at repair possibly due to myocardial fibrosis.[5,7,8,10,12,15]

Another type of atrial arrhythmia that can be present is focal atrial tachycardia. The focus is usually related to suture lines. The underlying mechanism can be either automatic, triggered automaticity, or microreentrant.[6,11,16,17]

Atrial fibrillation (AF) is a growing concern as patients with rTOF survive to older ages. After 55 years of age, AF is more prevalent than IART with a steeper rise in incidence compared with the general population. The incidence of AF is between 7% and 29% in different studies, depending on the length of the study and follow-up,[5,18] with paroxysmal or persistent forms occurring more frequently than permanent AF. Associated risk factors include low left ventricular ejection fraction and left atrial enlargement.

Associated vascular anomalies are common in ToF with coronary and arch anomalies being the most prevalent. Systemic venous anomalies are rare and reported to occur in 0.5%–4.5% of patients.[19,20] Interrupted inferior vena cava (IVC) is the most common systemic venous anomaly with two case series reporting 0.5%–1.5% incidence.[20,21] Other systemic venous anomalies include the presence of left superior vena cava draining to the coronary sinus (CS) and bilateral superior vena cava.[19,21] There have been case reports of complete absence of superior caval veins,[22] a retroaortic innominate vein,[20,23] absent innominate vein

with a levoatrial cardinal vein,[24] left superior vena cava with unroofed CS and atrial septal defect—Raghib's complex,[25,26] and portal venous atresia.[27]

Long-term treatment options to prevent recurrence of IART include use of antiarrhythmic drugs, pacemaker implantation to provide atrial antitachycardia pacing, catheter ablation, and surgical ablation.[12] In patients with frequent symptomatic IART, catheter ablation is preferable to long-term antiarrhythmic use. Acute success rate of ablation is approximately 90% with a recurrence rate of approximately 20%.[15,28] In patients where IART is not eliminated by the procedure, the frequency is usually reduced significantly, thus eliminating the need for long-term drug therapy. Experience with pharmacologic therapy had been less than satisfactory with one study reporting more than half will manifest drug-refractory or severely symptomatic IART.[29] However, this remains a good option for patients in whom catheter ablation is not feasible or unsuccessful.[30] Rhythm control is generally preferred over rate control. Antiarrhythmic agents that are typically used include β-blockers, digoxin, sotalol, amiodarone, class IC drugs, and dofetilide. A Cox-maze procedure can be considered for patients requiring surgical intervention for other hemodynamic reasons.

The majority of the IART reentrant circuits in rTOF involve the CTI.[14,16] The circuit frequently has a figure-of-eight or dual loop configuration,[31] with an outer loop around the atriotomy scar on the lateral RA wall.[28,32] Ablation strategies to effectively interrupt both circuits require creation of conduction block at the isthmus and at the narrow corridor between the lower edge of the atriotomy scar and the IVC.[11] In typical AFL, the CTI is frequently targeted by ablation of the slow zone of the circuit between the tricuspid valve and the IVC. The electrically inert tricuspid valve annulus is well established as the anterior boundary of the circuit.[32] The posterior boundary is less clearly defined but is typically thought to be the crista teminalis-Eustachian ridge. In the absence of an IVC, the hepatic vein orifice can act as an equivalent boundary. Others have suggested the crista terminalis-Eustachian ridge as another posterior boundary.

Ablation of the cavo-tricuspid isthmus is typically performed via a femoral approach with application of radiofrequency energy beginning at the ventricular end of the CTI and dragging the catheter toward the IVC to create a linear lesion through the isthmus. In this case, the presence of an interrupted IVC precludes traditional femoral approach to CTI ablation. The ablation was performed over a wide area of the lateral wall of the RA down onto the CTI and CS os; however, there was difficulty in maintaining catheter stability, thus resulting persistence of tachycardia circuit. It is unclear from the case, but an inferior-to-superior approach was likely done (femoral vein → azygos vein → left SVC → CS). The looping course of the catheter likely leads to catheter instability and difficulty in manipulation. **Other ways to approach the CTI in this case includes (1) superior approach** via **the jugular vein or the subclavian vein or by (2) transhepatic puncture into the suprahepatic veins as these directly connect to the RA in the absence of a right-sided IVC. There have been reported cases of successful CTI ablation in patients with interrupted IVC.**[33-37] In one case, a patient with interrupted IVC with preservation of the suprarenal segment of IVC had an ablation via a superior approach. A catheter inversion technique was utilized to align the catheter tip to the isthmus with improvement in catheter stability.[35] In cases with absence of suprarenal segment of the IVC, AFL can be terminated by creating a line from the tricuspid valve to the CS os[36] or from the tricuspid valve to the hepatic veins.[37] Both reported cases were approached superiorly from the right internal jugular vein.

Recommendations

1. **Another attempt at catheter ablation of the CTI utilizing a different approach.** A superior approach will be preferable; however, a transhepatic approach can be considered as well if catheter stability remains an issue. We also recommend discontinuing warfarin and achieving an INR <1.5 at the time of transhepatic access to decrease the risk of procedure-related liver hemorrhage and capsular hematoma.
2. **Consider creating a line of lesions from the tricuspid valve to the hepatic veins** as a line from the tricuspid valve to the CS failed to terminate the tachycardia. If performing a transhepatic puncture, contrast injection directly into the hepatic veins will help delineate the site of entrance into the RA and provide a helpful landmark.

TAKE-HOME POINTS (EDITORS)

1. In patients with biventricular hearts like ToF and IART, catheter ablation can be an excellent first option.
2. If catheter ablation fails due to technical reasons (such as abnormal venous anatomy), a repeat attempt with appropriate preprocedure planning and a different approach should be considered.

3. If multiple, technically adequate, catheter ablation attempts fail, drug therapy based on established guidelines should be considered.

REFERENCES

1. Villafañe J, Feinstein JA, Jenkins KJ, et al. Hot topics in tetralogy of Fallot. *J Am Coll Cardiol.* 2013;62:2155−2166.
2. Khairy P, Landzberg MJ, Gatzoulis MA, et al. Value of programmed ventricular stimulation after tetralogy of fallot repair: a multicenter study. *Circulation.* 2004;109:1994−2000.
3. Valente AM, Gauvreau K, Assenza GE, et al. Contemporary predictors of death and sustained ventricular tachycardia in patients with repaired tetralogy of Fallot enrolled in the INDICATOR cohort. *Heart.* 2014;100:247−253.
4. Dennis M, Moore B, Kotchetkova I, Pressley L, Cordina R, Celermajer DS. Adults with repaired tetralogy: low mortality but high morbidity up to middle age. *Open Heart.* 2017; 4:e000564.
5. Khairy P, Aboulhosn J, Gurvitz MZ, et al. Alliance for Adult Research in Congenital Cardiology (AARCC). Arrhythmia burden in adults with surgically repaired tetralogy of Fallot: a multi-institutional study. *Circulation.* 2010;122:868−875.
6. Janson CM, Shah MJ. Supraventricular tachycardia in adult congenital heart disease: mechanisms, diagnosis, and clinical aspects. *Card Electrophysiol Clin.* 2017;9:189−211.
7. Roos-Hesselink J, Perlroth MG, McGhie J, Spitaels S. Atrial arrhythmias in adults after repair of tetralogy of Fallot. Correlations with clinical, exercise, and echocardiographic findings. *Circulation.* 1995;91:2214−2219.
8. Ávila P, Oliver JM, Gallego P, et al. Natural history and clinical predictors of atrial tachycardia in adults with congenital heart disease. *Circ Arrhythm Electrophysiol.* 2017:10.
9. Triedman JK, Saul JP, Weindling SN, Walsh EP. Radiofrequency ablation of intra-atrial reentrant tachycardia after surgical palliation of congenital heart disease. *Circulation.* 1995;91:707−714.
10. Harrison DA, Siu SC, Hussain F, MacLoghlin CJ, Webb GD, Harris L. Sustained atrial arrhythmias in adults late after repair of tetralogy of fallot. *AJC.* 2001;87:584−588.
11. Sherwin ED, Triedman JK, Walsh EP. Update on interventional electrophysiology in congenital heart disease: evolving solutions for complex hearts. *Circ Arrhythm Electrophysiol.* 2013;6:1032−1040.
12. Walsh EP, Cecchin F. Arrhythmias in adult patients with congenital heart disease. *Circulation.* 2007;115:534−545.
13. Love BA, Collins KK, Walsh EP, Triedman JK. Electroanatomic characterization of conduction barriers in sinus/atrially paced rhythm and association with intra-atrial reentrant tachycardia circuits following congenital heart disease surgery. *J Cardiovasc Electrophysiol.* 2001;12:17−25.
14. Collins KK, Love BA, Walsh EP, Saul JP, Epstein MR, Triedman JK. Location of acutely successful radiofrequency catheter ablation of intraatrial reentrant tachycardia in patients with congenital heart disease. *AJC.* 2000;86: 969−974.

15. Triedman JK, Bergau DM, Saul JP, Epstein MR, Walsh EP. Efficacy of radiofrequency ablation for control of intraatrial reentrant tachycardia in patients with congenital heart disease. *J Am Coll Cardiol.* 1997;30:1032−1038.

16. de Groot NMS, Lukac P, Schalij MJ, et al. Long-term outcome of ablative therapy of post-operative atrial tachyarrhythmias in patients with tetralogy of Fallot: a European multi-centre study. *Europace.* 2012;14:522−527.

17. Seslar SP, Alexander ME, Berul CI, Cecchin F, Walsh EP, Triedman JK. Ablation of nonautomatic focal atrial tachycardia in children and adults with congenital heart disease. *J Cardiovasc Electrophysiol.* 2006;17:359−365.

18. Wu M-H, Lu C-W, Chen H-C, Chiu S-N, Kao F-Y, Huang S-K. Arrhythmic burdens in patients with tetralogy of Fallot: a national database study. *Heart Rhythm.* 2015; 12:604−609.

19. Dabizzi RP, Teodori G, Barletta GA, Caprioli G, Baldrighi G, Baldrighi V. Associated coronary and cardiac anomalies in the tetralogy of Fallot. An angiographic study. *Eur Heart J.* 1990;11:692−704.

20. Changela V, John C, Maheshwari S. Unusual cardiac associations with tetralogy of Fallot—a descriptive study. *Pediatr Cardiol.* 2010;31:785−791.

21. Cobanoglu A, Schultz JM. Total correction of tetralogy of Fallot in the first year of life: late results. *Ann Thorac Surg.* 2002;74:133−138.

22. Krasemann T, Kehl G, Vogt J, Asfour B. Unusual systemic venous return with complete absence of the superior caval veins. *Pediatr Cardiol.* 2003;24:397−399.

23. Balkman JD, Zahka KG, Gilkeson RC. Retroesophageal innominate vein in a tetralogy of Fallot patient. *Pediatr Cardiol.* 2010;31:733−734.

24. Fujiwara K, Naito Y, Komai H, et al. Tetralogy of Fallot with levoatrial cardinal vein. *Pediatr Cardiol.* 1999;20: 136−138.

25. Mallula KK, Patel ND, Abdulla R-I, Bokowski JW. Tetralogy of Fallot with left superior vena cava and coronary sinus atrial septal defect: a rare association. *Pediatr Cardiol.* 2015;36:1100−1101.

26. Jian Z, Li J, Xiao Y. Rare association of tetralogy of Fallot with partially unroofed coronary sinus and PLSVC: case report. *Thorac Cardiovasc Surg.* 2010;58:117−119.

27. Hishitani T, Hoshino K, Ogawa K, Koyanagi K, Nakamura Y. Perioperative course in two cases of tetralogy of fallot with portal venous atresia. *Pediatr Cardiol.* 2002; 23:545−547.

28. Walsh EP. Interventional electrophysiology in patients with congenital heart disease. *Circulation.* 2007;115: 3224−3234.

29. Biviano A, Garan H, Hickey K, Whang W, Dizon J, Rosenbaum M. Atrial flutter catheter ablation in adult patients with repaired tetralogy of Fallot: mechanisms and outcomes of percutaneous catheter ablation in a consecutive series. *J Interv Card Electrophysiol.* 2010;28:125−135.

30. Khairy P, Van Hare GF, Balaji S, et al. PACES/HRS expert consensus statement on the recognition and management of arrhythmias in adult congenital heart disease. *Heart Rhythm.* 2014;11:e102−e165.

31. Mah DY, Alexander ME, Cecchin F, Walsh EP, Triedman JK. The electroanatomic mechanisms of atrial tachycardia in patients with tetralogy of Fallot and double outlet right ventricle. *J Cardiovasc Electrophysiol.* 2011;22: 1013−1017.

32. Kalman JM, VanHare GF, Olgin JE, Saxon LA, Stark SI, Lesh MD. Ablation of "incisional" reentrant atrial tachycardia complicating surgery for congenital heart disease. Use of entrainment to define a critical isthmus of conduction. *Circulation.* 1996;93:502−512.

33. Guenther J, Marrouche N, Ruef J. Ablation of atrial flutter by the femoral approach in the absence of inferior vena cava. *Europace.* 2007;9:1073−1074.

34. Latcu DG, Bun S-S, Ricard P, Saoudi N. Hepatico-tricuspid isthmus ablation for typical-like atrial flutter by femoral approach in absence of the inferior vena cava: use of magnetic navigation and three-dimensional mapping with image integration. *Pacing Clin Electrophysiol.* 2012; 35:e312−e315.

35. Malavasi VL, Casali E, Rossi L, Grazia Modena M. Radiofrequency catheter ablation of common atrial flutter in a patient with anomalous inferior vena cava and azygos continuation. *Pacing Clin Electrophysiol.* 2005;28:733−735.

36. Kelesidis I, Palma E. *Catheter Ablation of Atrial flutter in a Patient with Azygos Continuation of the Inferior Vena Cava After Failed Surgical Cryolesions.* 2012:1−4.

37. Varma N, Gilkeson RC, Waldo AL. Typical counterclockwise atrial flutter occurring despite absence of the inferior vena cava. *Heart Rhythm.* 2004;1:82−87.

CHAPTER 4

Unrepaired Primum Atrial Septal Defect With Atrial Fibrillation and Broad Complex Tachycardia

Submitted by J.P. Bokma, MD, PhD

CASE SYNOPSIS

A 67-year-old man was referred to our hospital because of recurrent episodes of palpitations for the previous 3 years, which he described as irregular and fast. These episodes occurred several times per year. The palpitations usually started when he was at rest after a longer period of work or with stress. The diagnosis of atrial fibrillation was established and electric cardioversion was performed. A primum atrial septal defect (ASD) was diagnosed using transthoracic echocardiography. Considering the limited shunting and atrioventricular (AV) valve regurgitation, no intervention was performed.

The patient was then treated for several years with sotalol to prevent atrial fibrillation. A daily dosage of 240 mg was not tolerated because of increasing complaints of fatigue and exercise intolerance. A daily dosage of 120 mg was not sufficient to prevent recurrences. Within these recurrent episodes, the patient sometimes noticed a brief change in the palpitations. Suddenly the heart rhythm became fast and regular, during which the patient felt light-headed and needed to sit down. These episodes lasted no longer than approximately 20 s and he never lost consciousness.

He was admitted for atrial fibrillation to a community hospital. However, in preparing for cardioversion, the rhythm changed on the monitor, and patient described the known symptoms of light-headedness combined with fast regular palpitations. The monitor recording of that episode is shown in Fig. 4.1. During the symptoms, he appeared to have *recurrent and rapid (220/min) nonsustained monomorphic broad complex tachycardia (maximum 16 beats)*, which terminated

without intervention. During this broad complex tachycardia, there was a rightward shift of the QRS axis. Upon termination, he was again noted to be in atrial fibrillation.

After cardioversion during atrial fibrillation, sinus rhythm was restored. As the first diagnostic step, the congenital heart defect was reviewed in our hospital by transesophageal echocardiography to determine whether any intervention was needed for the underlying hemodynamic defect. During investigation, a primum ASD was observed with a left–right shunt limited to the atrial level (Fig. 4.2). The *magnitude of the shunt was small* and the left-sided AV valve regurgitation was considered mild to moderate. The ventricular septum was intact. Right ventricular function was mildly impaired.

As the next step, a cardiovascular magnetic resonance imaging (MRI) scan was performed. The right ventricular ejection fraction was 44% and left ventricular function was normal. There was no clear difference in stroke volumes. There were no signs of ischemia and the myocardium showed no late enhancement, suggesting no large ventricular scars that could act as substrates for ventricular tachycardia (VT). Overall, an ischemic origin of the VTs was felt to be unlikely, although the VT episodes occurred mainly during fast atrial fibrillation.

At exercise testing, nonsustained VT (maximum 22 beats, 220/min) and polymorphic premature ventricular complexes (PVCs) were observed. The nonsustained VT during exercise had a morphology similar to that of the nonsustained VTs previously observed during atrial fibrillation (Fig. 4.1). Owing to the

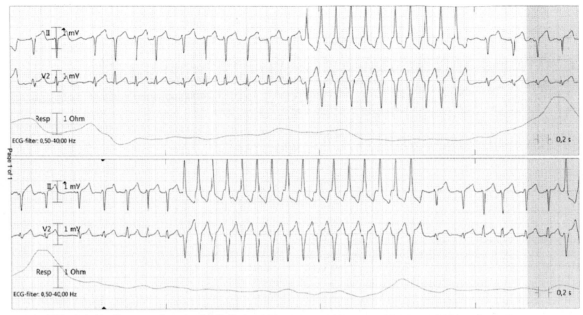

FIG. 4.1 Monitor recording of atrial fibrillation with monomorphic nonsustained ventricular tachycardia (220/min) of maximally 16 beats with rightward shift of the QRS axis.

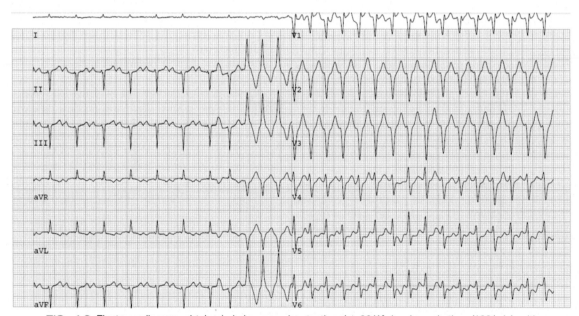

FIG. 4.2 Electrocardiogram obtained during exercise testing (at 96 W) in sinus rhythm (120/min) with broad-complex tachycardia (220/min) with QS pattern in V1 and rightward shift of the QRS axis.

persistent VT episodes with hemodynamic compromise, which were inadequately controlled with medication, an electrophysiologic study (EPS) was performed. During the EPS, PVCs were detected with a morphology similar to the clinical nonsustained VT, and *ablation of a left-sided septal substrate just below the AV valve* was successfully performed. However, PVCs with a different left bundle branch block (LBBB)-like configuration continued after ablation. An implantable cardioverter defibrillator (ICD) was implanted successfully afterward to prevent sudden cardiac death (SCD). There were no ventricular arrhythmias during the exercise testing performed after VT ablation, and our patient remained in sinus rhythm.

Questions

1. Given that he had an ASD and atrial fibrillation (aFib) would you manage the AFib any differently to what the referring team had done?
2. Was EPS definitely indicated for the VT?
3. Should an AFib ablation (pulmonary vein isolation vs. attempt to locate a focal origin) have been considered during the EPS?
4. Does this patient definitely need an ICD? Is there a role for a subcutaneous ICD (S-ICD)?
5. The ICD was placed transvenously. Given that there was an intracardiac shunt is there an increased risk of thromboembolism, and should that change the management approach (or is the Coumadin that the patient was presumably taking for the AFib sufficient)?

Consultant's Opinion #1

MADHUKAR S. KOLLENGODE, MD • DUY T. NGUYEN, MD

This is a case that highlights the nuanced nature of the management of electrophysiology issues for adult patients with unrepaired congenital heart disease (CHD). There is an increased incidence of atrial arrhythmias in patients with ASDs.[1,2] This is a consequence of long-standing hemodynamic overload resulting in atrial myocardial remodeling with increased myocyte size, interstitial fibrosis, and alterations in ultracellular structure predisposing to the development of atrial arrhythmias, in particular, atrial fibrillation (AFib).[1,2] Electrical remodeling has also been described, with increased P-wave duration and dispersion, as well as a lengthened atrial effective refractory period (AERP).[1] Although the majority of changes in patients with ASD are seen in right-sided chambers, a study evaluating patients with left-sided accessory pathways and ASD demonstrated lengthened AERP and enhanced inducibility of AFib. Importantly, despite the known remodeling and geometric distortion of the right ventricle associated with unrepaired ASD, there is no conclusive evidence of increased risk for ventricular arrhythmias.[1]

The first consideration is the *management of recurrent symptomatic AFib in this patient with unrepaired primum ASD. Therapy directed towards the restoration and maintenance of sinus rhythm is recommended.*[3] The long-term thromboembolic risk in this patient with simple nonvalvular CHD is not unlike that in the general population, and the decision to pursue anticoagulant therapy to prevent embolic complications should be guided by established scores for assessing risk such as the CHA_2DS_2-VASc.[4] This patient's CHA_2DS_2-VASc score of at least 1 is associated with low–moderate (0.9% per year) risk of embolic complications; either no antithrombotic therapy or treatment with an oral anticoagulant or aspirin may be considered.[5] We agree with the decision to initiate systemic anticoagulation, especially in the setting of recurrent AFib requiring cardioversion and the presence of an intracardiac shunt lesion. This can be accomplished with warfarin (international normalized ratio goals, 2.0–3.0), or by utilizing novel anticoagulants (NOACs) such as direct thrombin inhibitors or factor Xa inhibitors. *Management guidelines increasingly favor utilization of NOACs over warfarin, and in the absence of CHD-specific data, it is reasonable to consider NOACs in this patient with simple CHD and no hemodynamically significant valvular disease.*[4]

The ASD is hemodynamically insignificant (by MRI stroke volumes, no chamber enlargement), and normal right atrial size does not represent a risk factor for permanent AFib.[2] Initial rhythm control strategy for paroxysmal AFib utilizing Vaughan Williams class Ic agents, such as flecainide and propafenone (in the absence of significant structural heart disease or coronary artery disease), or class III agents, such as sotalol, dronedarone, or dofetilide, in conjunction with direct current (DC) cardioversion is reasonable.[5,6] We have had success with patients who did not tolerate sotalol but had less symptoms and good rhythm control on dofetilide, which is often better tolerated than other antiarrhythmics.[7] Catheter-based ablative therapy for rhythm control is useful for symptomatic paroxysmal AFib that is refractory or intolerant to at least one class I or III antiarrhythmic medication and is reasonably the first-line therapy for recurrent symptomatic paroxysmal AFib.[5] The success of AFib ablation in patients with CHD is lower; in a series of patients with predominantly simple CHD (ASDs in 61%), the success at 300 days was achieved in 42% compared with 53% of controls.[4] *In this patient with recurrent symptomatic paroxysmal AFib who was intolerant to therapeutic doses of sotalol, AFib ablation is reasonable; however, other antiarrhythmics with different side effect profiles may also be considered.*

The second issue is the diagnostic workup and management of symptomatic monomorphic wide complex regular tachycardia, which highlights the complexity of appropriate patient selection and risk stratification for ICD therapy in adult CHD (ACHD). Exercise-induced nonsustained VT has been reported in ~4% of asymptomatic middle-aged adults, with no increased mortality risk.[8] Hemodynamically tolerated VT in adults with CHD should be managed according to well-established adult guidelines, while taking into consideration CHD-specific issues.[4] Expert consensus guidelines for management of arrhythmias in patients with ACHD suggest considering EPS in those with palpitations suggestive of sustained arrhythmia when a conventional diagnostic workup is unrevealing, but these are based on limited clinical evidence.[4] In this situation, nonsustained monomorphic VT with hemodynamic compromise was reported during exercise testing, with replication of his clinical symptoms.

EPS with programmed ventricular stimulation, which is utilized for risk stratification in some patients with ACHD such as those with repaired tetralogy of Fallot, has been of little prognostic utility in other forms of CHD.[4] There is no known association between ASDs and increased risk of ventricular arrhythmias.[1] There are reports of SCD in patients with ASD, but the subgroup represented an older population with coexisting coronary disease.[9] *The presence of nonsustained VT in this adult is likely due to acquired factors and is unrelated to the hemodynamically insignificant ostium primum ASD.* Although ASD should be considered while making management decisions, risk stratification for SCD and ICD placement should focus on traditional risk factors. ICD therapy is far from benign and carries up to a 20% cumulative incidence of inappropriate shocks, as well as risks of device infection and lead malfunction.[8,10] In the absence of syncope, ventricular dysfunction, evidence of structural arrhythmogenic foci, or a family history of SCD, the placement of an ICD is rarely indicated.

EPS with programmed ventricular stimulation may be used to characterize arrhythmias and confirm a ventricular origin versus supraventricular tachycardia with aberrancy or occult accessory bypass tract, to document inducibility of VT, to guide catheter ablation, and to assess risks for recurrent VT or SCD to determine the need for ICD therapy.[8] The symptoms correlated with the presence of a monomorphic, rapid, wide complex tachycardia and thus *it was reasonable to proceed with EPS to identify and ablate the arrhythmogenic ventricular focus.*

VT was noninducible during EPS. Premature ventricular contractions with similar morphology to clinical VT were reportedly targeted. The inferiorly directed LBBB morphology VT with late precordial transition and predominantly negative deflection in lead I (Fig. 4.1) are features suggestive of an outflow tract origin, more likely right ventricular outflow tract. As an early intrinsic precordial transition in this patient is seen with sinus rhythm (Fig. 4.1, lead V2), compared with the later precordial transition of the VT, the ablated focus at a reported left-sided septal substrate below the outflow tract seems inconsistent with the clinical VT, as noted in the figures. Furthermore, the LBBB morphology's premature contractions reported following ablation are of unclear clinical significance and may be exits of different foci or related to the clinical VT and would themselves be amenable to catheter ablation. Inducibility of VT may depend on both sedation/anesthesia and concurrent pharmacologic and pacing modalities, which is generally required to ensure optimal abolition of the clinical VT. *In this patient, the role of ICD in the prevention of SCD remains unclear and hinges on the reported hemodynamic compromise.* There are risks of multiple ICD shocks for VT that may otherwise be targeted with ablation.

Lastly, we address the role of S-ICD rather than that of conventional transvenous ICD. Owing to a twofold increase in the risk of systemic thromboembolism in patients with conventional transvenous devices and intracardiac shunts, S-ICD is an appealing option in patients with ACHD.[11–14] He is on systemic anticoagulation and this will mitigate, although may not entirely abolish, his risks of paradoxic emboli with a transvenous system.[13,14] Additionally, venous cardiac access is often limited in patients with ACHD because of previous surgical treatments. S-ICD is a suitable alternative unless bradycardia therapy, cardiac resynchronization, or antitachycardia pacing are required.[8,13] In this patient with uncomplicated venous anatomy and a high likelihood of ongoing atrial arrhythmias (increasing risks of inappropriate shocks), as well as remaining ventricular arrhythmogenic foci that may respond to antitachycardia pacing maneuvers, S-ICD may not be an ideal choice when compared to continued anticoagulation and/or surgical closure. These concerns may also increase the threshold for which an ICD should be implanted.

SUMMARY

In this situation, paroxysmal symptomatic AFib should initially be managed with systemic anticoagulation, DC cardioversion, and pharmacologic rhythm control. Following therapeutic failure or medication intolerance, use of alternate antiarrhythmic agents or catheter ablation of AFib is a reasonable approach.

Nonsustained VT should prompt an investigation for underlying causes such as structural heart disease or coronary artery disease and is likely unrelated to the presence of an unrepaired ostium primum ASD. Consider initial therapy with β-blockers or antiarrhythmics. Following a negative noninvasive evaluation and breakthrough on medical therapy, EPS is the reasonable next step for both diagnostic and therapeutic objectives. ICD therapy should be considered for recurrent sustained VT on optimal medical therapy with hemodynamic concerns or evidence of significant structural heart disease, and risk stratification should be based on traditional risk factors for SCD.

REFERENCES

1. Chubb H, Whitaker J, Williams SE, et al. Pathophysiology and management of arrhythmias associated with atrial septal defect and patent foramen ovale. *Arrhythm Electrophysiol Rev.* 2014;3:168. Available at: http://www.radcliffecardiology.com/articles/pathophysiology-and-management-arrhythmias-associated-atrial-septal-defect-and-patent.
2. Blake GE, Lakkireddy D. Atrial septal defect and atrial Fibrillation: the known and unknown. *J Atr Fibrillation.* 2008;1:56–68.
3. Warnes CA, Williams RG, Bashore TM, et al. ACC/AHA 2008 guidelines for the management of adults with congenital heart disease: a report of the American College of Cardiology/American Heart Association Task Force on Practice Guidelines (writing committee to develop guidelines on the management of adults with congenital heart disease). *Circulation.* 2008;118: e714–833. Available at: http://www.ncbi.nlm.nih.gov/pubmed/18997169.
4. Khairy P, Van Hare GF, Balaji S, et al. PACES/HRS expert consensus statement on the recognition and management of arrhythmias in adult congenital heart disease. *Hear Rhythm.* 2014;11:e102–e165. Available at: http://linkinghub.elsevier.com/retrieve/pii/S154752711400513X.
5. January CT, Wann LS, Alpert JS, et al. 2014 AHA/ACC/HRS guideline for the management of patients with atrial fibrillation: executive summary: a report of the American College of Cardiology/American Heart Association Task Force on Practice Guidelines and the Heart Rhythm Society. *J Am Coll Cardiol.* 2014;64:2245–2280.
6. Armin Barekatain M, Mehdi Razavi M. Antiarrhythmic therapy in atrial fibrillation: indications, guidelines, and safety. *Tex Heart Inst J.* 2012;39(4):532–534.
7. Lafuente-Lafuente C, Mouly S, Longás-Tejero MA, Mahé I, Bergmann J-F. Antiarrhythmic drugs for maintaining sinus rhythm after cardioversion of atrial fibrillation. *Arch Intern Med.* 2006;166:719. Available at: http://archinte.jamanetwork.com/article.aspx?doi=10.1001/archinte.166.7.719.
8. Priori SG, Blomström-Lundqvist C, Mazzanti A, et al. 2015 ESC guidelines for the management of patients with ventricular arrhythmias and the prevention of sudden cardiac death. *Eur Heart J.* 2015;36:2793–2867. Available at: https://academic.oup.com/eurheartj/article-lookup/doi/10.1093/eurheartj/ehv316.
9. Koyak Z, Harris L, De Groot JR, et al. *Sudden Cardiac Death in Adult Congenital Heart Disease.* 2012:1944–1955.
10. van der Heijden AC, Borleffs CJW, Buiten MS, et al. The clinical course of patients with implantable cardioverter-defibrillators: extended experience on clinical outcome, device replacements, and device-related complications. *Heart Rhythm.* 2015;12:1169–1176. Available at: http://www.ncbi.nlm.nih.gov/pubmed/25749138.

11. Khairy P, Landzberg MJ, Gatzoulis MA, et al. Transvenous pacing leads and systemic thromboemboli in patients with intracardiac shunts: a multicenter study. *Circulation.* 2006; 113:2391–2397.
12. Moore JP, Mondésert B, Lloyd MS, et al. Clinical experience with the subcutaneous implantable cardioverter-defibrillator in adults with congenital heart disease. *Circ Arrhythm Electrophysiol.* 2016;9:1–8.
13. Chubb H, O'Neill M, Rosenthal E. Pacing and defibrillators in complex congenital heart disease. *Arrhythm Electrophysiol Rev.* 2016;5:57–64. Available at: http://www.ncbi.nlm.nih.gov/pubmed/27403295.
14. DeSimone CV, Friedman PA, Noheria A, et al. Stroke or transient ischemic attack in patients with transvenous pacemaker or defibrillator and echocardiographically detected patent foramen ovale. *Circulation.* 2013; 128(13):1433–1441. Available at: http://circ.ahajournals.org/content/early/2013/08/14/CIRCULATIONAHA.113.003540.short.

Consultant's Opinion #2

KRISHNAKUMAR NAIR, MBBS, CCDS, CCEP • LOUISE HARRIS, MBCHB, FRCP(C)

This is an unusual case of a patient presenting with an atrial arrhythmia labeled as atrial fibrillation leading to diagnosis of an undetected CHD of moderate complexity[1] and subsequent development of VT.

There are multiple points for discussion. As the longevity of patients with CHD increases, the prevalence of arrhythmias increases. In fact, arrhythmias are the most frequent reason for hospital admission in adult patients with CHD.[2,3] Although ASDs usually have a benign course in childhood and may remain undiagnosed as in this patient, atrial arrhythmias have been increasingly noted in older patients.[4,5] Atrial flutter is the commonest arrhythmia seen in younger patients; however, atrial fibrillation is commoner in the older age group.[6] Overall, ASD is associated with an increased incidence of AFib regardless of therapy, especially in patients older than 40 years.[7,8]

In ACHD, arrhythmias are often the first indication of hemodynamic change.[9–11] A full workup is required to ensure that shunt closure is not required. In this patient the magnitude of the shunt and the left AV valve regurgitation was found not significant enough to require surgical intervention. Transcatheter device closure of the ASD is also not feasible in view of its primum location.

The second issue is the strategy for atrial arrhythmia management in this patient. The patient was cardioverted and then maintained on sotalol. Two separate meta-analyses reported all-cause mortality was significantly higher with sotalol than with controls.[12,13] Use of sotalol is now a class IIB indication for maintenance of sinus rhythm in ACHD with normal ventricular function as per the guidelines.[1] It is important to monitor corrected QT interval and to check if renal function is adequate (not known for this patient).[14] The risk of torsade has been found to be <0.5% for a total dose of 320 mg.[14]

Amiodarone is the most effective antiarrhythmic medication for maintaining sinus rhythm[14] *and for chronic suppression of ventricular arrhythmias in CHD.*[1] Use of a rhythm control strategy utilizing cardioversion with or without amiodarone is reasonable in newly diagnosed atrial fibrillation, especially if the atria are not significantly dilated (which is not known for this patient). *Of note, antiarrhythmic agents such as amiodarone and sotalol with potential toxicities should be prescribed only when a rhythm control strategy is pursued.*

However, an important consideration in this case is the possibility of the atrial arrhythmia being an intra-atrial reentrant tachycardia (IART). This suspicion is based on the electrocardiographic signals seen before and after the broad QRS tachycardia recorded on the monitor just before cardioversion in Fig. 4.1. In Fig. 4.1 the atrial rhythm is clearly nonsinus with varying QRS morphology and varying T waves possibly due to superimposed flutter waves and there is a suggestion of organized atrial activity during the pause (see arrows).

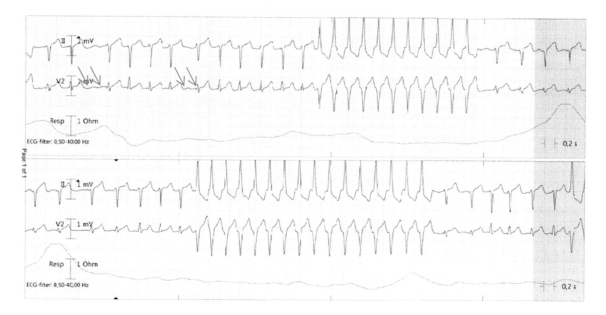

Of note, it is often difficult to identify IART in CHD because of low-amplitude flutter waves. Although recognition of IART is often challenging, it is important because it may readily lend itself to ablation. A baseline 12-lead ECG in sinus rhythm would possibly help make the differentiation.

Catheter ablation is now a safe and effective treatment option in atrial flutter in ACHD,[9,15,16] especially in a relatively simple CHD such as an ASD.

Success rates of radiofrequency ablation in ACHD depend on the anatomic complexity of the defect and vary between 72% and 77%.[9,17–19]

In this patient with a left to right shunt and likely right-sided chamber enlargement, atrial fibrillation is likely to have biatrial substrates and a pulmonary vein isolation alone may not suffice; however, there is only limited data on the subject. The evidence for pulmonary vein isolation in CHD is not very encouraging. In one study of pulmonary vein isolation in 36 patients with simple CHD (61% ASD), a success rate of 42% at 300 days and 27% at 4 years was obtained as compared with the 53% and 36%, respectively, in 355 controls without CHD.[20]

The third issue is the diagnosis and management of the symptomatic broad QRS tachycardia that emerged after the dose of sotalol was reduced and needed cardioversion. The differential diagnosis of regular broad QRS tachycardia includes VT, supraventricular tachycardia (including atrial flutter with 1:1 AV conduction) and

aberrancy, preexcited tachycardias, paced rhythm, and rarely artifacts. Clearly defined QRS complexes are seen ruling out artifacts. The broad QRS tachycardia is followed by a pause and then an atrial arrhythmia. No baseline preexcitation is seen ruling out broad preexcited tachycardia. *The most likely diagnosis of the broad QRS tachycardia here is VT.* However, the baseline rhythm seems to be IART.

Risk stratification of the VT includes ventricular function and substrate assessment by imaging, exercise stress testing, and EPS. Imaging (in the form of transesophageal echocardiography and MRI) in this case was negative for wall motion and scar. In addition, imaging and sometimes hemodynamic testing (not performed here) are needed for surgery/intervention for the underlying substrate, including shunt and valve-related issues. Exercise stress testing is important to rule out ischemia and to look for inducibility of VT.

Inducible sustained VT at programmed ventricular stimulation has been shown to be an independent risk factor for clinical VT and SCD in patients with tetralogy of Fallot and risk factors such as left ventricular systolic or diastolic dysfunction, nonsustained VT, QRS duration >180 ms, and extensive right ventricular scarring.[21,22] EPSs have been shown to be of little value in patients who have undergone atrial switch surgery for classic transposition of great arteries.[23] However, there is no data on the value of this investigation in most other CHDs including ASDs. *In this patient with structural heart disease, as the VT was fast and the patient was symptomatic with light-headedness, an EPS is reasonable.* However, there are no systematic studies on catheter ablation of VT in this population. The main purposes of the EPS would be to attempt radiofrequency ablation of VT and to determine the need for an ICD. In this patient, it is unclear if a pace mapping approach or an activation mapping approach was used for PVC mapping. The pace mapping approach is limited because of the large virtual electrode that is obtained during local capture pacing. It is unclear if induction of VT was performed during the study. Conceivably, if VT was inducible before ablation and clearly noninducible after ablation, an ICD could have been avoided in this patient with normal biventricular function and no scar but with structural heart disease.

The fourth issue is the safety of a transvenous defibrillator (ICD) in a patient with an atrial shunt. As per the guidelines, endocardial leads are generally contraindicated (class III indication) in patients with intracardiac shunts.[1] In a multicenter retrospective cohort study of 202 patients with intracardiac shunts, which included 64 patients with transvenous leads, transvenous leads remained an independent predictor of systemic thromboemboli (hazard ratio, 2.6; $P = .0265$) in multivariate stepwise regression analyses. Having had aspirin or warfarin prescribed was not protective in this study.[24]

Our recommendation would have been the use of an S-ICD if the VT could not be successfully ablated because this patient does not have any indications for pacing and has a primum ASD that cannot be closed by a device.

REFERENCES

1. Kirsh JA, Walsh EP, Triedman JK. Prevalence of and risk factors for atrial fibrillation and intra-atrial reentrant tachycardia among patients with congenital heart disease. *Am J Cardiol.* 2002;90:338–340.
2. Philip F, Muhammad KI, Agarwal S, Natale A, Krasuski RA. Pulmonary vein isolation for the treatment of drug-refractory atrial fibrillation in adults with congenital heart disease. *Congenit Heart Dis.* 2012;7:392–399.
3. Katritsis DG. Transseptal puncture through atrial septal closure devices. *Heart Rhythm.* 2011;8:1676–1677.
4. Gatzoulis MA, Freeman MA, Siu SC, Webb GD, Harris L. Atrial arrhythmia after surgical closure of atrial septal defects in adults. *N Engl J Med.* 1999;340(11):839–846.
5. Egeblad H, Berning J, Efsen F, Wennevold A. Non-invasive diagnosis in clinically suspected atrial septal defect of secundum or sinus venosus type. Value of combining chest X-ray, phonocardiography, and M-mode echocardiography. *Br Heart J.* 1980;44(3):317–321.
6. Khairy P, Van Hare GF, Balaji S, et al. PACES/HRS expert consensus statement on the recognition and management of arrhythmias in adult congenital heart disease: developed in partnership between the Pediatric and Congenital Electrophysiology Society (PACES) and the Heart Rhythm Society (HRS). Endorsed by the governing bodies of PACES, HRS, the American College of Cardiology (ACC), the American Heart Association (AHA), the European Heart Rhythm Association (EHRA), the Canadian Heart Rhythm Society (CHRS), and the International Society for Adult Congenital Heart Disease (ISACHD). *Heart Rhythm.* 2014;11(10):e102–e165.
7. Khairy P, Landzberg MJ, Gatzoulis MA, et al. Epicardial Versus ENdocardial pacing and Thromboembolic Events Investigators. Transvenous pacing leads and systemic thromboemboli in patients with intracardiac shunts: a multicenter study. *Circulation.* 2006;113(20):2391–2397.
8. Kaemmerer H, Fratz S, Bauer U, et al. Emergency hospital admissions and three-year survival of adults with and without cardiovascular surgery for congenital cardiac disease. *J Thorac Cardiovasc Surg.* 2003;126:1048.
9. Philip F, Muhammad KI, Agarwal S, Natale A, Krasuski RA. Pulmonary vein isolation for the treatment of drug-refractory atrial fibrillation in adults with congenital heart disease. *Congenit Heart Dis.* 2012;7:392–399.
10. Lafuente-Lafuente C, Longas-Tejero MA, Bergmann JF, Belmin J. Antiarrhythmics for maintaining sinus rhythm after cardioversion of atrial fibrillation. *Cochrane Database Syst Rev.* 2012;5:CD005049.
11. Freemantle N, Lafuente C, Mitchell S, Eckert L, Reynolds M. Mixed treatment comparison of dronedarone, amiodarone, sotalol, flecainide, and propafenone, for the management of atrial fibrillation. *Europace.* 2011;13:329–345.
12. Kaemmerer H, Bauer U, Pensl U, et al. Management of emergencies in adults with congenital cardiac disease. *Am J Cardiol.* 2008;101:521–525.
13. Khairy P. Programmed ventricular stimulation for risk stratification in patients with tetralogy of Fallot: a Bayesian perspective. *Nat Clin Pract Cardiovasc Med.* 2007;4:292–293.
14. Khairy P, Landzberg MJ, Gatzoulis MA, et al. Value of programmed ventricular stimulation after tetralogy of Fallot repair: a multicenter study. *Circulation.* 2004;109:1994–2000.
15. VanHare GF, Lesh MD, Stanger P. Radiofrequency catheter ablation of Supraventricular arrhythmias in patients with congenital heart disease: results and technical considerations. *J Am Coll Cardiol.* 1993;22:883–890.
16. Kanter RJ, Papagiannis J, Carboni MP, Ungerleider RM, Sanders WE, Wharton JM. Radiofrequency catheter ablation of supraventricular tachycardia substrates after Mustard and Senning operations for d-transposition of the great arteries. *J Am Coll Cardiol.* 2000;35:428–441.
17. Drago F, Russo MS, Marazzi R, Salerno-Uriarte JA, Silvetti MS, DePonti R. Atrial tachycardias in patients with congenital heart disease: a minimally invasive simplified approach in the use of three-dimensional electroanatomic mapping. *Europace.* 2011;13:689–695.

18. Triedman JK, Jenkins KJ, Colan SD, Saul JP, Walsh EP. Intra-atrial reentrant tachycardia after palliation of congenital heart disease: characterization of multiple macroreentrant circuits using fluoroscopically based three-dimensional endocardial mapping. *J Cardiovasc Electrophysiol.* 1997;8:259−270.
19. deGroot NM, Atary JZ, Blom NA, Schalij MJ. Long-term outcome after ablative therapy of postoperative atrial tachyarrhythmia in patients with congenital heart disease and characteristics of atrial tachyarrhythmia recurrences. *Circ Arrhythm Electrophysiol.* 2010;3:148−154.
20. Khairy P, Harris L, Landzberg MJ, et al. Sudden death and defibrillators in transposition of the great arteries with

intra-atrial baffles: a multicenter study. *Circ Arrhythm Electrophysiol.* 2008;1:250−257.
21. Contractor T, Levin V, Madapati R. Drug therapy in adult congenital heart disease. *Card Electrophysiol Clin.* 2017; 9(2):295−310 [Review].
22. Kanter RJ, Garson Jr A. Atrial arrhythmias during chronic follow-up of surgery for complex congenital heart disease. *Pacing Clin Electrophysiol.* 1997;20:502−511.
23. Khairy P, Dore A, Talajic M, et al. Arrhythmias in adult congenital heart disease. *Expert Rev Cardiovasc Ther.* 2006; 4:83−95.
24. Khairy P, Balaji S. Cardiac arrhythmias in congenital heart diseases. *Indian Pacing Electrophysiol J.* 2009;9:299−317.

CHAPTER 5

Ebstein Anomaly After Tricuspid Valve Replacement Needing Pacemaker Implantation

Case submitted by Christopher J. McLeod, MBChB, PhD

CASE REPORT

A 61-year-old man with a history of Ebstein anomaly underwent valve repair with concomitant intraoperative ablation of an accessory pathway and right atrial maze procedure in 1997 at age 41.

This was followed by tricuspid valve replacement in 2001 with a 35-mm Carpentier-Edwards bioprosthesis.

Owing to recurrent symptomatic paroxysmal atrial fibrillation, he then underwent a successful pulmonary vein isolation (PVI) procedure in 2004. The electrophysiologic study performed at that time revealed severe sinus node dysfunction with intact atrioventricular (AV) conduction; however, he was asymptomatic. It was also noted that the tricuspid valve prosthesis was implanted proximal to the coronary sinus.

The patient now presents with frequent severe near-syncopal episodes with evidence of sinoatrial exit block and episodes of high-grade AV block on ambulatory monitoring (Fig. 5.1). Given the symptomatic conduction system disease, permanent pacemaker implantation was recommended.

The patient is an overweight gentleman with a body mass index of 27. He has no hypertension and his resting heart rate is 52 beats per minute. On examination, he has normal carotid and jugular venous findings. The cardiac examination reveals a moderate right ventricular (RV) heave with a regular heart rate and no murmurs.

His electrocardiogram (ECG) reveals a sinus bradycardia with ventricular rate of 45 beats per minute and a right bundle branch block with a QRS duration of 156 ms, with a PR interval of 136 ms (Fig. 5.1). The chest radiograph is in shown in Fig. 5.2. The transthoracic echo identifies normal left ventricular (LV) size

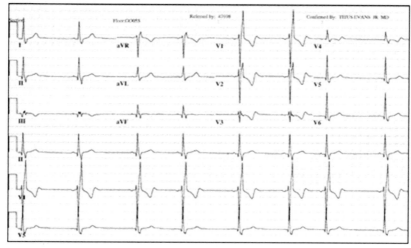

FIG. 5.1

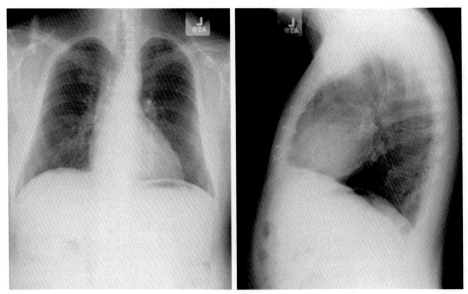

FIG. 5.2

and function with no regional wall abnormalities. The RV is moderately enlarged with moderate systolic dysfunction; the mean gradient across the tricuspid valve prosthesis was 3 mmHg at a heart rate of 42 beats per minute with trace tricuspid regurgitation.

Although permanent pacemaker implantation has been recommended, the type of pacemaker/pacing system has not been decided upon. For many patients with multiple prior sternotomies and a bioprosthetic tricuspid valve, it has been a preference to avoid placing a pacemaker lead through the bioprosthetic leaflets so as to preserve valve function.

Questions

1. Should he have implantation of a transvenous or an epicardial pacemaker?
2. Could this be intra-atrial block that masquerades as a block at the AV nodal level?

Consultant Opinion #1

NARAYANSWAMI SREERAM, MD • DANIEL STEVEN, MD

The patient presents with symptomatic bradyarrhythmia. The ECG and Holter traces confirm episodes of sinoatrial exit block and high-grade AV block. In association with the frequent episodes of near syncope, the indication for implantation of a permanent pacemaker seems given.

Progressive conduction system disease is part of the disease process in a variety of structural heart lesions, including Ebstein anomaly, and may be inherent to the disease or acquired as a result of multiple surgical procedures. Our patient has undergone previous surgery for tricuspid valve regurgitation and a surgical right atrial maze procedure. The commonest indications for permanent pacing in adults with structural heart disease are sinus node dysfunction and AV block acquired outside the acute surgical setting.[1,2] Our patient appears to have developed both these pathologic conditions. *It is possible that the intra-atrial block, resulting in part from the previous right atrial maze procedure, may be masquerading as an episodic AV block as seen on the Holter recording. This, however, should not influence the choice of permanent pacemaker but necessitates implantation of a ventricular lead.*

The choice of optimal technique and the route for permanent pacing in this patient are complicated by three factors: Ebstein anomaly with a history of surgery and evidence of persistent RV dysfunction, a bioprosthetic tricuspid valve, and its implanted location upstream from the coronary sinus. *Patients with operated structural heart disease and residual hemodynamic sequelae benefit from retaining AV synchrony, necessitating the consideration of a dual chamber pacing system in this patient.* In general, it is preferable not to have a permanent pacing lead passing through the prosthetic valve in order to prevent the development of unacceptable tricuspid valve insufficiency (which was likely the primary indication for bioprosthetic tricuspid valve implantation in this patient). This is particularly important in the setting of Ebstein anomaly, where RV function is likely to remain compromised, regardless of previous surgical repair. A possible option in the setting of replacement of the tricuspid valve in a patient with a preexisting endocardial ventricular pacing lead would have been to allow the lead to be placed exterior to the sewing ring of the valve, but this was not a consideration here, as the patient did not have symptomatic bradyarrhythmia or a preexisting endocardial pacing lead at the time of valve surgery.

In the recent years, there has been considerable controversy regarding the optimal ventricular pacing site. Several large studies in adults and children have established that chronic RV pacing is associated with LV dyssynchrony, dysfunction, and structural alterations in the LV that may be progressive.[3–6] Although this is probably of particular importance to children, who will require lifelong pacing over several decades, several studies have established that a relevant proportion of patients with Ebstein anomaly have preexisting structural and functional abnormalities affecting the LV. Structural alterations include LV noncompaction, mitral valve prolapse, and LV fibrosis.[7,8] Both systolic and diastolic dysfunction of the LV have been reported in Ebstein anomaly, and some of these functional alterations persist and may progress despite surgical procedures in the right side of the heart.[9,10] The ideal pacing technique would therefore be dual chamber pacing with a right atrial and a LV lead. In this patient,

access to the coronary sinus, and therefore the possibility of transvenous LV pacing, is precluded by the location of the tricuspid valve bioprosthesis. Permanent pacing would therefore have to be accomplished by the use of an epicardial LV lead, accepting the fact that epicardial systems are less durable and have a shorter lifespan than transvenous systems. The choice of location for the atrial lead also needs to be carefully considered. Owing to the previous surgical procedures (right atrial maze and tricuspid valve replacement), there is a considerable risk that poor atrial thresholds may be obtained from epicardial atrial sites caused by scar tissue from prior surgery. *It may be necessary therefore to implant an endocardial atrial lead in combination with the epicardial LV pacing lead.*

Permanent pacing in adults with structural heart disease also presents unique problems, both procedure related and at follow-up. Surgical access is likely to be more complicated, and the incidence of acute complications such as bleeding, pocket infection, and pneumothorax is higher. Failed or difficult lead placement is common in this setting, with increasing difficulty being associated with a higher number of prior surgical procedures.[1,2] Such procedural difficulties and failures occur more frequently in Ebstein anomaly than in other structural lesions.[1] Late complications such as early battery depletion, pacemaker migration, and erosion are also more frequently observed in the setting of permanent epicardial pacing in this patient population.[2]

Lead failures, defined as a failure to reliably capture or sense the ventricle or atrium, and lead dislodgement or fracture are commonly encountered with epicardial ventricular leads. The presence of Ebstein anomaly has been noted to be an independent risk factor for lead failure in one study, regardless of epicardial or endocardial location and whether the lead was implanted in the RV or LV. It has been suggested that this may be a unique feature of this anomaly and may be the result of an inherent tendency to fibrosis around the lead tip at the site of implantation.[1]

In summary, the rather unique postsurgical anatomy of this patient necessitates the choice of a suboptimal dual chamber pacing system, with an anticipated higher rate of acute and follow-up complications. A final consideration would be the transvenous implantation of a leadless single chamber pacemaker. There are few reports on the use of such a system in adults with complex structural heart disease and little follow-up data on their performance in this patient population.[11,12] There is a small risk of cardiac perforation, and this may be relevant in the setting of Ebstein anomaly and a thinned-out RV.

Considering that the patient is still relatively young and fit, this would not be the procedure of choice but may be considered in the future.

REFERENCES

1. McLeod CJ, Attenhofer CH, Warnes CA, et al. Epicardial versus endocardial permanent pacing in adults with congenital heart disease. *J Interv Card Electrophysiol.* 2010; 28:235–243.
2. Opic P, van Kranenburg M, Yap S-C, et al. Complications of pacemaker therapy in adults with congenital heart disease: a multicenter study. *Int J Cardiol.* 2013;168: 3212–3216.
3. Sweeney MO, Hellkamp AS, Ellenbogen KA, et al. Mode Selection Trial Investigators. Adverse effect of ventricular pacing on heart failure and atrial fibrillation among patients with normal baseline QRS duration in a clinical trial of pacemaker therapy for sinus node dysfunction. *Circulation.* 2003;107:2932–2937.
4. Moak JP, Hasbani K, Ramwell C, et al. Dilated cardiomyopathy following right ventricular pacing for AV block in young patients: resolution after upgrading to biventricular pacing systems. *J Cardiovasc Electrophysiol.* 2006;17: 1068–1071.
5. Janousek J, van Geldorp IE, Krupickova S, et al. Permanent cardiac pacing in children: choosing the optimal pacing site. A multicenter study. *Circulation.* 2013;127:613–623.
6. Karpawich PP, Rabah R, Haas JE. Altered cardiac histology following apical right ventricular pacing in patients with congenital atrioventricular block. *Pacing Clin Electrophysiol.* 1999;22:1372–1377.
7. Daliento L, Angelini A, Ho SY, et al. Angiographic and morphologic features of the left ventricle in Ebstein's malformation. *Am J Cardiol.* 1997;80:1051–1059.
8. Saxena A, Lee AH, Fong LV. Functional and histologic abnormalities of the left ventricle in Ebstein's anomaly of the tricuspid valve. *Indian Heart J.* 1993;45:135–136.
9. Inai K, Nakanishi T, Mori Y, Tomimatsu H, Nakazawa M. Left ventricular diastolic dysfunction in Ebstein's anomaly. *Am J Cardiol.* 2004;93:255–258.
10. Benson LN, Child JS, Schwaizer M, Perloff JK, Schelbert HR. Left ventricular geometry and function in adults with Ebstein's anomaly of the tricuspid valve. *Circulation.* 1987;75:353–359.
11. Ferrero P, Yeong M, D'Elia E, Duncan E, Stuart AG. Leadless pacemaker implantation in a patient with complex congenital heart disease and limited vascular access. *Indian Pacing Electrophysiol J.* 2016;16:201–204.
12. Wilson DG, Morgan JM, Roberts PR. "Leadless" pacing of the left ventricle in adult congenital heart disease. *Int J Cardiol.* 2016;209:96–97.

Consultant Opinion #2

HENRY CHUBB, MBBS, PHD • ERIC ROSENTHAL, MD FRCP

INTRODUCTION

In general, the need for device implantation or renewal in patients with adult congenital heart disease (ACHD) should not be considered as a "stand-alone device procedure."[1] It should prompt a multidisciplinary meeting with ACHD surgeons, cardiologists, and electrophysiologists to consider the impact of the device in the specific anatomy and in respect of potential concomitant or future catheter interventions or cardiac surgery. Although updating the imaging is always important, some pacemaker systems will render the patient ineligible for magnetic resonance imaging (MRI) scanning in the future and so the opportunity to perform a cardiac MRI should be considered before device implantation. Currently, epicardial leads and most coronary sinus (LV) leads are not MRI compatible.

This patient has had a good result from his bioprosthesis and antitachycardia surgery. He now presents with evidence of both sinoatrial disease and atrioventricular disease manifesting in near syncope. He has had a previous sternotomy for a valve repair, and the type of pacing system needs to be considered. It would appear that no other procedures are considered to be imminent, and the choice of system is predominantly affected first by the presence of a bioprosthetic tricuspid valve that is functioning well and second by previous sternotomy.

PERMANENT PACING IMPLANTATION METHODS

Although a single chamber ventricular pacemaker may be enough to prevent syncopal pauses, a dual chamber system will enable reliable atrioventricular synchrony and be more effective if his sinoatrial disease progresses as it is likely to do. There is the small possibility that a single lead atrial system would suffice (see response to question 2) but this is unlikely. The main concern is regarding the placement of the ventricular lead, which include several options.

Transvenous Ventricular Pacing
Coronary sinus pacing
The coronary sinus would be the first choice in patients with a prosthetic tricuspid valve so as to avoid any valve leaflet dysfunction and not interfere with subsequent surgical or percutaneous replacement.[2] An additional benefit would be reduction in LV dysfunction in patients who needed continuous ventricular pacing; this is not the case for our patient but the pacing burden may increase with time.

For this patient, it has been documented that the coronary sinus is not available, but this option should nonetheless be explored before dismissal—referral to the PVI procedural note from 2004 is not sufficient, as access may have been attempted only with larger or nonsteerable catheters. The original operation note should be consulted, and further imaging (e.g., computed tomography [CT]) should be considered in the event of any doubt. In addition, a left-sided superior vena cava to coronary sinus has been described in patients with Ebstein anomaly, and this should also be excluded because its presence would allow ventricular pacing without crossing the tricuspid valve prosthesis.[3] Angiography in the coronary sinus may identify coronary veins draining directly to the right atrium. Manipulating a guide wire through the coronary sinus and into the right atrium would allow the wire to be snared in the right atrium and exteriorized to place a coronary sinus lead over the guide wire circuit (with or without coronary venoplasty) into the coronary venous system, which would allow ventricular pacing without crossing the tricuspid valve. Such connections are unlikely to be seen with CT scanning.[4]

Transvalvular pacing
The placement of a pacing lead across a valve prosthesis is not ideal, but in some cases, it is unavoidable. The long-term impact of the presence of pacing lead upon valve function has not been well described but can only be detrimental. McCarthy and colleagues identified the presence of pacing to increase the incidence of severe tricuspid prosthesis regurgitation from 23% to 42% of

subjects at 5 years, but the type, positioning, and timing of the ventricular pacing leads were not detailed.[5] Cooper and colleagues described in more detail the placement of a pacing lead across a tricuspid valve prosthesis (two mechanical and two bioprosthetic), and this was well tolerated by patients with bioprosthetic valves, albeit with short follow-up.[6] If transvalvular pacing is necessary, the use of a SelectSecure 4F lead (Medtronic) across the bioprosthesis is likely to minimize any valve dysfunction[7] and allows for easier extraction.[8]

Future considerations would include the eventuality that further valve replacement may be required. Intraoperative removal of the transvenous lead should be achievable, and permanent epicardial leads should be placed if a good epicardial site is identified. If not, temporary epicardial pacing would be required, with later placement of a new transvenous system (ideally via coronary sinus at that stage). If a percutaneous valve-in-valve[9] is possible, then the SelectSecure lead will need extracting so as not to be trapped between the two valves followed by placement of a new system at the same sitting, or later if the patient is not pacemaker dependent at that time.

If the decision is made to place a transvalvular lead, the lead should be targeted to the true septum or His bundle below the bioprosthesis or RV apex[10] in order to minimize any LV dysfunction. The RV is not dysfunctional, so dual site ventricular pacing or free wall RV pacing is not required to resynchronize the RV.[11]

His bundle pacing
Pacing of the compact AV node or the bundle of His in the right atrium has been well described, screwing the lead into the membranous septum.[12] This would avoid both crossing the bioprosthesis and ventricular dyssynchrony. There have been no published reports on the use of His bundle pacing in patients with tricuspid valve bioprosthesis, but the theory is attractive if a suitable location could be found. Prior or simultaneous electroanatomic mapping may be useful in searching for appropriate sites in the immediate vicinity of the valve.

Leadless Pacemaker
The long-term data regarding leadless pacemakers is limited but could provide a relative simple pacing solution. Two leadless pacemakers are currently available: the Nanostim LP (St. Jude Medical)[13] and the Micra transcatheter pacing system (Medtronic).[14] The Nanostim is 42 mm in length with maximum diameter 6 mm and delivered via 18F sheath, whereas the Micra is 26 mm in length with maximum diameter 6.7 mm and delivered via a 23F internal diameter (27F external diameter) steerable catheter. Both these pacemakers are

currently limited to single chamber functionality only (VVIR), and the main concerns regard those of cardiac perforation and vascular access. In a patient with Ebstein anomaly, and potentially thin RV wall, careful evaluation before implantation is required and CT may represent the best imaging modality for delineation of wall thickness. Positioning in the apical septum is likely to be required for a Nanostim device; however, there may be difficulty in finding sufficient trabeculation within the RV to anchor the passive tines of the Micra.

In the longer term, the battery lifespan of the leadless pacing device remains to be determined, but has been estimated at 10–15 years.[15] For this patient, it would be anticipated that the pacing burden could be kept low unless there is further deterioration in the conduction system and this would also minimize the impact of the anticipated pacing dyssynchrony. However, the device should be implanted with the expectation that it will not be retrievable following endothelialization.

Epicardial Ventricular Pacing

While possible with all anatomies, previous surgical scarring may make it difficult to find a suitable site that gives low thresholds and does not cause ventricular dyssynchrony. Extensive scarring is likely to preclude the use of minimally invasive surgical techniques.[16]

Historic concerns regarding lead longevity and high thresholds have been largely overcome with the use of bipolar steroid-eluting leads.[17] However repeated sternotomies render epicardial placement of pacing leads less attractive, and, in general, this approach would be reserved for obligatory sternotomy for additional intracardiac procedures. Multidisciplinary discussion among the surgeon, implanting physician, and imaging teams would be important to delineate the relative risk of epicardial versus endocardial approaches for the placement of the ventricular lead.

INTRA-ATRIAL BLOCK VERSUS ATRIOVENTRICULAR NODAL LEVEL BLOCK

Could he have only sinus node disease with intra-atrial delayed or blocked conduction due to the right atrial maze? Would a site in the right atrium allow atrial pacing that conducts normally to the AV node?

The P-wave morphology on the 12-lead ECG is within normal limits for sinus nodal origin (positive in II, III, and aVF; positive then negative in V1[18]) and, furthermore, is not prolonged. Significant lengthening of the P wave would be anticipated in the case of severe intra-atrial block at rest. The ambulatory monitoring (Fig. 5.3, 4 p.m.) demonstrates P waves marching

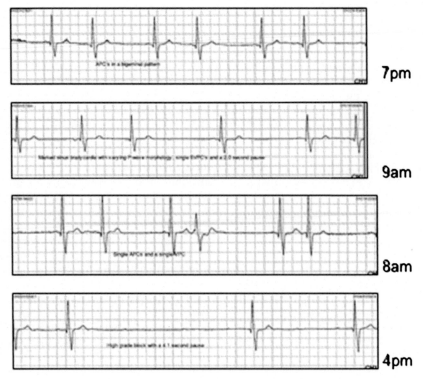

FIG. 5.3

through with a similar morphology and rate to baseline; it is unlikely that atrial conduction disease will have developed to an extent sufficient to cause intermittent intra-atrial block in the absence of P-wave morphology alteration.

However, it is important to be wary of the potential for severe atrial disease. The patient has had a previous right-sided maze procedure, and the right atrium has been exposed to chronic volume and pressure overload, promoting structural remodeling that will include fibrosis and myocyte hypertrophy.[19] *Electroanatomic mapping of the right atrium at the time of lead implantation would clarify the extent of atrial myopathy, and limited electrophysiologic study would confirm or refute the extent of AV nodal disease.* Although unlikely, normal AV nodal conduction properties (note that it was normal at the time of PVI in 2004) and extensive atrial scar could possibly lead to the identification of intra-atrial block as the cause of AV dissociation, potentially allowing atrial pacing alone to avoid the abovementioned considerations.

Regardless, electroanatomic mapping should be considered to assist in the identification of a suitable site for long-term atrial pacing, and a septal atrial pacing site (using an active lead) may be preferred to reduce intra-atrial conduction time and enhance AV synchrony in the presence of residual intrinsic ventricular conduction.[20] This patient is likely to require an increasing degree of atrial pacing as sinus nodal dysfunction progresses, and an AAI(R)↔DDD(R) mode switch algorithm (e.g., Managed Ventricular Pacing [Medtronic] or RYTHMIQ [Boston Scientific]) will be useful in the minimization of ventricular pacing. However, AV synchrony would be lost with AAI pacing in the presence of severe conduction delay.

SUMMARY

If a single chamber system is considered enough, just to prevent pauses, then the leadless pacemaker would be the least invasive, would not affect the tricuspid prosthesis, and would be MRI compatible. For a dual chamber endocardial system, a SelectSecure lead across the prosthetic valve would allow a simple procedure and a more versatile system that is also MRI compatible but with potential for a more complicated procedure in the future. Epicardial pacing would be appropriate if the patient agrees to redo sternotomy or thoracotomy but neither a single nor dual chamber system would be MRI compatible currently. Electroanatomic mapping (assessing intra-atrial block, His pacing options) and coronary sinus venography to enable lead placement into a coronary vein without crossing the tricuspid valve are not

only likely to be challenging and time-consuming but also the most sophisticated approaches to the problem. Only certain LV lead configurations would be MRI compatible currently. Finally, a frank discussion with the patient after an ACHD multidisciplinary meeting to complete the decision making is required.

TAKE-HOME POINTS (EDITORS)

1. The presence of a prosthetic tricuspid valve is a relative but not absolute contraindication to endocardial pacing.
2. Epicardial pacing is a good option but does involve more surgery.
3. Innovative endocardial approaches, such as the leadless pacemaker, can be considered depending on the indication to pace.
4. Hybrid procedures (part endocardial and part epicardial) and newer leads (lumenless leads) can be used in some patients.

REFERENCES

1. Chubb H, O'Neill M, Rosenthal E. Pacing and defibrillators in complex congenital heart disease. *Arrhythmia Electrophysiol Rev.* 2016;5(1):57−64.
2. Grimard C, Clémenty N, Fauchier L, Babuty D. Ventricular pacing through coronary sinus in patients with tricuspid prosthesis. *Ann Thorac Surg.* 2010;89:e51−e52. Elsevier Inc.
3. Marianeschi SM, McElhinney DB, Reddy VM, Silverman NH, Hanley FL. Alternative approach to the repair of Ebstein's malformation: intracardiac repair with ventricular unloading. *Ann Thorac Surg.* 1998;66:1546−1550. Elsevier.
4. Furniss GO, Liang M, Jimenez A, Harding S. Wire externalisation for left ventricular lead placement in cardiac resynchronisation therapy: a step-by- step guide. *Heart Lung Circ.* 2015;44:1094−1103.
5. McCarthy PM, Bhudia SK, Rajeswaran J, et al. Tricuspid valve repair: durability and risk factors for failure. *J Thorac Cardiovasc Surg.* 2004;127:674−685.
6. Cooper JP, Jayawickreme SR, Swanton RH. Permanent pacing in patients with tricuspid valve replacements. *Br Heart J.* 1995;73:169−172.
7. Antonelli D, Adam Freedberg N. Endocardial ventricular pacing through a bioprosthetic tricuspid valve. *Pacing Clin Electrophysiol.* 2007;30:271−272.
8. Shepherd E, Stuart G, Martin R, Walsh MA. Extraction of SelectSecure leads compared to conventional pacing leads in patients with congenital heart disease and congenital atrioventricular block. *Heart Rhythm.* 2015;12:1227−1232.
9. Milburn K, Bapat V, Thomas M. Valve-in-valve implantations: is this the new standard for degenerated bioprostheses? Review of the literature. *Clin Res Cardiol Springer Berlin Heidelberg.* 2014;103:417−429.

10. Janousek J, van Geldorp IE, Krupickova S, et al. Permanent cardiac pacing in children: choosing the optimal pacing site: a multicenter study. *Circulation*. 2013;127:613–623.

11. Kubuš P, Materna O, Tax P, Tomek V, Janoušek J. Successful permanent resynchronization for failing right ventricle after repair of tetralogy of Fallot. *Circulation*. 2014;130: e186–e190.

12. Mulpuru SK, Cha YM, Asirvatham SJ. Synchronous ventricular pacing with direct capture of the atrioventricular conduction system: functional anatomy, terminology, and challenges. *Heart Rhythm*. 2016;13:2237–2246. Elsevier.

13. Reddy VY, Exner DV, Cantillon DJ, et al. Percutaneous implantation of an entirely intracardiac leadless pacemaker. *N Engl J Med*. 2015;373:1125–1135.

14. Ritter P, Duray GZ, Steinwender C, et al. Early performance of a miniaturized leadless cardiac pacemaker: the Micra Transcatheter Pacing Study. *Eur Heart J*. 2015;36: 2510–2519.

15. Clarke TSO, Zaidi AM, Clarke B. Leadless Pacemakers: practice and promise in congenital heart disease. *J Congenit Cardiol*. 2017;1:4.

16. Costa R, Scanavacca M, da Silva K. Novel approach to epicardial pacemaker implantation in patients with limited venous access. *Heart Rhythm*. 2013;10:1646–1652.

17. Tomaske M, Gerritse B, Kretzers L, et al. A 12-year experience of bipolar steroid-eluting epicardial pacing leads in children. *Ann Thorac Surg*. 2008;85:1704–1711.

18. Kistler PM, Roberts-Thomson KC, Haqqani HM, et al. P-wave morphology in focal atrial tachycardia. Development of an algorithm to predict the anatomic site of origin. *J Am Coll Cardiol*. 2006;48:1010–1017.

19. Ueda A, Adachi I, McCarthy KP, Li W, Ho SY, Uemura H. Substrates of atrial arrhythmias: histological insights from patients with congenital heart disease. *Int J Cardiol*. 2013;168:2481–2486. Elsevier Ireland Ltd.

20. Khairy P, van Hare GF, Balaji S, et al. PACES/HRS expert consensus statement on the recognition and management of arrhythmias in adult congenital heart disease. *Heart Rhythm*. 2014;11:e1–e63.

CHAPTER 6

Transposition With Atrial Switch and Risk of Sudden Death

Submitted by Marc G. Cribbs, MD, FACC

CASE SYNOPSIS

LB is a 26-year-old male with a history of dextro-transposition of the great arteries (DTGA) and intact ventricular septum. Desaturation and restriction of atrial level flow was almost immediately apparent and balloon atrial septostomy was performed just hours after he was born. At 3 months of age, he underwent a Senning-type atrial switch operation.

One month after surgery, he was admitted with an atrial tachycardia for which he was started on propranolol. The arrhythmia improved and regular follow-up demonstrated normal sinus rhythm with no evidence of pathologic tachycardia. LB maintained close congenital cardiology follow-up until he was 15 years of age and was then lost to follow-up.

At age 26 years, he presented with the New York Heart Association (NYHA) class IV heart failure. He was admitted to the CCU and the adult congenital heart disease (ACHD) team was consulted. He described a 6-month history of progressive shortness of breath, fatigue, three- to four-pillow orthopnea, and paroxysmal nocturnal dyspnoea. He also complained of a 10- to 15-pound weight loss over the previous 3 months because of nausea and early satiety. Most notable was a history of palpitations that had preceded all these symptoms. The palpitations were initially noted as infrequent episodes of "rapid heart rate" that, over time, became more and more frequent. There was no history of syncope. There was also no history of drug, tobacco, or alcohol use.

A transthoracic echocardiogram suggested severe biventricular dysfunction and moderate tricuspid insufficiency; however, the images were of poor quality. A cardiac MRI later confirmed severe systemic right ventricular (RV) dysfunction (right ventricular ejection fraction [RVEF], 20%), severe pulmonic left ventricular dysfunction (left ventricular ejection fraction, 22%), moderate systemic tricuspid insufficiency,

and no evidence of systemic or pulmonary venous baffle dysfunction. With this and the palpitation history in mind, LB was taken to the electrophysiology (EP) laboratory where an atrioventricular nodal reentry tachycardia (AVNRT) was mapped and successfully ablated. Hemodynamic assessment at the time of EP study revealed a cardiac index of 2.1 L/min/m². He was initiated on intravenous milrinone, gradually transitioned to conventional oral medications, and discharged home 3 weeks later with NHYA class II−III symptoms.

For the next 2 months, the patient maintained close ACHD follow-up and adherence to all medications. Follow-up rhythm monitoring (Holter as well as a 30-day event monitor) demonstrated no evidence of arrhythmia, rare premature atrial contractions, and a single 8-beat run of nonsustained ventricular tachycardia (VT). Again there was no syncope. Subsequent imaging with transthoracic echocardiography, however, demonstrated no improvement in cardiac function and his exertional shortness of breath and fatigue returned. He was readmitted, this time to the Heart Failure and Transplant Service. A right heart catheterization subsequently demonstrated a cardiac index of 1.5 L/min/m², modestly elevated filling pressures (wedge pressure, 15−19 mmHg), and no evidence of baffle dysfunction. Given this, heart transplant evaluation was started. The ACHD team was also consulted regarding prophylactic implantable cardioverter defibrillator (ICD) placement in this patient with severe biventricular dysfunction.

Questions

1. What should be the next step in his treatment?
2. Is there place for an ICD at this time?
3. Should it be a subcutaneous ICD (S-ICD) or a transvenous single, dual, or biventricular ICD?
4. Does he need any treatment such as specific medications or ablation for the nonsustained VT?

Consultant Opinion #1

JEREMY MOORE, MD

This is an interesting case with several important EP considerations unique to the ACHD population, specifically to those with DTGA palliated by the Mustard or Senning operation. *The first issue to be examined is the unexplained development of severe biventricular dysfunction in this patient, with the possible contribution of an undiagnosed supraventricular tachycardia.* The phenomenon of tachycardia-induced cardiomyopathy is well described and is a fully reversible form of congestive heart failure.[1] This process is characterized by incessant or nearly incessant tachycardia with the insidious progression of heart failure. Although there are no systematic studies of tachycardia-induced cardiomyopathy in the ACHD population, anecdotally, these cases usually stem from initially subclinical atrial arrhythmias such as intra-atrial reentrant tachycardia or atrial fibrillation. Although certainly incessant or nearly incessant AVNRT could in theory result in cardiomyopathy, this form of tachycardia tends to be paroxysmal in nature and rarely leads to cardiomyopathy. On the other hand, supraventricular arrhythmia that arises as a result of ventricular dysfunction is well described in the ACHD literature.[2,3] Because AVNRT[4] and progressive ventricular dysfunction are both common after surgically repaired DTGA, it is likely that the AVNRT discovered in this patient is an incidental finding.

The second issue here is this patient's need for an ICD. Sudden death risk following the DTGA Mustard or Senning operation is one of the highest in the ACHD population, equaling approximately 0.5% per patient-year.[5] The risk tends to be bimodal with an early peak after repair, followed by a second peak in adulthood that corresponds with the progressive decline in systemic RV function. Risk factors are multiple and include atrial tachyarrhythmia, ventricular dysfunction, tricuspid regurgitation, increasing age, and electrocardiographic findings such as QRS duration (140 ms serving as a useful discriminant value).[6–10] Unlike other forms of congenital heart disease, there is limited utility for programmed stimulation in the risk stratification process.[9,11] Importantly, β-blocker administration

has been shown to be protective against sudden cardiac death in this population.[9]

Currently, the only available guidelines for ICD placement in the setting of DTGA after Mustard or Senning operation are a result of expert consensus, generally supported by limited clinical evidence.[12] Such guidelines suggest that ICD therapy may be reasonable with an RVEF <35%, especially if accompanied by additional risk factors such as complex ventricular arrhythmias, unexplained syncope, NYHA functional class II or III symptoms, QRS duration ≥140 ms, or severe systemic atrioventricular (AV) valve regurgitation.

An important consideration when planning ICD placement for patients with congenital heart disease is the presence of an intracardiac shunt, which can as much as double the rate of systemic thromboembolism after implantation.[13] Also, the presence of severe pulmonary hypertension with subsequent mitral regurgitation can result in further clinical deterioration. In either of these scenarios, S-ICD could be considered to avoid potential complications associated with conventional ICD.[14] Importantly, lack of bradycardia pacing and cardiac resynchronization therapy (CRT) capability is an important limitation to S-ICD, and this especially applies to the present case where both the functionalities may be important.[14]

The final issue is the risks versus benefits of CRT in this situation. CRT for congenital heart disease has been shown to be beneficial in many circumstances. Patients with chronic ventricular pacing are most likely to benefit, in whom the electrical delay is, in part, iatrogenic and ubiquitous. For others, especially those with systemic RV morphology as in the present case, the benefits of CRT are less clear. Although mechanical dyssynchrony as observed by echocardiography is extremely common among patients with DTGA after a Mustard or Senning operation, CRT is of limited to no use unless accompanied by markers of electrical delay.[15] For this reason the QRS duration is of paramount importance. Current guidelines emphasize complete right bundle branch block with a QRS duration of at least 150 ms before contemplation of CRT for these patients.[12] This degree of QRS prolongation has been shown to be present in approximately 7% of ACHD patients with DTGA after Mustard or Senning operation and thus may apply here.[16]

Importantly, CRT is necessarily invasive in the DTGA group as the coronary venous system draining the systemic RV is rarely, if ever, accessible by the transvenous route. Most centers prefer to place a dual chamber pacing system first, followed by an epicardial lead for resynchronization of the RV. The epicardial lead is typically placed on the RV free wall via a right thoracotomy. Ideally, the epicardial lead is placed at the site of the latest RV activation. This can be assessed at the time of pacemaker implantation by 3D mapping or alternatively in the operating room with a roving electrode. A more empirical, anatomic approach in which the lead is placed directly across the tricuspid valve annulus when the valve is viewed *en face* may achieve the widest separation in the two ventricular leads and optimal resynchronization performance.[17]

RECOMMENDATION

Proceed with ICD implantation with CRT-defibrillator device if QRS duration is prolonged, i.e., >150 ms, approaching the RV free wall via surgical thoracotomy. Consider S-ICD if intracardiac shunt or severe pulmonary hypertension is present, but only with normal QRS duration and no significant bradycardia. No medical therapy other than β-blockade is recommended for the finding of nonsustained VT, given the available evidence.

REFERENCES

1. Gopinathannair R, Etheridge SP, Marchlinski FE, Spinale FG, Lakkireddy D, Olshansky B. Arrhythmia-induced cardiomyopathies: mechanisms, recognition, and management. *J Am Coll Cardiol.* 2015;66:1714—1728.
2. Gewillig M, Cullen S, Mertens B, Lesaffre E, Deanfield J. Risk factors for arrhythmia and death after Mustard operation for simple transposition of the great arteries. *Circulation.* 1991;84:III187—192.
3. Puley G, Siu S, Connelly M, et al. Arrhythmia and survival in patients >18 years of age after the mustard procedure for complete transposition of the great arteries. *Am J Cardiol.* 1999;83:1080—1084.
4. Kanter RJ, Papagiannis J, Carboni MP, Ungerleider RM, Sanders WE, Wharton JM. Radiofrequency catheter ablation of supraventricular tachycardia substrates after Mustard and Senning operations for d-transposition of the great arteries. *J Am Coll Cardiol.* 2000;35:428—441.
5. Silka MJ, Hardy BG, Menashe VD, Morris CD. A population-based prospective evaluation of risk of sudden cardiac death after operation for common congenital heart defects. *J Am Coll Cardiol.* 1998;32:245—251.
6. Sarkar D, Bull C, Yates R, et al. Comparison of long-term outcomes of atrial repair of simple transposition with implications for a late arterial switch strategy. *Circulation.* 1999;100:II176—181.
7. Gatzoulis MA, Walters J, McLaughlin PR, Merchant N, Webb GD, Liu P. Late arrhythmia in adults with the mustard procedure for transposition of great arteries: a surrogate marker for right ventricular dysfunction? *Heart.* 2000;84:409—415.
8. Dos L, Teruel L, Ferreira IJ, et al. Late outcome of Senning and Mustard procedures for correction of transposition of the great arteries. *Heart.* 2005;91:652—656.
9. Khairy P, Harris L, Landzberg MJ, et al. Sudden death and defibrillators in transposition of the great arteries with intra-atrial baffles: a multicenter study. *Circ Arrhythm Electrophysiol.* 2008;1:250—257.
10. Schwerzmann M, Salehian O, Harris L, et al. Ventricular arrhythmias and sudden death in adults after a Mustard operation for transposition of the great arteries. *Eur Heart J.* August 2009;30:1873—1879.
11. Kertesz NJ, Ackley T, Daniels CJ, et al. ICDs fro primary prevention in d-TGA status post intra-atrial baffle repair: is the cure worse than the disease? *Heart Rhythm.* 2011;8: S98.
12. Khairy P, Van Hare GF, Balaji S, et al. PACES/HRS expert consensus statement on the recognition and management of arrhythmias in adult congenital heart disease: executive summary. *Heart Rhythm.* 2014;11: e81—e101.
13. Khairy P, Landzberg MJ, Gatzoulis MA, et al. Transvenous pacing leads and systemic thromboemboli in patients with intracardiac shunts: a multicenter study. *Circulation.* May 23, 2006;113:2391—2397.
14. Moore JP, Mondésert B, Lloyd MS, et al. Clinical experience with the subcutaneous implantable cardioverter-defibrillator in adults with congenital heart disease. *Circ Arrhythm Electrophysiol.* 2016;9:e004338.
15. Chow PC, Liang XC, Lam WW, Cheung EW, Wong KT, Cheung YF. Mechanical right ventricular dyssynchrony in patients after atrial switch operation for transposition of the great arteries. *Am J Cardiol.* 2008;101:874—881.
16. Diller GP, Okonko D, Uebing A, Ho SY, Gatzoulis MA. Cardiac resynchronization therapy for adult congenital heart disease patients with a systemic right ventricle: analysis of feasibility and review of early experience. *Europace.* 2006;8:267—272.
17. Janousek J, Tomek V, Chaloupecky VA, et al. Cardiac resynchronization therapy: a novel adjunct to the treatment and prevention of systemic right ventricular failure. *J Am Coll Cardiol.* 2004;44:1927—1931.

Consultant Opinion #2

RONALD KANTER, MD

Diagnostic and management decisions for this patient include considerations that are both generalizable to adults having unexplained systolic dysfunction and clinical heart failure and specific to those who have undergone Mustard or Senning operation (atrial switch procedures) for DTGA. First, it is surprising that such a patient would be apparently well through the age of 15 years and then deteriorate so severely by the age of 26 years. Tachycardia-induced cardiomyopathy comes to mind first, and in the population who have undergone atrial switch, intra-atrial reentry tachycardia (IART) is usually the culprit.[1] As maintenance of this tachycardia is less autonomically influenced than AV node–dependent tachycardias, its potential for persistence over time is great. Also, because the atrial rate is usually 200–300 bpm, patients may be asymptomatic so long as they have 3–4:1 AV conduction and notice palpitations only during catecholamine stress and 1–2:1 conduction. However, this consideration appears to be moot, as IART was neither observed clinically nor induced during EP testing. The diagnosis of AV nodal reentry, although not uncommon in this patient group,[2] would not be expected to be incessant, and paroxysmal episodes would affect myocardial function only briefly. Therefore, other contributory factors, which may be relevant to post–heart transplant care, should be thoroughly investigated. Hypertension and obesity seem to be especially detrimental to systemic RV function over time.[3] Lifestyle issues, especially recreational drug use and chronic alcohol intake, should also be investigated. Finally, residual baffle leaks and paradoxic embolization to the coronary artery system are possible.

Unlike adults having structurally normal hearts and either ischemic or nonischemic cardiomyopathy,[4,5] risk factors for sudden death—and, thus, opportunities for primary prevention—are poorly understood those with congenital heart disease. Therefore, people who care for adults with congenital heart disease have traditionally relied upon data from the structurally normal population to make recommendations. An RVEF of <35% has been especially popular to determine ICD implantation and has been supported by a consensus statement.[6] That said, reports have provided some additional guidance in the patients who have undergone atrial switch. Previous atrial tachyarrhythmias,[7,8] prior VT/sudden cardiac arrest,[9] absence of chronic therapy with β-blocking drugs,[9] older age at surgery,[8] associated structural lesions (such as subpulmonic stenosis),[10] NYHA class >III,[10] impaired RV function,[10] and QRS duration >140 ms[10] have been identified as associations with increased risk in reports of 5–47 affected patients. Our patient, LB, has ample risk factors. The decision to place a transvenous ICD versus S-ICD is based on the need for bradycardia pacing, the potential benefit of biventricular pacing, baffle obstruction, and the existing baffle leaks with the potential for right-to-left shunts. These patients therefore require thorough evaluation for associated defects. If bradycardia or biventricular pacing is deemed appropriate, catheter-based interventions to treat baffle leaks or obstruction may then be necessary before placement of intracardiac hardware. Early experience with S-ICDs in the congenital heart population is favorable, including a multi-institutional experience that included two patients, following atrial switch operation.[11]

RV dysfunction following atrial switch procedures has been shown to be associated with late gadolinium enhancement by cardiac MRI, which in turn is associated with intraventricular RV conduction delay, especially of the free wall.[12] Selecting patients for attempted CRT is not trivial because it nearly always requires open chest surgery for RV lead placement, usually near the acute margin. Favoring such an approach might be a QRS duration (>140 ms)[10] or proof of mechanical delay by speckle tracking techniques. Speckle tracking techniques to determine ventricular longitudinal strain has been adapted to the systemic RV[13] and successfully applied to patients who have undergone Mustard or Senning operation to identify those who ultimately benefitted from CRT.[14] The authors used the "classic pattern" to identify patients having the dyssynchrony phenotype that is amenable to therapy.[15] If the patient is a candidate for CRT, a hybrid approach is usually used, wherein the left ventricular lead is transvenous and the surgically placed RV lead is tunneled to a left subclavicular pocket. This minimizes the need for extensive surgical dissection and may enable a limited thoracotomy/sternotomy for RV lead placement.

Recommendations regarding EP evaluation/therapies:

1. Perform speckle tracking for RV mechanics.
2. Assess for sinoatrial node or AV conduction disease (presumed negative from history).
3. If "classic pattern" is present or there is severe RV conduction delay (QRS duration, >140 ms), then complete evaluation/treatment of baffle leaks/obstruction. Then proceed to placement of biventricular ICD using hybrid approach.
4. If QRS duration is <140 ms and "classic pattern" is absent, then place S-ICD.
5. Initiate carvedilol, metoprolol, or bisoprolol therapy.

TAKE-HOME POINTS (EDITORS)

In a patient with systemic ventricular dysfunction who has undergone atrial switch (Mustard/Senning operation)

1. consider persistent or recurrent tachyarrhythmia as a potential cause of the ventricular dysfunction;
2. if the QRS duration is prolonged then consider biventricular pacing using a hybrid approach;
3. if the QRS duration is narrow, there is no benefit to CRT and, as long as there is no indication to pace, a S-ICD is the best option;
4. antiarrhythmic agents other than β-blockers have little benefit in the treatment of nonsustained VT.

REFERENCES

18. Baysa SJ, Olen M, Kanter RJ. Arrhythmias following the Mustard and Senning operations for dextro-transposition of the great arteries. Clinical aspects and catheter ablation. In: Balaji S, Mandapati R, Shivkumar K, eds. *Cardiac Electrophysiology Clinics*. Philadelphia: Elsevier; 2017:255−272. Cardiac Arrhythmias in Adults with Congenital Heart Disease; Vol. 9.
19. Kanter RJ, Papagiannis J, Carboni MP, Ungerleider RM, Sanders WE, Wharton JM. Radiofrequency catheter ablation of supraventricular tachycardia substrates after mustard and Senning operations for d-transposition of the great arteries. *J Am Coll Cardiol.* 2000;35:428−441.
20. Tabtabai S, Yeh DD, Stefanescu A, Kennedy K, Yeh RW, Bhatt AB. National trends in hospitalizations for patients with single-ventricle anatomy. *Am J Cardiol.* 2015;116: 773−778.
21. Moss AJ, Zareba W, Hall WJ, et al. Prophylactic implantation of a defibrillator in patients with myocardial and reduced ejection fraction. *N Engl J Med.* 2002;346: 877−883.
22. Bardy GH, Lee KL, Mark DB, et al. Amiodarone or an implantable cardioverter-defibrillator for congestive heart failure. *N Engl J Med.* 2005;352:225−237.
23. Khairy P, Van Hare GF, Balaji S, et al. PACES/HRS expert consensus statement on the recognition and management of arrhythmias in adult congenital heart disease. *Heart Rhythm.* 2014;11:e102−e165.
24. Kammeraad JA, van Deurzen CH, Sreeram N, et al. Predictors of sudden cardiac death after Mustard or Senning repair for transposition of the great arteries. *J Am Coll Cardiol.* 2004;44:1095−1102.
25. Wheeler M, Grigg L, Zentner D. Can we predict sudden cardiac death in long-term survivors of atrial switch surgery for transposition of the great arteries? *Congen Heart Dis.* 2014;9:326−332.
26. Khairy P, Harris L, Landzberg MJ, et al. Sudden death in transposition of the great arteries with intra-atrial baffles: a multicenter study. *Circ Arrhythm Electrophysiol.* 2008;1: 250−257.
27. Schwerzmann M, Salehian O, Harris L, et al. Ventricular arrhythmias and sudden death in adults after a Mustard operation for transposition of the great arteries. *Eur Heart J.* 1873-1879;2009:30.
28. Moore JP, Mondesert B, Lloyd MS, et al. Clinical experience with the subcutaneous implantable cardioverter-defibrillator in adults with congenital heart disease. *Circ Arrhythm Electrophysiol.* 2016;9.
29. Babu-Narayan SV, Goktekin O, Moon JC, et al. Late gadolinium enhancement cardiovascular magnetic resonance of the systemic right ventricle in adults with previous atrial redirection surgery for transposition of the great arteries. *Circulation.* 2005;111:2091−2098.
30. Forsha D, Risum N, Kropf PA, et al. Right ventricular mechanics using a novel comprehensive three-view echocardiographic strain analysis in a normal population. *J Am Soc Echocardiogr.* 2014;27:413−422.
31. Forsha D, Risum N, Smith PB, et al. Frequent activation delay-induced mechanical dyssynchrony and dysfunction in the systemic right ventricle. *J Am Soc Echocardiogr.* 2016;29:1074−1089.
32. Risum N, Jons C, Olsen NT, et al. Simple regional strain pattern analysis to predict response to cardiac resynchronization therapy: rationale, initial results, and advantages. *Am Heart J.* 2012;163:697−704.

CHAPTER 7

Ebstein Anomaly With Atrial Tachycardia

Case submitted by James Oliver, MBChB, PhD, MRCP

CASE SYNOPSIS

Diagnoses

Ebstein anomaly of the tricuspid valve (TV).

TV repair with right atrial (RA) cryoablation and epicardial pacemaker, February 2015.

TV replacement, March 2016.

Very troublesome atrial tachyarrhythmia with multiple direct current (DC) cardioversions and ablations.

Type 2 diabetes.

Gout.

Varicose veins.

Initial Assessment, 2011

The patient is a 49-year-old male seen in our center for the first time in October 2011 following referral from his local cardiologist. He had been under follow-up at another center for a number of years. He is working as an electrician and is a keen body builder.

He described increasing breathlessness over the previous 12 months. He reported occasional dizziness, mainly related to eating and very occasional palpitations. He was on simvastatin for hypercholesterolemia and metformin for type 2 diabetes. His other medical problems are gout and varicose veins.

At initial assessment, he was normally saturated at rest; heart rate, 60 bpm; and BP, 140/88 mmHg, with a soft flow murmur at the left sternal edge.

Electrocardiography (ECG): SR and PR 234 ms and QRS 142 ms (right bundle branch block). ECG was not submitted, as its quality has degraded.

Transthoracic echocardiography showed severe tricuspid regurgitation (TR) with flow reversal in hepatic veins and dilated right ventricle (RV).

Assessment 2013–14

The patient did not attend a number of office visits in 2011/12 and was seen again in March 2013 when he felt more breathless and dizzy. Dizziness was more prominent after exercise. Palpitations were lasting up to 15 s. He was advised to cut down alcohol consumption (he was drinking 20 pints of beer over a 3-day weekend). Jugular venous pulse was just visible at the root of the neck. His weight was 110 Kg. The systolic murmur was soft and liver was not palpable.

Findings of a 24-h Holter monitor were unremarkable. Sinus throughout in first-degree heart block and there were occasional supraventricular and ventricular ectopics.

Bicycle cardiopulmonary exercise (CPEX) test: completed 9.5 min of a 20-W ramp. The test was stopped because it was felt that he had gone into supraventricular tachycardia (on review, this was not convincing—it looked on review to be a gradual onset sinus tachycardia). At this point, his Vo_2 was 14.2 mL/Kg/min. No desaturation was observed.

MRI examination during November 2013 showed RV end-diastolic volume, 454 mL (195 mL/m^2); RV end-systolic volume, 222 mL; and RV ejection fraction, 51%. Septal leaflet of TV displaced 56 mm. Severe TR with an estimated regurgitation fraction of 63%. RA dilated (97 cm^2). Left side of the heart was normal, and there was no other abnormality. No evidence of a shunt was seen.

He underwent an electrophysiologic (EP) study under local anesthesia on March 6, 2014. The report included the following.

Atrial tachycardia (AT) induced using catheter manipulation. Cycle length (CL), 308 ms (but with some variability). Variable atrioventricular (AV) conduction (ventricular rate never above 90 bpm). Patient was asymptomatic. Accelerated following atrial burst pacing to 220 ms. Eventually terminated with atrial burst at 180 ms.

Diagnostic catheterization showed a mean RA pressure of 10 mmHg (with peak of 23 mmHg due to TR); a RV pressure of 32 mmHg, with end-diastolic pressure of 3; and a right pulmonary artery pressure of 32/5 mmHg, with a mean of 16 mmHg.

Summary

No evidence of accessory pathway conduction.

No AV nodal reentry tachycardia.

Inducible AT with variable AV block.

Normal pulmonary artery pressures.

An ablation was not attempted because there was a provisional plan for him to undergo surgery.

The CPEX test was repeated in April 2014. He managed 7 min of the Bruce protocol and made a good effort (maximal test). His Vo_2 max was 15.9 mL/Kg/min; heart rate, 72 bpm baseline, 147 bpm at peak; blood pressure (BP), 110/80 mmHg baseline, 160/80 mmHg at peak.

Subsequent coronary angiography showed very mild left anterior descending artery atheroma, and he was accepted for TV surgery with concomitant RA cryoablation.

FIRST EPISODE OF CLINICALLY EVIDENT ATRIAL ARRHYTHMIA, SEPTEMBER 2014

The patient was seen in clinic in September 2014, before he had undergone surgery, when he gave a history of being significantly more easily breathless with chest discomfort and an increased heart rate. His jugular venous pressure was elevated to 4 cm, and there was a small amount of ankle edema. ECG showed atrial flutter with a ventricular rate of 70 bpm. He had been started on furosemide and was anticoagulated with warfarin. There was a mild abnormality of the liver function tests suggestive of hepatic congestion. He underwent successful DC cardioversion. Given the forthcoming surgery, baseline first-degree heart block, and slow ventricular response in atrial flutter, a regular antiarrhythmic was not prescribed.

FIRST OPERATION—FEBRUARY 2015, SUBSEQUENT EPISODES OF ATRIAL FLUTTER

In February 2015, surgery was performed and consisted of TV repair, RA cryoablation, and permanent epicardial dual chamber pacemaker implantation. Mild to moderate residual TR was noted at intraoperative transesophageal echocardiography and was accepted.

Early after operation, he was back in atrial flutter with an intrinsic ventricular rate of 65 bpm. It was not possible to pace-terminate via the pacemaker. He was discharged on bisoprolol and amiodarone. Six weeks after discharge, he remained in atrial flutter and

was <0.1% atrial and ventricular paced. A further attempt to pace-terminate the flutter was not successful and he underwent a successful DC cardioversion.

In May 2015, he presented again with atrial flutter and a further DC cardioversion was performed.

He was keen to stop amiodarone (there were also mildly deranged thyroid function tests) and this was discontinued after uptitrating bisoprolol in July 2015.

A further DC cardioversion was performed in August 2015 and he was changed from bisoprolol to sotalol 80 mg BD.

RECURRENCE OF SEVERE TRICUSPID REGURGITATION NOTED OCTOBER 2015

In October 2015, he was 97% atrially and 100% ventricularly paced. Transthoracic echocardiography suggested recurrence of severe TR, and he described becoming breathless and tired very easily. He had not noticed any symptomatic improvement following his surgery.

A further DC cardioversion was performed in November 2015.

A further EP study and ablation was performed in December 2015. Transesophageal echocardiography at the time confirmed severe TR. The EP study found the following.

The patient had an inducible atrial flutter, CL 460 ms, and attempted pace termination was unsuccessful, although he managed to accelerate tachycardia. There was significant scar laterally and posteriorly and it identified an area of scar anterolaterally running inferiorly from the region of superior vena cava (SVC)/RA junction.

A line of block was created from scar anterior and inferior to lateral TV annulus with progressive lengthening of CL from 460 to 580 ms (rate 103) with 1:1 conduction. In all, a 10cm burn was performed.

There was spontaneous cessation of tachycardia into sinus bradycardia with a long PR interval. The study concluded that the flutter was significantly modified with ablation, with remaining tachycardia of CL 580 ms (rate 103), and a decision was made to not pursue it further.

TRICUSPID VALVE REPLACEMENT, MARCH 2016, FURTHER TROUBLESOME ATRIAL FLUTTER

He was keen to undergo any procedure that might improve his symptoms and underwent redo sternotomy with a 33-mm Hancock II porcine biological TV replacement in March 2016. Consideration was given to perform a bidirectional cavopulmonary shunt at the time, given the poor RV function, but he came off bypass easily and this was not felt necessary at the time.

He again presented in May 2016 with atrial flutter and a further EP study was performed acutely. An ablation was performed with an extension of the linear lesion between the TV annulus and the inferior vena cava, as well as areas of fractionated atrial electrograms in the inferior portion of the RA. The tachycardia ceased during the procedure and could not be reinduced. A few weeks later, there had been no recurrence of atrial arrhythmia and he was 88% atrially paced and 98% ventricularly paced.

In July 2016, at a routine clinic review, he was again found to be in atrial flutter and a further EP study and ablation was performed. This time a PentaRay catheter was used to create geometry and timing map. The patient was in AT with a CL of 390 ms at the beginning of the case. The earliest signals were in the atrial appendage with early signals meeting late signals around the base of the appendage and SVC. A voltage map in this region suggested a scar laterally (atriotomy) and a scar around the base of the atrial appendage. A discontinuous area of scar was seen in posterior RA, with isthmus of active tissue with perfect return cycle on entrainment.

A line of lesions was created from SVC posterior to TV annulus with a change in tachycardia CL to 440 ms. A limited remap showed the RA appendage outside the circuit but now with interesting electrograms in inferolateral RA with concealed entrainment and a perfect return cycle.

Further ablation in a low lateral RA position linking scars and then a further burn across a line of double potentials was done with cessation of tachycardia.

However, there was further induction of tachycardia with burst atrial pacing with a different CL from previous tachycardia (280–300 ms) suggesting an RA focus. So further lesions were placed to extend the lateral line inferior and anterior to further scar.

OCTOBER 2016, REMAINS LIMITED, LIKELY VENTRICULAR TACHYCARDIA ON EXERCISE

In October 2016, he continued to report severe exercise limitation. His TV prosthesis had good function, and there was felt to be a small improvement in RV systolic function, although this remains significantly impaired. At this stage, he was still on sotalol and was restarted on a diuretic.

At a CPEX test, he made a good effort and exercised for almost 7 min of the Bruce protocol, stopping because of dizziness and breathlessness. Vo_2 max was 18.6 mL/Kg/min (improved when compared with the CPEX test result before his first operation). During the exercise test, he went into broad-complex tachycardia, which was felt likely to be ventricular tachycardia (VT, 150 bpm), reverting to a paced rhythm when he stopped exercising. His pacemaker was reprogrammed to detect ventricular high rates of 145 bpm and more.

Because of concerns of developing faster VT, a subcutaneous ICD was implanted, after ensuring suitability.

QUESTIONS

1. What is his risk for sudden death and does he definitely need an implantable cardioverter defibrillator (ICD)?
2. Are there any other options for managing his rhythm problems?

Consultant's Opinion #1

SANTABHANU CHAKRABARTI, MBBS, MD, FRCPC, FRCP (EDIN), FRCPCH, FACC, FHRS, DARRYL WAN MD AND COLLEAGUES

This case describes the follow-up events of a 49-year-old man with Ebstein anomaly with other comorbidities including diabetes and dyslipidemia presenting with right-side heart failure due to severe TR. The patient underwent several EP studies and ablation of various RA arrhythmia circuits with good acute success but suboptimal medium-term outcomes. The patient required redo TV surgery and developed significant RV dysfunction and exercise-induced VT.

WHAT IS HIS RISK FOR SUDDEN DEATH AND DOES HE DEFINITELY NEED AN ICD?

Individuals with congenital heart disease (CHD) have a higher risk of sudden cardiac death (SCD) than the general population.[1] In the CHD group, patients with systemic RV, single ventricle, and tetralogy of Fallot are deemed to have higher risk of SCD.[2] The risk of SCD in Ebstein anomaly is not well defined; however, SCD has been reported in Ebstein anomaly.[3–5] On the other hand, severe RV or left ventricular systolic dysfunction in CHD is a risk factor for SCD.[6] The patient had normal biventricular systolic dysfunction on MRI. However, with progression of time, he has had significant RV dysfunction and sustained VT and hence, *he would meet the criteria for ICD implantation.*

ARE THERE ANY OTHER OPTIONS FOR MANAGING HIS RHYTHM PROBLEMS?

This patient has sinus bradycardia with bifascicular conduction delay, VT, and multiple atrial arrhythmias, which resulted in hemodynamic decompensation. Medical therapy is the first line of therapy with pacemaker and ICD support. Ongoing β-blocker therapy for prevention of arrhythmia and slowing of AV node conduction is another good option. *The use of amiodarone for both AT and VT will be a good choice as the second-line therapy, in addition to β-blocker use.*

Subcutaneous ICD (S-ICD) needs to be used after careful consideration in this clinical scenario, as it has been associated with increased inappropriate shock compared with transvenous ICD. However, *an S-ICD is attractive in this patient, as he has had multiple TV surgeries and epicardial pacing.*[7]

If the atrial arrhythmias become severe, the use of any other antiarrhythmic agent apart from amiodarone has to be considered with extreme caution in view of the significantly dysfunctional RV and structural heart disease. AV node ablation may be considered as the last resort because the LV systolic function is preserved but performing AV node ablation in the setting of two previous TV replacements may be challenging from a femoral approach owing to the difficulty in mapping the His bundle area.

A subsequent pacing strategy if/when the LVEF deteriorates may involve using cardiac resynchronization with an epicardial LV lead or His bundle pacing. In view of the two previous pericardiotomies obtaining access to an optimum basal LV pacing site for epicardial lead placement is likely to be challenging. On the other hand, placing an endocardial His bundle lead around the operated TV annulus in Ebstein anomaly would be difficult as well. Furthermore, pacing artifacts from an epicardial LV lead or His bundle lead may interfere with optimum S-ICD detection.

Therefore, it is sensible to consider rate control for AT as long it is tolerated well. Repeat ablation for AT or VT should be offered with force sensing technology and 3D mapping.

REFERENCES

1. Walsh EP. Sudden death in adult congenital heart disease: risk stratification in 2014. *Heart Rhythm.* 2014;11(10): 1735–1742.
2. Silka MJ, Hardy BG, Menashe VD, Morris CD. A population-based prospective evaluation of risk of sudden cardiac death after operation for common congenital heart defects. *J Am Coll Cardiol.* 1998;32(1):245–251.
3. Cipolletta L, Luzi M, Piangerelli L, Guerra F, Capucci A. Entirely subcutaneous implantable defibrillator: safest option in a young girl with ventricular tachycardia and Ebstein anomaly. *Circ Arrhythm Electrophysiol.* 2014;7(2):358–359.
4. Chen SSM, Sheppard MN. Sudden cardiac death in Ebstein's malformation due to a cardiac haemangioma. *Eur Heart J.* 2011;32(19):2364.
5. Nikolić BP, Lovrić D, Puljević D, et al. Cardiac arrest in a patient with Ebstein's anomaly without accessory pathways. *Coll Antropol.* 2013;37(4):1357–1359.
6. Khairy P. Ventricular arrhythmias and sudden cardiac death in adults with congenital heart disease. *Heart Br Card Soc.* 2016;102(21):1703–1709.
7. Moore JP, Mondésert B, Lloyd MS, et al. Clinical experience with the subcutaneous implantable cardioverter-defibrillator in adults with congenital heart disease. *Circ Arrhythm Electrophysiol.* 2016;9(9).

Consultant's Opinion #2

EDWARD P. WALSH, MD

Ebstein anomaly can be associated with a wide assortment of atrial and ventricular arrhythmias.[1,2] Some of these are intrinsic to the malformation itself (e.g., accessory AV pathways, atriofascicular fibers, reentrant VT in the atrialized ventricular muscle), whereas others arise from the insidious process of degenerative remodeling caused by the hemodynamic burden of TV dysfunction, RV enlargement, and surgical scarring (e.g., atrial macroreentrant circuits, atrial fibrillation, myopathic VTs). This case presents a challenging example of the latter category in a middle-aged man who underwent TV surgery late in life at a time when degenerative remodeling was likely to be far advanced. ATs were the dominant problem outlined in the case material, but there is also more recent concern raised for the possibility of VT.

I shall begin by addressing the AT. The EP study conducted in June 2014 was helpful in ruling out abnormal conduction pathways and establishing primary AT as the principle issue. A sustained AT was mechanically induced with catheter manipulation at that study and attempts to overdrive pace for termination resulted in shifts to other AT CLs, which immediately indicates this was not a straightforward single-circuit substrate. Formal mapping was not performed because he was being considered for surgery that would involve an RA maze lesion set. Before this surgery, he presented with a clinical episode of sustained AT that was described as atrial flutter. The ECG provided for the September 2014 episode has features that make me suspicious if this was actually a more complex AT, with variations in the P-wave shape and axis indicating multiple circuits or possibly even atrial fibrillation. During the surgery in February 2015, he underwent tricuspid valvuloplasty along with RA cryoablation and epicardial dual chamber pacemaker placement. Details of the cryoablation lesions were not provided, but presumably, this involved the cavotricuspid isthmus as well as the lateral wall connecting the atriotomy to one or both vena cavae. Unfortunately, neither the valve repair nor the RA maze provided long-term benefit. Despite therapy with multiple drugs, including amiodarone, he subsequently required multiple cardioversions for recurrent AT episodes. At the second EP study in December 2015, a slow AT with CL >400 ms was induced, once

again with occasional shifts in CLs during attempts to pace-terminate, suggesting a complex substrate, and irrigated ablation within the RA slowed the circuit but never achieved complete termination. He subsequently had a bioprosthetic TV replacement to address progressive regurgitation, but postoperatively still had AT that required two additional ablation sessions with extensive RA lesions. The clinical narrative does not specify whether he still has AT episodes after ablation while taking sotalol, but it sounds as if the primary cardiologists are concerned that AT is still not completely controlled.

Description of the catheter ablations in this case confirms that elegant mapping and aggressive ablation techniques were appropriately employed during all procedures. No doubt the RA is markedly dilated and likely quite thickened in this case. Despite our best efforts, mapping is often incomplete in this setting, and regions labeled as scar may in fact contain small conduction channels that can be difficult to detect. Furthermore, despite the use of irrigation, radiofrequency lesions may not achieve complete transmural injury when atrial muscle becomes very thick. This challenge is especially relevant to patients who have undergone an atriopulmonary Fontan operation[3] but may be operative in a case like this as well. Similar to some patients who have undergone the Fontan operation, surgical resection of large regions of redundant atrial free-wall tissue may be required to eliminate all relevant conduction corridors that can contribute to reentrant circuits. A case like this may be further complicated by AT involving left atrial tissue or even atrial fibrillation. The ECG from 2014 raises the possibility in my mind that atrial fibrillation may be operative in at least some of the arrhythmia recurrences. At my center, we have performed biatrial maze procedures with pulmonary vein isolation for certain patients undergoing the cone procedure for Ebstein anomaly whenever we suspect the risk of atrial fibrillation is high, and the results have been encouraging thus far.[4] I am not proposing reoperation solely for atrial muscle resection or biatrial maze after the fact for this particular patient, but if he ever requires reoperation on the TV in the future, I would certainly incorporate these maneuvers into the surgery. *At present, I would lean toward repeat catheter ablation procedures as necessary, using high-density mapping with a PentaRay catheter, as was described in the July 2016 session, and ablate all suspicious areas as aggressively as possible. Personally, I have little confidence in pharmacologic therapy for achieving complete control in this type of AT, although it may attenuate the problem to some degree.*

More recently, the possibility of VT was raised in this case. Patients with Ebstein anomaly are indeed at risk for this complication, and ECG recordings during a 2016 exercise test raised the suspicion for this patient when a wide-QRS tachycardia at 150 bpm was observed that differed from the QRS at baseline (which was presumably a ventricular paced QRS). It is hard for me to draw firm conclusions about the tachycardia mechanism based only on the two ECGs provided. Recording quality is not optimal. I cannot be sure I see pacing spikes on the baseline recording, and details of the transition between the baseline QRS and the tachycardia QRS were not provided. Were any data recorded from the pacemaker leads to clarify atrial rhythm during this event? Does he ever conduct through his AV node when catecholamine levels are elevated, and if so, what does the QRS look like? Nevertheless, in the absence of firm data, my best speculation is that this was actually not monomorphic VT but quite possibly a conducted AT event. I have two reasons for this speculation. First, the event has a pattern of right bundle branch block across the precordial leads and this is not entirely dissimilar to his ECG from 2014. Second, most of the documented monomorphic VTs in patients with Ebstein anomaly have been mapped to the diaphragmatic surface of the RV where ventricular muscle is most atrialized and tends to generate a left bundle branch block pattern.[2,5] For the purpose of this discussion, I will allow that this might have been a true VT because I do not have firm data to say otherwise, but if the primary cardiologists are in fact unsure themselves about the mechanism, I would propose doing atrial and ventricular stimulation through the pacemaker to see if this pattern could be recreated for diagnostic purposes. *If in fact this is VT, I agree it is a high-risk situation that deserves consideration of an ICD. Putting a transvenous lead through a reconstructed or a prosthetic valve in a patient like him is clearly not desirable. An S-ICD system would be a reasonable (if not preferred) alternative, assuming QRS sensing is suitable.*

TAKE-HOME POINTS (EDITORS)

1. Severe RV or left ventricular dysfunction and sustained VT should be an indication for ICD placement in patients with severe forms of CHD.
2. Avoid placing pacing or defibrillation leads through prosthetic AV valves.
3. In patients with severe recurrent atrial arrhythmias despite multiple therapies (drugs, catheter ablation, and surgery), it is important to keep considering repeat catheter ablation procedures with alternative technology as and when they become available.
4. Similarly, consideration should be given to referral to more specialized centers in such cases
5. VT in patients with Ebstein anomaly commonly arises from the diaphragmatic aspect of the atrialized RV and should be considered for catheter ablation.

REFERENCES

1. Sherwin ED, Triedman JK, Walsh EP. Update on interventional electrophysiology in patients with congenital heart disease: evolving solutions for complex hearts. *Circ Arrhythm Electrophysiol.* 2013;6:1032−1040.
2. Shivapour JK, Sherwin ED, Alexander ME, et al. Utility of preoperative electrophysiologic studies in patients with Ebstein's anomaly undergoing the Cone procedure. *Heart Rhythm.* 2014;11:182−186S.
3. Walsh EP. Interventional electrophysiology in patients with congenital heart disease. *Circulation.* 2007;115:3224−3234.
4. Vogel M, Marx GR, Tworetzky W, et al. Ebstein's malformation of the tricuspid valve: short-term outcomes of the "cone procedure" versus conventional surgery. *Congenit Heart Dis.* 2012;7:50−58.
5. Obioha-Ngwu O, Milliez P, Richardson A, Pittaro M, Josephson ME. Ventricular tachycardia in Ebstein's anomaly. *Circulation.* 2001;104:E92−E94.

CHAPTER 8

Resynchronization Therapy and Sudden Death Management in Congenitally Corrected Transposition

Submitted by Damien Cullington, MBChB (Hons), MD, MRCP, FESC

CASE DETAILS

History of Presenting Medical Complaint

A 38-year-old man presented to his local hospital with a 9-month history of expectorating small volumes of hemoptysis preceded by exertional dyspnoea for 4—5 months. He also gave a history of two brief episodes of dizziness but no syncope. He was referred following a recording of his 12 lead ECG which showed complete heart block (CHB) (Fig. 8.1).

Echo demonstrated that he had congenitally corrected transposition of the great arteries (ccTGA) with a mildly dilated systemic right ventricle (RV) with severely impaired function and moderate systemic tricuspid valve (TV) regurgitation into a dilated left atrium. The subpulmonic, morphologic left ventricle (LV) was also severely impaired with trivial mitral regurgitation. There was no ventricular septal defect. There was a small atrial shunt with left to right flow.

He initially underwent implantation of dual chamber pacemaker. A transesophageal echo was performed under general anesthesia at the same time as pacemaker implantation and cardiac catheterization. This showed that there was moderate systemic right ventricular impairment, moderate-to-severe systemic tricuspid regurgitation, and severely impaired subpulmonic left ventricular function.

He was then readmitted with decompensated heart failure. This admission was preceded by 10 days of worsening shortness of breath, abdominal discomfort, and anorexia. He had hepatorenal decompensation with ALT 830 iu/L (<40) (normal values in brackets); ALP 119 iu/L (30—130); Bilirubin 53 umol/L (2—21); Urea 19 mmol/L (2.5—7.8); Creatinine 179 umol/L (64—104); and eGFR 37 mL/min/1.73 m^2. He was diuresed and commenced on dobutamine. His clinical condition marginally improved. Symptomatically he remained in NYHA III off inotropes, but he was accepted for an assessment at our local cardiac transplant center due to our concerns of his declining status. After continued diuresis and further optimization of his medical therapy, he continued to improve, with a reduction in his pulmonary artery pressure (PAP) and was deemed too fit for cardiac transplantation.

He is now stable on medical treatment and is symptomatically NYHA class II. He has had no further admissions due to decompensated heart failure for over 12 months. His hemoptysis has entirely resolved with reduction in his pulmonary pressures. A recent cardiopulmonary exercise test (Jan 2017) using bike ergometry at 15 W ramp staging remeasured his peak VO$_2$ at 19.7 mL/kg/min at an respiratory exchange ratio (RER) of 1.56. He exercised for 13 min 2 s.

Admission Blood Tests (Normal Values Given in Brackets)

Hb 173 g/L (135—180); WCC 8.7 10^9/L (4.00—11.00); Plt 197 10^9/L (150—400)

NTproBNP levels
2013 ng/L (11/01/16)
157 ng/L (25/10/16)
Current
Hb 115 g/L (135—180);
Sodium 140 mmol/L (133—146);
Potassium 4.9 mmol/L (3.5—5.3);
Urea 10.9 mmol/L (2.5—7.8);
Creatinine 123 umol/L (64—104).

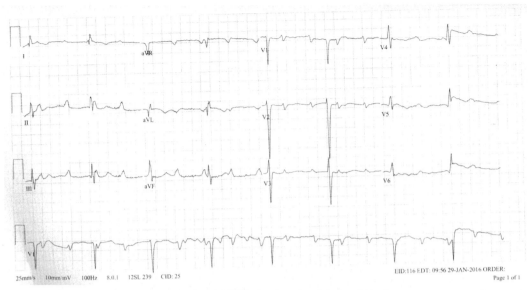

FIG. 8.1   12 Lead ECG showing complete heart block.

Observations

On initial presentation:
    Blood pressure 147/100;
    Heart rate 60 per minute;
    Saturations in room air 97%.

Past Medical History and Medication (Prior to Initial Admission)

Gout—treated with allopurinol

Current Medications (2017)

Spironolactone 25 mg od
    Digoxin 125 mcg od
    Bumetanide 2 mg twice daily
    Entresto 50 mg twice daily
    Carvedilol 12.5 mg twice daily
    Metformin 500 mg od
    Edoxaban 30 mg od

Social History

Nonsmoker and no alcohol intake.
    Father of five children.
    Works as a charity worker.

Electrocardiogram

Admission 12 lead ECG showed CHB with a junctional escape rhythm at a rate of 50 per minute (see traces) (Fig. 8.1).

CT Pulmonary Angiogram

Dilated pulmonary arteries. No pulmonary embolism to account for raised pulmonary artery pressure.

Cardiac Catheterization

Right PAP 62/40 mmHg; Left PAP 67/28 mmHg; Aortic pressure 63/35 mmHg.

Cardiac Catheterization—Post Diuresis at Transplant Center

Right atrial pressure 5 mmHg; PAP 43/13 mmHg; mean PAP 25 mmHg; wedge pressure 17 mmHg with V wave to 21 mmHg; cardiac index 2.2 L/min/m^2; pulmonary vascular resistance 2.2 Woods Units; transpulmonary gradient 8 mmHg.

Dual Chamber Pacemaker (ECG)

An endocardial dual chamber pacemaker with leads to the right atrium and the morphologic LV was implanted and set to pace in dual chamber (DDD) mode at 60—150bpm. With atrial tracking and ventricular pacing the BP was greatly improved (89—90 systolic) (Figs. 8.2—8.4).

Because of the readmission with recurrent congestive heart failure he underwent upgrade to a biventricular-implantable cardiac defibrillator. (Chest X-ray Figure, EMGs and biventricular paced ECG, coronary sinus selected shots—Figs. 8.5—8.7A and B)

He now has episodes of nonsustained ventricular tachycardia (NSVT) seen on device follow-up plus

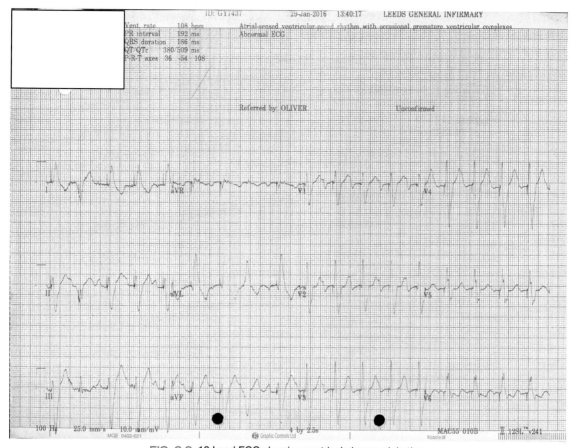

FIG. 8.2 12 Lead ECG showing ventricularly paced rhythm.

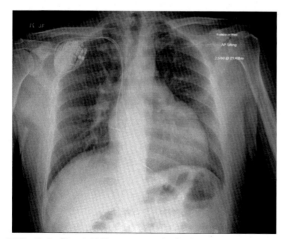

FIG. 8.3 Chest X-Ray - post dual chamber pacemaker implant.

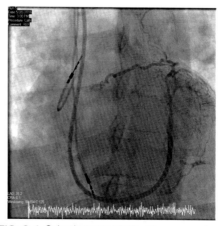

FIG. 8.4 Selective venography of coronary sinus.

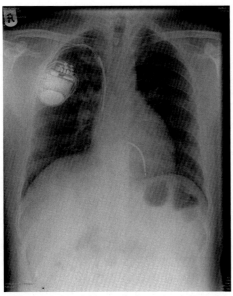

FIG. 8.5 Chest X-ray - post biventricular-ICD implant.

episodes of atrial fibrillation (AF) so he was commenced on a direct oral anticoagulant.

Questions

1. How would one risk stratify a patient with ccTGA (or perhaps a patient with a systemic RV) to mitigate against the risk of sudden cardiac death (SCD)?
2. What is the role of electrophysiology (EP) studies, signal-averaged ECG, and perhaps heart rate turbulence (HRT) and also of how useful is imaging to assist in risk stratification?
3. What is the role of biventricular pacing in patients with ccTGA? Should he have directly had a biventricular-implantable cardiac defibrillator without the intervening step of a dual chamber pacemaker?
4. What should be done with his current tachyarrhythmias?

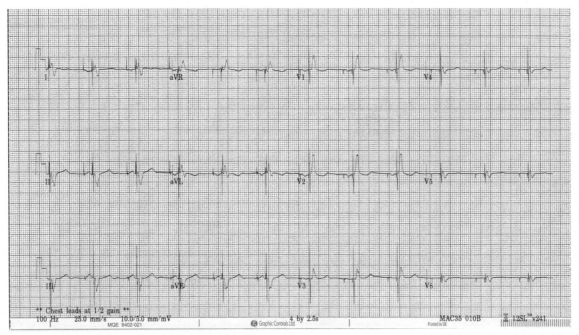

FIG. 8.6 12 Lead ECG following upgrade of PPM to biventricular pacemaker showing atrial and biventricular pacing.

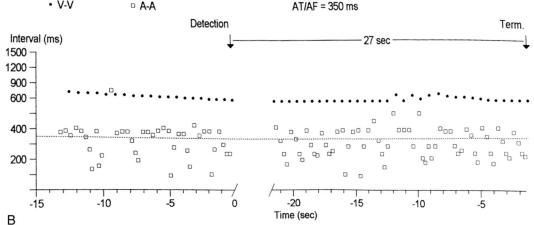

FIG. 8.7 Intracardiac electrograms of BIV-ICD showing non sustained ventricular tachycardia (top traces) and atrial fibrillation (bottom traces) Figs 8.7A&B.

Consultant Opinion #1

OKTAY TUTAREL, MD, FESC • GABRIELE HESSLING, MD

This is an interesting case of a patient first diagnosed with ccTGA with CHB and biventricular failure at the age of 38 years.

Patients with isolated ccTGA [i.e., without associated congenital heart defects (CHDs)] may go unrecognized until the third or fourth decade of life due to lack of symptoms. Survival into the sixth or seventh decade of life has been reported.[1] Long-term outcome is mainly defined by associated anomalies, arrhythmias, systemic atrioventricular (AV) valve regurgitation, and systemic right ventricular failure.[2]

Interestingly, this patient presented not only with impairment of the systemic RV but also of the subpulmonic LV. This is unusual and needs further investigation. One possible cause is the development of pulmonary hypertension, which has been reported in patients with complete transposition of the great arteries (TGA)[3] The mean PAP in this patient was 25 mmHg after treatment for heart failure. Coronary artery disease could also be a cause of ventricular dysfunction and coronary angiography might be advisable. Additionally, an MRI would also be valuable for further assessment. On a side note—as adult congenital heart disease (ACHD) patients often need an MRI for diagnostic reasons—the implementation of MRI-approved devices is recommended.

The issue of risk stratification for SCD in patients with ccTGA is challenging. While progressive failure of the systemic RV was reported as the most common cause of death in patients with ccTGA,[4] sudden death is also encountered. Tachyarrhythmia risk, implantable cardioverter-defibrillator (ICD) implant risks, long-term outcomes, and rates of appropriate and inappropriate ICD therapies are not well studied and characterized in this patient population. **While it is reasonable to implant an ICD for secondary prevention, there is no good evidence for directing our therapy to primary prevention of SCD.** Furthermore, up to 20% of SCDs in CHD may be due to nonarrhythmic causes such as cerebral or pulmonary embolism and aortic or aneurysmal rupture not amenable to ICD therapy.[5] Nonetheless, SCD in an otherwise clinically asymptomatic ccTGA patient was observed at an unexpectedly high rate in one of the largest series (1 death

per 109 patient-years).[6] In that study, the authors could not identify any clinical predictors of SCD.

We have more data in patients after atrial switch operation for complete TGA. Although these patients have other associated complications and are not an ideal comparison cohort for ccTGA patients, both cohorts have a systemic RV.[6] In one study, sustained VT/SCD was more likely to occur in patients with associated anomalies and impaired systemic ventricular function. Patients with a QRS duration ≥140 ms were at the highest risk.[7] In a Dutch study, symptoms of arrhythmias or heart failure at most recent follow-up and a history of documented supraventricular arrhythmias were the best predictors, whereas Holter ECG was not predictive for SCD.[8] In a multicenter study of patients with TGA and atrial switch with an ICD, supraventricular arrhythmias seemed to be implicated in the etiology of VT, while treatment with β-blockers was protective.[9] Inducible VT at an EP study did not predict future events.[9] In a recent study including patients with ccTGA (n = 25) and TGA after atrial switch operation (n = 63), it was reported that right ventricular end-diastolic volume index measured by MRI or CT and peak systolic blood pressure (SBP) on exercise testing were the best predictors of adverse clinical events (including death, worsening heart failure, and arrhythmias).[10] These predictors were similar in those with ccTGA and those with TGA and an atrial switch operation.[10]

Rydman et al. reported that systemic right ventricular fibrosis detected by MRI was associated with clinical outcomes, mainly supraventricular arrhythmias, in TGA patients after an atrial switch operation.[11] Therefore, imaging with late gadolinium enhancement could play a more prominent role for risk assessment in the future. While signal-averaged ECGs have been proposed as useful markers in patients after right ventriculotomy,[12] its role in ccTGA patients is not well defined.

Current guidelines state that ICD therapy may be reasonable in adults with a systemic right ventricular ejection fraction <35%, particularly in the presence of additional risk factors such as complex ventricular arrhythmias, unexplained syncope, NYHA functional class II or III symptoms, QRS duration ≥140 ms, or

severe systemic AV valve regurgitation.[5] Technical challenges of ICD implantation may arise especially in ccTGA patients and residual intracardiac shunts or dextrocardia. These should also be accounted for when considering ICDs for primary prevention in patients with ccTGA.[2]

Deterioration in systemic ventricular function has been reported following univentricular pacing in ccTGA patients.[13,14] It was proposed that all patients with ccTGA who develop CHB should undergo primary biventricular pacing to prevent late systemic ventricular dysfunction.[13] **Current guidelines recommend that CRT can be useful for adults with a systemic right ventricular ejection fraction below 35%, at least NYHA functional class II and complete right bundle branch block with a QRS complex >150 ms (spontaneous or paced).**[5] Furthermore, CRT can be useful in adults with CHD, a systemic ventricular ejection fraction <35%, an intrinsically narrow QRS complex, and at least NYHA class II symptoms who undergo device implantation or device replacement if a requirement for a significant amount (>40%) of ventricular pacing is anticipated.[5] Keeping in mind the anatomic variations of the coronary sinus in ccTGA patients, primary biventricular pacing may be reasonable. **Nonetheless, ventricular function should be monitored closely after pacing is initiated.**

Episodes of AF and of NSVT were detected on the patient's ICD follow-up. Rhythm control is generally recommended as the initial strategy for patients with moderate or complex forms of CHD. The loss of sinus rhythm, even with a controlled heart rate, can have an important adverse impact both on hemodynamics and ventricular function in ACHD patients.[5]

Antiarrhythmic drugs have been, for a long time, the only treatment used in CHD patients but not always with success. Koyak et al. investigated the efficacy of antiarrhythmic drugs in 92 CHD patients (68% atrial fibrillation). Class III drugs (amiodarone) were the most effective to prevent recurrences but at the same time were the drugs with the most side effects (thyroid toxicity).[15] Specific recommendations for AF ablation in CHD population have not yet been developed due to scarcity of published data. Philip et al. reported their experience in a cohort of 36 ACHD patients, but there were no ccTGA patients in this report.[16] In their patient population, a single pulmonary vein isolation was successful in 42% of patients at 300 days of follow-up with success rates, left atrial size, and complication rates similar in the CHD and the non-CHD group. Catheter ablation for AF might therefore be discussed with the patient, especially if his or her AF episodes are highly symptomatic.

Data about VT ablation in ccTGA patients are scarce. Corresponding to other entities of nonischemic cardiomyopathy, the substrate in nonoperated systemic RVs might be complex and variable, thereby limiting ablation success.[17] Regarding our patient, from findings in the TGA/atrial switch population, **no medical therapy other than β-blockade seems to be recommendable for the finding of NSVT.**[9]

REFERENCES

1. Graham TP Jr, Bernard YD, Mellen BG, et al. Long-term outcome in congenitally corrected transposition of the great arteries: a multi-institutional study. *J Am Coll Cardiol.* 2000;36:255−261.
2. Stout KK, Broberg CS, Book WM, et al. Chronic heart failure in congenital heart disease: a Scientific Statement from the American Heart Association. *Circulation.* 2016;133:770−801.
3. Lammers AE, Bauer UM. Pulmonary hypertension after timely arterial switch operation in children with simple transposition of the great arteries: a new disease entity? *Heart.* 2017 Aug;103(16):1227−1228.
4. Connelly MS, Liu PP, Williams WG, Webb GD, Robertson P, McLaughlin PR. Congenitally corrected transposition of the great arteries in the adult: functional status and complications. *J Am Coll Cardiol.* 1996;27:1238−1243.
5. Khairy P, Van Hare GF, Balaji S, et al. PACES/HRS Expert Consensus Statement on the Recognition and management of arrhythmias in adult congenital heart disease: developed in partnership between the Pediatric and Congenital Electrophysiology Society (PACES) and the Heart Rhythm Society (HRS). Endorsed by the governing bodies of PACES, HRS, the American College of Cardiology (ACC), the American Heart Association (AHA), the European Heart Rhythm Association (EHRA), the Canadian Heart Rhythm Society (CHRS), and the International Society for Adult Congenital Heart Disease (ISACHD). *Heart Rhythm.* 2014;11:e102−e165.
6. McCombe A, Touma F, Jackson D, et al. Sudden cardiac death in adults with congenitally corrected transposition of the great arteries. *Open Heart.* 2016;3:e000407.
7. Schwerzmann M, Salehian O, Harris L, et al. Ventricular arrhythmias and sudden death in adults after a Mustard operation for transposition of the great arteries. *Eur Heart J.* 2009;30:1873−1879.
8. Kammeraad JA, van Deurzen CH, Sreeram N, et al. Predictors of sudden cardiac death after Mustard or Senning repair for transposition of the great arteries. *J Am Coll Cardiol.* 2004;44:1095−1102.
9. Khairy P, Harris L, Landzberg MJ, et al. Sudden death and defibrillators in transposition of the great arteries with intra-atrial baffles: a multicenter study. *Circ Arrhythm Electrophysiol.* 2008;1:250−257.
10. van der Bom T, Winter MM, Groenink M, et al. Right ventricular end-diastolic volume combined with peak systolic

blood pressure during exercise identifies patients at risk for complications in adults with a systemic right ventricle. *J Am Coll Cardiol.* 2013;62:926–936.

11. Rydman R, Gatzoulis MA, Ho SY, et al. Systemic right ventricular fibrosis detected by cardiovascular magnetic resonance is associated with clinical outcome, mainly new-onset atrial arrhythmia, in patients after atrial redirection surgery for transposition of the great arteries. *Circ Cardiovasc Imaging.* 2015:8.

12. Perloff JK, Middlekauf HR, Child JS, Stevenson WG, Miner PD, Goldberg GD. Usefulness of post-ventriculotomy signal averaged electrocardiograms in congenital heart disease. *Am J Cardiol.* 2006;98: 1646–1651.

13. Hofferberth SC, Alexander ME, Mah DY, Bautista-Hernandez V, del Nido PJ, Fynn-Thompson F. Impact of pacing on systemic ventricular function in L-transposition of the great arteries. *J Thorac Cardiovasc Surg.* 2016;151:131–138.

14. Yeo WT, Jarman JW, Li W, Gatzoulis MA, Wong T. Adverse impact of chronic subpulmonary left ventricular pacing on systemic right ventricular function in patients with congenitally corrected transposition of the great arteries. *Int J Cardiol.* 2014;171:184–191.

15. Koyak Z, Kroon B, de Groot JR, et al. Efficacy of antiarrhythmic drugs in adults with congenital heart disease and supraventricular tachycardias. *Am J Cardiol.* 2013; 112:1461–1467.

16. Philip F, Muhammad KI, Agarwal S, Natale A, Krasuski RA. Pulmonary vein isolation for the treatment of drug-refractory atrial fibrillation in adults with congenital heart disease. *Congenit Heart Dis.* 2012;7:392–399.

17. Muser D, Santangeli P, Castro SA, et al. Long-term outcome after catheter ablation of ventricular tachycardia in patients with nonischemic dilated cardiomyopathy. *Circ Arrhythm Electrophysiol.* 2016;9.

Consultant Opinion #2

FRANK ZIMMERMANN, MD

The case presented is a good illustration of the long-term sequelae of ccTGA. One of the challenges in this population is that individuals may live for many years with relatively good health only to develop progressive heart failure and arrhythmias later in life.

The first question is how to risk stratify a patient with ccTGA to mitigate against the risk for SCD. A number of small series have reported on the risk for SCD in ccTGA. In patients with d-transposition of the great arteries (dTGA) and systemic RV following the Mustard or Senning procedure (Mustard/Senning), the risk for SCD is estimated to be between 2% and 15%.[1] Connelly et al., reported an 8% incidence of SCD in 52 adults with ccTGA.[2] In another series of 39 patients with ccTGA, the incidence of SCD was 12.8% giving a hazard ratio of 1 per 109 patient-years.[1] An important finding in these studies is that the risk of death from progressive systemic ventricular dysfunction or severe TV regurgitation is far greater than that from SCD in this population.

There is currently little data regarding risk stratification for SCD in ccTGA. In a large cohort of adults with CHD, factors associated with SCD among ccTGA patients (27 SCD cases vs. 52 controls) were heart failure symptoms, AF/flutter, and impaired systemic ventricular function by univariate analysis.[3] This is similar to the findings in a series of patients with dTGA following Mustard/Senning.[4] In another single-center review of patients with dTGA following the Mustard procedure, the incidence of sustained VT or SCD was 9% and was associated with older age, reduced systolic RV function, and QRS duration >140 ms[5]

The role for noninvasive testing to further refine risk stratification for SCD in ccTGA is unclear. Holter monitoring for atrial or ventricular arrhythmias or the development of AV block is important for routine management.[6] HRT determined from Holter recordings is a reflection of cardiac autonomic function. Impairment in HRT has been shown to be predictive of VT and sudden death in those with chronic heart failure or following myocardial infarction.[7,8] HRT has been shown to predict SCD in a small cohort of operated and unoperated patients with CHD.[9] HRT indices are also found to be impaired in tetralogy of Fallot patients following surgical repair.[10] Larger studies will be needed to further assess the predictive value of this parameter in ccTGA.

Cardiac MR has an important role for defining anatomy and determining RV systolic function in CHD.[11,12] Additional assessment of myocardial scar or fibrosis can also be performed. A study of patients with ccTGA or dTGA following Mustard/Senning found that MRI-derived RV end-diastolic volume index and peak SBP on exercise testing were predictors of arrhythmias, heart failure, and death.[13]

The role of invasive electrophysiology study testing (EPS) in asymptomatic individuals with a systemic RV has not been shown to predict future events. In a study of 37 patients with dTGA following Mustard/Senning and ICD placement, none with inducible VT at EPS received an appropriate shock, while 37.5% with no inducible VT at EPS did have an appropriate shock.[14] At this time, EPS is currently not recommended for further risk stratification in asymptomatic patients with dTGA following Mustard/Senning.[6]

Indications for primary prevention ICD use in ccTGA and long-term outcomes are not well described. The low rate of appropriate ICD shocks in patients with dTGA following Mustard/Senning of 0.5% for primary prevention makes this a challenging situation.[14] **The current recommendation (Class 2B, level of evidence C) is that ICD therapy may be reasonable in adults with systemic RV ejection fraction <35%, particularly in the presence of additional risk factors such as complex ventricular arrhythmias, unexplained syncope, NYHA functional class II or III symptoms, QRS duration >140 ms, or severe systemic AV valve regurgitation.**[6]

The role for cardiac resynchronization therapy (CRT) in systemic RV has been evolving. Small retrospective case series have suggested a benefit for CRT with a systemic RV.[15] There are mixed results regarding the degree of improvement with CRT for systemic RV compared with systemic LV.[16,17] The potential detrimental effects of ventricular pacing for CHB seen in adults with normal anatomy have also been described in those with a systemic RV.[18] Thus, there may be a role for primary CRT in those with systemic RV who require ventricular pacing due to CHB. In a series of 53 patients with ccTGA requiring ventricular pacing for CHB, 52% of those with univentricular pacing developed severe systemic ventricular dysfunction compared with none of those who received primary CRT.[19]

Specific to this case is that there is a >twofold increased risk for systemic thromboembolism with transvenous pacing/defibrillator leads in the presence of an intracardiac shunt.[20] **Therefore, assessment and potential intervention to eliminate intracardiac shunts should be considered prior to placement of transvenous pacemaker/defibrillator leads.**

Arrhythmia management in ACHD patients is important for symptomatic relief as well as possible reduction of the risk for SCD. In patients with a pacemaker or ICD, atrial arrhythmias can be addressed with antitachycardia pacing, often with the addition of an AV nodal blocking agent.[14,21] Antiarrhythmic medical therapy can be initiated with a strategy of rate or rhythm control. If rhythm control is preferred, Class I antiarrhythmic medications should be avoided in the setting of systemic or subpulmonary ventricular dysfunction. Amiodarone or dofetilide could be considered for treatment of symptomatic atrial arrhythmias in the setting of ventricular dysfunction.[6] Treatment of ventricular arrhythmias could also be addressed with antitachycardia pacing.[22] The use of β-blockers has been shown to decrease the incidence of ventricular arrhythmias in dTGA s/p Mustard.[14]

Recommendations

1. The patient was likely a candidate for ICD implantation at the time of pacemaker placement due to severe RV dysfunction (EF was not mentioned) and moderate TV regurgitation although this is a Class IIb recommendation.
2. Transcatheter device closure of the atrial-level shunt prior to placement of transvenous pacing/defibrillator leads would decrease the risk for systemic thromboembolism.
3. Biventricular ICD placement could have been considered at the time of the initial implant due to the concern for worsening ventricular function with univentricular pacing in systemic RV.
4. Antiarrhythmic therapy with metoprolol rather than carvedilol could be considered as this would have the dual role of AV node blockade (rate control of nonsustained atrial arrhythmias) and the potential to diminish the frequency of ventricular arrhythmias and risk for SCD in the setting of a systemic RV.

TAKE-HOME POINTS (EDITORS)

1. Whenever possible, use only MRI-compatible devices in patients with CHD.
2. CRT should be considered as an important therapeutic option in patients with systemic ventricular failure.
3. All intracardiac shunts should be eliminated prior to placement of an endocardial device.
4. In ACHD patients who do not respond to pharmacologic therapy for AF, catheter ablation of either all

pulmonary veins or culprit veins should be considered.

5. β blocker therapy should be considered in all ACHD patients with systemic ventricular dysfunction and NSVT.

REFERENCES

1. McCombe A, et al. Sudden cardiac death in adults with congenitally corrected transposition of the great arteries. *Open Heart.* 2016;3(2):e000407.
2. Connelly MS, et al. Congenitally corrected transposition of the great arteries in the adult: functional status and complications. *J Am Coll Cardiol.* 1996;27(5):1238−1243.
3. Koyak Z, et al. Sudden cardiac death in adult congenital heart disease. *Circulation.* 2012;126(16):1944−1954.
4. Kammeraad JA, et al. Predictors of sudden cardiac death after Mustard or Senning repair for transposition of the great arteries. *J Am Coll Cardiol.* 2004;44(5):1095−1102.
5. Schwerzmann M, et al. Ventricular arrhythmias and sudden death in adults after a Mustard operation for transposition of the great arteries. *Eur Heart J.* 2009;30(15):1873−1879.
6. Khairy P, et al. PACES/HRS expert consensus statement on the recognition and management of arrhythmias in adult congenital heart disease: developed in partnership between the Pediatric and Congenital Electrophysiology Society (PACES) and the Heart Rhythm Society (HRS). Endorsed by the governing bodies of PACES, HRS, the American College of Cardiology (ACC), the American Heart Association (AHA), the European Heart Rhythm Association (EHRA), the Canadian Heart Rhythm Society (CHRS), and the International Society for Adult Congenital Heart Disease (ISACHD). *Heart Rhythm.* 2014;11(10):e102−e165.
7. Francis J, Watanabe MA, Schmidt G. Heart rate turbulence: a new predictor for risk of sudden cardiac death. *Ann Noninvasive Electrocardiol.* 2005;10(1):102−109.
8. Koyama J, et al. Evaluation of heart-rate turbulence as a new prognostic marker in patients with chronic heart failure. *Circ J.* 2002;66(10):902−907.
9. Lammers A, et al. Impaired cardiac autonomic nervous activity predicts sudden cardiac death in patients with operated and unoperated congenital cardiac disease. *J Thorac Cardiovasc Surg.* 2006;132(3):647−655.
10. Davos CH, et al. Heart rate turbulence in adults with repaired tetralogy of Fallot. *Int J Cardiol.* 2009;135(3):308−314.
11. Marcotte F, et al. Evaluation of adult congenital heart disease by cardiac magnetic resonance imaging. *Congenit Heart Dis.* 2009;4(4):216−230.
12. Dodge-Khatami A, et al. Comparable systemic ventricular function in healthy adults and patients with unoperated congenitally corrected transposition using MRI dobutamine stress testing. *Ann Thorac Surg.* 2002;73(6):1759−1764.
13. van der Bom T, et al. Right ventricular end-diastolic volume combined with peak systolic blood pressure during exercise identifies patients at risk for complications in adults with a systemic right ventricle. *J Am Coll Cardiol.* 2013;62(10):926−936.
14. Khairy P, et al. Sudden death and defibrillators in transposition of the great arteries with intra-atrial baffles: a multicenter study. *Circ Arrhythm Electrophysiol.* 2008;1(4):250−257.
15. Janousek J, et al. Cardiac resynchronization therapy: a novel adjunct to the treatment and prevention of systemic right ventricular failure. *J Am Coll Cardiol.* 2004;44(9):1927−1931.
16. Janousek J, et al. Cardiac resynchronisation therapy in paediatric and congenital heart disease: differential effects in various anatomical and functional substrates. *Heart.* 2009;95(14):1165−1171.
17. Dubin AM, et al. Resynchronization therapy in pediatric and congenital heart disease patients: an international multicenter study. *J Am Coll Cardiol.* 2005;46(12):2277−2283.
18. Yeo WT, et al. Adverse impact of chronic subpulmonary left ventricular pacing on systemic right ventricular function in patients with congenitally corrected transposition of the great arteries. *Int J Cardiol.* 2014;171(2):184−191.
19. Hofferberth SC, et al. Impact of pacing on systemic ventricular function in L-transposition of the great arteries. *J Thorac Cardiovasc Surg.* 2016;151(1):131−138.
20. Khairy P, et al. Transvenous pacing leads and systemic thromboemboli in patients with intracardiac shunts: a multicenter study. *Circulation.* 2006;113(20):2391−2397.
21. Stephenson EA, et al. Efficacy of atrial antitachycardia pacing using the Medtronic AT500 pacemaker in patients with congenital heart disease. *Am J Cardiol.* 2003;92(7):871−876.
22. Kalra Y, et al. Antitachycardia pacing reduces appropriate and inappropriate shocks in children and congenital heart disease patients. *Heart Rhythm.* 2012;9(11):1829−1834.

CHAPTER 9

Postmaze Atrial Tachycardia
Case Submitted by: Berardo Sarubbi, MD, PhD

CASE SYNOPSIS

AR was the only daughter of normal parents, with no family history of cardiac abnormalities.

A cardiac murmur was heard at 8 days. At 3 years, palpation confirmed a thrill, and investigations confirmed the presence of a huge ostium secundum atrial septal defect with moderate pulmonary stenosis.

At the age of 10 years she underwent an uncomplicated atrial septal defect closure and pulmonary valvotomy.

She remained well until she was admitted, aged 32 years, in a peripheral hospital, for a first episode of atrial fibrillation. Severe pulmonary regurgitation was noted at the time.

When she was 34 years old, she suffered repeated episodes of atrial fibrillation and atrial flutter, which were hard to control despite various antiarrhythmic treatments (propafenone or sotalol alone, than amiodarone alone and in combination with propranolol).

When she was 36 years old, she underwent radiofrequency catheter ablation (RFCA) for atrial fibrillation consisting of pulmonary vein isolation. However, she soon had recurrences despite ongoing treatment with amiodarone.

She was referred to our cardiac tertiary center when she was 44 years old and underwent surgical operation for pulmonary valve replacement and surgical ablation of atrial arrhythmias through a tailored approach. She was discharged with sotalol treatment, which was discontinued 6 months after the operation.

She remained free of palpitations with routine periodic follow-up until age 48 when she suffered a new occurrence of atrial arrhythmias with no associated hemodynamic impairment.

At admission to our department, she reported dyspnea only with moderate to severe exertion.

Physical examination was remarkable only for a grade 1−2/6 systolic murmur at the left sternal border. Transcutaneous oxygen saturation was 99% and arterial blood pressure was 110/70 mmHg.

Electrocardiogram showed a narrow QRS tachycardia with a mean HR of 105 bpm and slight irregularity in the RR interval. Negative P-waves were seen in II, III, and aVF leads, with 2:1 atrioventricular (AV) conduction, leading to a diagnosis of intraatrial reentrant tachycardia (Fig. 9.1).

Transthoracic echocardiogram revealed normal left ventricular dimensions and normal global left ventricular systolic function (left ventricular end-diastolic diameter [LVEDD] 45 mm; left ventricular ejection fraction [LVEF] 60%), along with moderate biatrial enlargement (Left atrial volume index [LAESV A-L index] 36 ml/m2 BSA), right ventricular hypertrophy and moderate dilation (right ventricular end-diastolic diameter [RVEDD] 42 mm), mild right ventricular dysfunction (TAPSE:14 mm), and severe pulmonary regurgitation. There was no right ventricular outflow tract obstruction.

After a detailed 3-D electroanatomic activation mapping (EnSite NavX Velocity technology), the patient underwent RFCA using a multielectrode dedicated catheter (Intella Tip Mifi XP Boston Scientific 8F 8 mm).

Three-dimensional mapping showed that the intraatrial reentry tachycardia involved a circuit around an atriotomy scar along the lateral right atrium wall (Fig. 9.2 and 9.3), so it was decided to perform the extension of surgically created lines of conduction between the caval veins in a manner that could divide any corridors of myocardial tissue needed to sustain reentry. During radiofrequency application the arrhythmia stopped (Fig. 9.4) and it was not possible to induce it again. A complete bidirectional conduction block was then demonstrated across the ablated region.

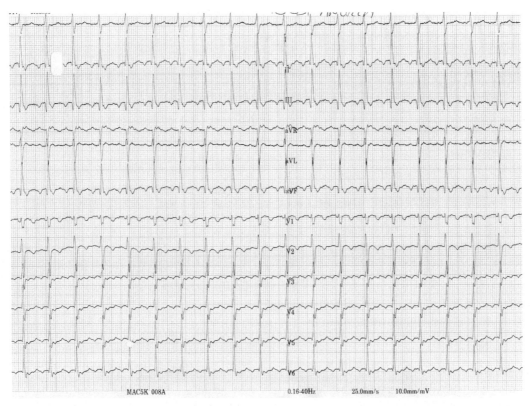

FIG. 9.1 Electrocardiogram traces showing intraatrial reentry tachycardia with a 2:1 relationship between atrial and ventricular activity, mean HR of 105bpm. Note negative P-waves in II, III and aVF leads

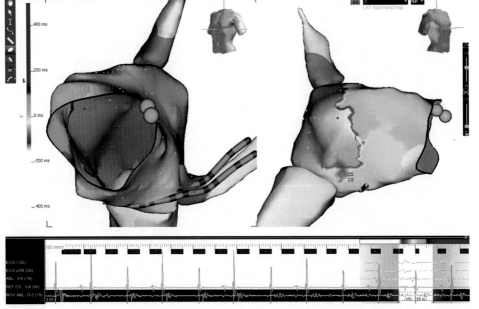

FIG. 9.2 An activation map obtained through electroanatomic mapping with the use of the EnSite NavX Velocity technology. This map highlights the isthmus between the inferior and the superior cava veins, not completely closed during previous surgical ablation, which provided to be a critical part of the tachycardia circuit.

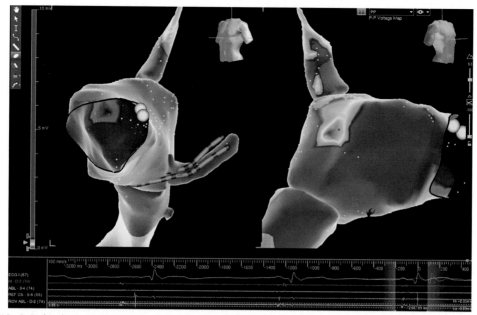

FIG. 9.3 A voltage map obtained through electroanatomic mapping with the use of the EnSite NavX Velocity technology.

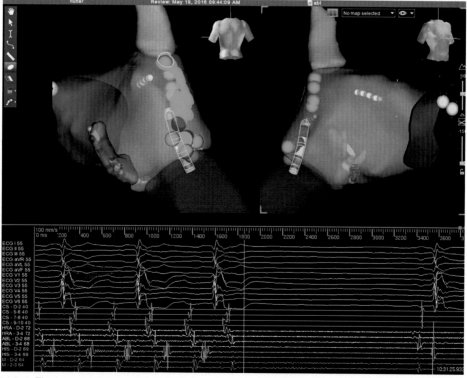

FIG. 9.4 Electroanatomic mapping with the use of the EnSite NavX Velocity technology. The ablation line, between cava veins successfully eliminated the arrhythmia, as shown by the electrocardiogram traces and intracavitary electrograms.

Questions

1. Timing and indications for catheter ablation in patient with congenital heart disease and severe hemodynamic impairment
2. Antiarrhythmic treatment for prevention of atrial arrhythmias
3. Indications for oral anticoagulation and eventual use of new oral anticoagulants
4. Indications for surgical ablation for atrial tachycardias
5. Rate control of atrial arrhythmias versus rhythm control in patients with congenital heart disease

Consultant's Opinion # 1

FRANK FISH, MD

CLINICAL QUESTIONS

1. **Timing and indications for RFCA in patients with congenital heart disease and severe hemodynamic impairment**—Atrial arrhythmias are often poorly tolerated in patients with postsurgical congenital heart disease. As a consequence, the goal of therapy should be rhythm control rather than rate control, whenever possible.[1]

   Catheter ablation probably represents the treatment of choice for atrial tachycardia in this population in whom antiarrhythmic therapy often proves unsatisfactory.[2] Antiarrhythmic therapy may also carry risks in patients with associated abnormalities in sinus or AV node conduction, those with ventricular dysfunction, and those prone to associated electrolyte disturbances.

   When such patients require surgical treatment for associated structural abnormalities, it may be reasonable to consider intraoperative ablation to target such abnormalities. However, multiple potential circuits may be responsible for arrhythmias in such patients, which may involve regions of slow conduction related to the cavo-tricuspid valve isthmus, an atriotomy scar, abnormal conduction across the crista terminalis, and reentry around an atriotomy patch.[3,4] **It is therefore often advisable to perform electrophysiology study and detailed mapping and RFCA preoperatively.** When appropriate, additional intraoperative cryoablation to consolidate RFCA lesions might be considered.

   While RFCA should be considered early in the course of treatment for atrial tachycardias, there is less experience to guide the optimal timing (or technical approach) for atrial fibrillation in adult congenital heart disease (ACHD) patients. However, it is important to recognize that atrial tachycardia is often incorrectly characterized as atrial fibrillation due to the frequent absence of classic "flutter" waves and frequently variable ventricular response. If the diagnosis is unclear, it is important to perform electrophysiologic testing to attempt induction and characterization of the tachycardia mechanism, especially before contemplating on RFCA to target atrial fibrillation (as occurred in this case) or surgical maze procedure.

2. **Antiarrhythmic treatment for prevention of atrial arrhythmias**—When antiarrhythmic therapy is contemplated, the choices for atrial arrhythmias in adult CHD patients may include Class I agents (flecainide or propafenone) or Class III agents (sotalol or dofetilide, dronedarone, amiodarone). [1]

   In many instances, it may be necessary to slow the ventricular response with the addition of a β-blocker or a calcium channel blocker. This may be especially important in the ACHD patients whose atrial rates tend to be slower than typical atrial flutter and may display more robust AV node conduction, predisposing them to 1:1 AV conduction during tachycardia.

   Class IC agents probably carry increased risk for those patients with impaired ventricular function as well as those with associated (recognized or occult) coronary artery disease and should be avoided in such patients. Because they slow conduction velocity and thus prolong the tachycardia cycle length, they slow the tachycardia in the atrium, which can lead to conduction of more beats to the ventricle (thus, for example, a patient with an atrial rate of 300 with 2:1 block would have a ventricular rate of 150, whereas slowing the atrial rate to 200 could lead to 1:1 conduction and a ventricular rate of 200, which would be less well tolerated by the patient).

Class III agents are therefore generally preferred in ACHD patients, acting to prolong refractoriness and thus limit the excitable gap of the reentrant circuit without substantial effect on the atrial rate itself. However, sotalol may be poorly tolerated in patients with moderate-severe ventricular dysfunction or those with impaired AV conduction, and dofetilide may be a preferred choice in such cases. Dronedarone is not recommended in patients with congestive heart failure or significant ventricular function due to concerns of increased mortality.[5]

Amiodarone may offer the best potential for efficacy but carries the potential for side effects including thyroid dysfunction, pulmonary fibrosis, and hepatotoxicity with long-term use.

In selected patients with infrequent tachycardia episodes, there may be a role for episodic ("pill-in-the-pocket") therapy. This might include administration of oral diltiazem at first onset of symptoms to limit AV conduction while patients seek medical attention (it must be explicitly explained that this is a short-term temporizing measure only, and attenuation of symptoms should not be presumed to reflect tachycardia termination). Additionally, successful termination of atrial tachycardia with acute oral administration of sotalol has been described. [6]

3. **Indications for oral anticoagulation and eventual use of new oral anticoagulants**—Although some data exist in the ACHD population,[7] the role for chronic anticoagulation in ACHD patients with atrial arrhythmias is largely extrapolated from the extensive body of data for stroke prevention in adults with atrial fibrillation.[8] However, there may be important differences. Many (but not all) ACHD patients may be acutely aware of the onset of their tachycardia. In such patients, it may be reasonable to forego chronic anticoagulation and begin anticoagulation with a newer anticoagulation agent at the onset of symptoms (possibly concurrent with an agent to slow AV conduction). However, such an approach may be inappropriate in patients who have previously presented with atrial tachycardia discovered incidentally during routine evaluation or when presenting with hemodynamic deterioration without acute palpitations. Likewise, the addition of a chronic AV-slowing agent may hinder the patient's recognition of future tachycardia recurrences.

Although adult studies suggest improved safety and efficacy of the newer oral anticoagulants compared with warfarin,[9-12] there are limited data in their use in ACHD patients. The most recent consensus statement in ACHD patients suggested warfarin remains the standard therapy but acknowledged the newer agents might be considered in patients with simple forms of CHD and no significant valve disease or mechanical valve.[4] However, experience is being accrued, and multicenter collaborative efforts are underway to review the experience of these agents in ACHD patients.

4. Indications for surgical ablation for atrial tachycardias—The role for surgical ablation rather than catheter ablation is dependent on multiple factors, including the patient's anatomy, the operation being planned, the institutional experience of the surgical and ablation teams, and the availability of intracardiac mapping and other advanced intraoperative techniques such as hybrid epicardial-endocardial approach.[13] As noted earlier, if surgical ablation is contemplated, it is often advisable to perform preoperative electrophysiology study and mapping to better define the region or regions to be targeted. In the case of Fontan conversion to extracardiac conduit, intraoperative cryoablation should be routinely performed, although the best placement of cryolesions may vary according to the anatomy and type of previous Fontan connection. Although the approach pioneered by Mavroudis and Deal included a Cox III maze targeting atrial fibrillation,[14] there are little data to support routine preemptive treatment of atrial fibrillation at the time of Fontan conversion. The potential impairment of left atrial transport function with this approach and adverse consequences on the Fontan circulation may represent a more significant concern than late presentation with atrial fibrillation. Indeed, while there may be a notion that Fontan revision represents the "last chance" to intervene due to loss of direct vascular access to the atria, experience is growing in ablation after ECC-Fontan.[15]

5. **Rate control of atrial arrhythmias** versus **rhythm control in patients with congenital heart disease**—As noted earlier, patients with ACHD may be more prone to hemodynamic compromise due to their arrhythmias, making rate control an unattractive option. This can be the result of overt issues such as residual structural impairments (e.g., as semilunar or AV valve dysfunction) or the adverse impact on passive transpulmonary flow in the Fontan circulation with loss of 1:1 AV synchrony. In other instances, even patients with a seemingly good surgical result may suffer occult diastolic dysfunction, affecting their ability to tolerate their arrhythmia. Congestive heart failure may develop chronically or even acutely in ACHD patients in whom seemingly effective rate control has been maintained. **Thus, rhythm control is usually preferable, ideally by**

catheter ablation alone, or in combination with antiarrhythmic therapy or antitachycardia pacing when appropriate.

REFERENCES

1. Khairy P, Van Hare GF, Balaji S, et al. PACES/HRS Expert consensus statement on the recognition and management of arrhythmias in adult congenital heart disease: developed in Partnership between the Pediatric and congenital electrophysiology Society (PACES) and the heart rhythm Society (HRS). Endorsed by the Governing Bodies of PACES, HRS, the American College of Cardiology (ACC), the American heart association (AHA), the European heart rhythm association (EHRA), the Canadian heart rhythm Society (CHRS), and the International Society for adult congenital heart disease (ISACHD). *Heart Rhythm Heart Rhythm*. 2014:102—165.
2. Koyak Z, Kroon B, de Groot JR, et al. Efficacy of antiarrhythmic drugs in adults with congenital heart disease and supraventricular tachycardia. *Am J Cardiol*. 2013;112:1461—1467.
3. Lukac P, Pedersen AK, Mortensen PT, et al. Ablation of atrial tachycardia after surgery for congenital and acquired heart disease using an electroanatomic mapping system: which circuits to expect in which substrate? *Heart Rhythm*. 2005;2:64—72.
4. Peichl P, Kautzner J, Cihak R, Vancura V, Bytesni J. Clinical application of electroanatomical mapping in the characterization of "incisional" atrial tachycardias. *Pacing Clin Electrophysiol*. 2004;26:420—442.
5. Kober L, Torp-Pedersen C, McMurray JJ, et al. Increased mortality after dronedarone therapy for severe heart failure. *N Engl J Med*. 2008;358:2678—2687.
6. Rao SO, Boramanand NK, Burton DA, Perry JC. Atrial tachycardias in young adults and adolescents with congenital heart disease: conversion using single dose oral sotalol. *Int J Cardiol*. 2009;136:253.
7. Hoffmann A, Chockalingam P, Balint OH, et al. Cerebrovascular accidents in adult patients with congenital heart disease. *Heart*. 2010;96:1223—1226.
8. Anderson JL, Halperin JL, Albert NM, et al. Management of patients with atrial fibrillation (compilation of 2006 ACCF/AHA/ESC and 2011 ACCF/AHA/HRS recommendations): a report of the American College of Cardiology/American heart association Task Force on practice Guidelines. *J Am Coll Cardiol*. 2013;61:1935—1944.
9. Connolly SJ, Ezekowitz MD, Yusuf S, et al. Dabigatran versus warfarin in patients with atrial fibrillation. *N Engl J Med*. 2009;361:1139—1151.
10. Granger CB, Alexander JH, McMurray JJ, et al. Apixaban versus warfarin in patients with atrial fibrillation. *N Engl J Med*. 2011;365:981—992.
11. Patel MR, Mahaffey KW, Garg J, et al. Rivaroxaban versus warfarin in nonvalvular atrial fibrillation. *N Engl J Med*. 2011;365:883—891.
12. Giugliano RP, Ruff CT, Braunwald E, et al. Edoxaban versus warfarin in patients with atrial fibrillation. *N Engl J Med*. 2013;369:2093—2104.
13. Bulava A, Mokracek A, Hanis J, Eisenberger M, Kurfirst V, Dusek L. Correlates of arrhythmia recurrence after hybrid Epi- and endocardial radiofrequency ablation for persistent atrial fibrillation. *Circ Arrhythm Electrophysiol*. 2017;10(8):e005273.
14. Deal BJ, Costello JM, Webster G, Tsao S, Backer CL, Mavroudis C. Intermediate-term outcome of 140 consecutive fontan conversions with arrhythmia operations. *Ann Thorac Surg*. 2016;101(2):717—724.
15. Moore JP, Shannon KM, Fish FA, et al. Catheter ablation of supraventricular tachyarrhythmia after extracardiac Fontan surgery. *Heart Rhythm*. 2016;13(9):1891—1897.

Consultant's Opinion #2

DAVID J. BRADLEY, MD

This is a case of an adult patient with what might be considered repaired simple congenital heart disease: pulmonary stenosis (PS) and ostium secundum atrial septal defect (ASD). More than 20 years after initial surgical repair at 10 years of age, atrial arrhythmias—atrial flutter and atrial fibrillation (AF)—become problematic, and along with pulmonary valve replacement (PVR), require numerous treatments, the last being a successful ablation for intraatrial reentry tachycardia (IART).

A bulleted summary of her diagnoses and their treatments is as follows:

1. Atrial septal defect, ostium secundum, large
   a. Diagnosed by murmur in infancy
   b. Repaired at 10 years of age

2. Moderate valvar pulmonary stenosis
   a. Valvotomy at 10 years of age with ASD closure
3. Severe pulmonary regurgitation, identified at 32 years of age
   a. PVR, age 44
4. Atrial arrhythmias: intraatrial reentry tachycardia and possible atrial fibrillation
   a. Onset at 34 years of age
   b. Refractory to β blocker, propafenone, sotalol, and amiodarone
   c. Pulmonary vein isolation using non-3-D mapping at 36 years old
   d. Surgical LA maze at time of PVR age 44
   e. Control on sotalol thereafter
   f. Recurrence at 48 years of age
   g. Successful ablation using 3-D mapping, age 48 years

DISCUSSION

Before addressing the discussion questions for this case, a few comments are in order. Details of the initial arrhythmia at age 34 are incomplete, but it is described as "atrial fibrillation and flutter." (Because of the possibility that it is not typical, isthmus-dependent atrial flutter, the more inclusive term for atrial macroreentry, intraatrial reentry tachycardia, or IART, will be used in this discussion.) It is slightly unusual for a patient with purely right-sided lesions to present with atrial fibrillation as the first arrhythmia. The left atrial size is normal and her young age argues against AF; in the absence of diagnostic tracings, this may instead have been IART. IART is commonly misdiagnosed by non-CHD physicians as AF because IART may not have classic flutter waves, may be conducted irregularly, and presents for CHD patients in clinical units such as emergency departments more accustomed to AF. Alternatively, if AF was truly the rhythm, it may have been a secondary to an initial IART. The initial LA maze procedure may not have achieved much for rhythm control. Now, to the questions:

1. **Timing and indications of RFCA in CHD and severe hemodynamic impairment**—Atrial arrhythmias in the adult with repaired CHD are a challenge to manage with medications, and while ablation, too, is technically difficult, it provides definitive treatment with fewer side effects and no reliance on patient compliance. **For this reason, not only ablation but also the use of 3-D mapping are Class I treatments in the 2014 consensus statement on arrhythmia management in adult CHD (cited later). These must be performed in an** established center of excellence, and, if and when successful, can result in incremental or total arrhythmia relief for years. The detail provided in the description of the ablation procedure, the coherence of the maps, and the arrhythmia termination attest to the experience of the final treating team. Especially if an IART was the root cause of her early presentations, this team would have served her well with an ablation as first-line therapy.

2. **Antiarrhythmic treatment for prevention of atrial arrhythmias**—This case demonstrates some of the limitations to medical therapy for atrial arrhythmia. The series of unsuccessful courses of medication by this patient represents innumerable visits, hospitalizations, and cardioversions, a frustrating process for patient and clinician alike. Various factors further impair their incomplete effectiveness under the best of circumstances. One reason for failure of medications is subtherapeutic dosing. Taking the example of d-sotalol, a common initial dose is 80 mg twice daily. Initiation of this medication is usually undertaken during a 72-h inpatient stay to observe QT intervals and guard for proarrhythmia. Up-titration requires the same again. A fair trial of this medication is therefore extremely cumbersome. Class 1 C medications, appropriate in this case, are felt less suitable for the patient with congestive heart failure symptoms or ventricular scarring. A second reason for medication failure is poor patient adherence, either due to difficulty obtaining or paying for the medication or a false sense that it is not needed. Side effects, usually of fatigue or malaise, are common with higher doses of β blocker, sotalol, and amiodarone. Proarrhythmia is a serious concern that requires careful selection and monitoring of patients at initiation, a broad topic that will not be explored here. Amiodarone deserves special mention. While it is clearly the most effective choice, its wide array of potential adverse effects makes it unfavorable long term in children and young adults. Amiodarone should be considered a short-term therapy except when alternatives have been exhausted. In summary, single-medication management is effective in fewer than half of adult CHD patients with troublesome atrial arrhythmias.

3. **Indications for oral anticoagulation including new oral anticoagulants**—The mainstay of oral anticoagulation, warfarin, now has viable alternatives in the "novel oral anticoagulant" (NOAC) category, agents which do not reduce the production of clotting factors but are direct inhibitors of thrombin.

Long-term anticoagulation is appropriate for the CHD patient with recurrent episodes of atrial arrhythmia or whose arrhythmia is chronic. For younger patients with clear symptoms upon tachycardia initiation who need infrequent cardioversion, it is still reasonable to withhold chronic anticoagulation, but if these become frequent, or if there is evidence of asymptomatic events, anticoagulation should be initiated, according to the CHA2DS2-VASc scoring system. **The NOACs have a higher cost than warfarin but require no ongoing testing and are increasingly favored over warfarin in the CHD population. Caution, however, should be taken in the most complex forms of CHD as data regarding their safety and efficacy are unavailable.**

4. **Indications for surgical ablation for atrial tachycardias**—Despite the success and minimally invasive nature of catheter approaches, there is a place for surgical ablation for atrial arrhythmias in CHD. There are few situations where its risks and morbidity are justified as the sole operation. But when additional hemodynamic lesions are being addressed and the rhythm has posed a management challenge as in this patient, it can be beneficial. For recurrent atrial fibrillation, a Cox III maze operation coupled with cavo-tricuspid isthmus ablation has established benefit. Results are somewhat dependent on center experience. Right atrial modified maze operations are potentially very effective, and lesion sets for the Fontan population and others are available in the literature. They are most effective when (1) addressing reentrant (rather than focal) arrhythmia, (2) informed by preoperative catheter-based mapping to establish key ablation zones, and (3) preceded by a formal conversation between cardiothoracic surgeon and congenital electrophysiologist with a detailed knowledge of the anatomy and surgical records.

5. **Rate versus rhythm control for management of atrial arrhythmias in CHD.** Whereas chronic management of AF and atrial flutter in adults with normal hearts usually consists of rate control, CHD patients appear to benefit significantly from correction of the rhythm, and significant effort should be made to achieve this. Even in patients with surgically modified atria such as those after Mustard and Fontan palliation, AV synchrony and physiologic heart rates seem beneficial. There remain no prospective comparisons of rate- versus rhythm-control strategies; the above conclusions are, however, widely appreciated by clinicians who manage such patients.

FURTHER READING

1. Freemantle N, Lafuente-Lafuente C, Mitchell S, Eckert L, Reynolds M. Mixed treatment comparison of dronedarone, amiodarone, sotalol, flecainide, and propafenone, for the management of atrial fibrillation. *Europace.* 2011;13(3):329–345. https://doi.org/10.1093/europace/euq450.
2. Khairy P, Van Hare GF, Balaji S, et al. PACES/HRS Expert consensus statement on the recognition and management of arrhythmias in adult congenital heart disease. *Hear Rhythm.* 2014;11(10):e102–e165. https://doi.org/10.1016/j.hrthm.2014.05.009.
3. January CT, Wann LS, Alpert JS, et al. 2014 AHA/ACC/HRS Guideline for the management of patients with atrial fibrillation. *J Am Coll Cardiol.* 2014;64(21):e1–e76. https://doi.org/10.1016/j.jacc.2014.03.022.
4. Kim HL, Bin Seo J, Chung WY, Kim SH, Kim MA, Zo JH. The incidence and predictors of overall adverse effects caused by low dose amiodarone in real-world clinical practice. *Korean J Intern Med.* 2014;29(5):588–596. https://doi.org/10.3904/kjim.2014.29.5.588.
5. Labombarda F, Hamilton R, Shohoudi A, et al. Increasing Prevalence of atrial fibrillation and Permanent atrial arrhythmias in congenital heart disease. *J Am Coll Cardiol.* 2017;70(7):857–865. https://doi.org/10.1016/j.jacc.2017.06.034.
6. Vorperian VR, Havighurst TC, Miller S, January CT. Adverse effects of low dose amiodarone: a meta-analysis. *J Am Coll Cardiol.* 1997;30(3):791–798. https://doi.org/10.1016/S0735-1097(97)00220-9.
7. Walsh EP, Cecchin F. Arrhythmias in adult patients with congenital heart disease. *Circulation.* 2007;115(4):534–545. https://doi.org/10.1161/CIRCULATIONAHA.105.592410.

CHAPTER 10

Fontan Patient With Brady and Tachyarrhythmia Issues

Case Submitted by Vivienne Ezzat, MBChB

CASE SYNOPSIS

A 34-year-old man was referred to the congenital heart disease arrhythmia service in 2015. Original diagnoses were tricuspid atresia and pulmonary stenosis. Previous interventions were a left modified Blalock-Taussig shunt in 1980 as an infant; atriopulmonary Fontan operation in 1983 (aged 3 years) with subsequent conversion to an intracardiac total cavopulmonary connection (TCPC) fenestrated (4 mm) lateral tunnel, resection of right atrium (RA) wall, and Gor-Tex enlargement of left pulmonary rtery (LPA) in 1995 (aged 15 years). Following this he was cyanosed with baseline saturations on air of 90%–93%, desaturating to ∼84% on exercise. Cardiac catheterization in 2001 showed a patent bidirectional Glenn with good size pulmonary arteries; the inferior vena cava (IVC) tunnel was patent and dilated at 7 cm, with rapid filling of the levo phase, excluding pulmonary vein compression. Pressures were as follows: left ventricle (LV)—86/5 mmHg, IVC 9/6 mean 8 mmHg, superior vena cava (SVC) mean 9 mmHg, LPA mean 8 mmHg, right pulmonary artery (RPA) 8 mmHg, LPA to PA pullback—no gradient, LV to Ao pullback—no gradient; saturations: SVC 77%, IVC 84%, RPA 80%, LPA 77%. Left ventriculography—preserved systolic function.

The patient began to develop symptoms of palpitations in 2002 with documented atrial tachycardia and went on to have electrophysiologic (EP) studies with radiofrequency catheter ablation in 2002, 2004, and 2005. He was noted to be in a persistent atrial tachycardia on each occasion and for all procedures a 3D electroanatomic mapping system was used. The procedures were not performed in the same regional center in which he was being seen for his congenital heart disease. Examples of his tachycardia are shown in Fig. 10.1.

The first procedure performed in 2002 was the ablation of a macroreentrant tachycardia within the pulmonary venous atrium accessed via the fenestration and comprised of a circuit in the morphologic left atrium, using the mitral valve annulus and an area of scar on the posterior wall. Tachycardia was slowed but not terminated with ablation and still inducible at the end of the case. He was discharged on amiodarone, which initially maintained sinus rhythm; however, by the end of 2003, he again developed a persistent atrial tachycardia.

His second procedure was performed in 2004. The pulmonary venous atrium was again accessed via the lateral tunnel fenestration. Two tachycardia were seen—one with a cycle length of 240 ms, the other faster but with a similar appearance on 12 lead ECG. There were large areas of the atrium electrically dissociated from the tachycardia circuit which occupied the anterior and lateral parts of the native right atrium. This appeared to have an area of scar as its central obstacle and was terminated during the creation of a linear lesion from the scar to a line of double potentials in the posterolateral aspect of the right atrium and believed to represent the suture lines of the lateral tunnel. At the end of the case, sustained tachycardia could not be induced (including with isoprenaline).

In 2005 a third procedure was performed. Under conscious sedation, it was noted at this time that the pressure within the lateral tunnel was 19 mmHg. Mapping of the lateral tunnel and systemic venous atrium revealed focal activation arising from the inferior part of the residual interatrial septum. Ablation here slowed and subsequently terminated the tachycardia; however, there was transient atrioventricular (AV) block after the ablation. A second tachycardia was then ablated in a similar area to the circuit seen in 2004, on the lateral wall of the pulmonary venous (morphologic right) atrium. At the end of the case the patient was in Mobitz type I (Wenckebach) second-degree heart block, which subsequently resolved to first-degree heart block (Fig. 10.2), and by the time of discharge the PR interval was reported as being within normal limits.

In 2002

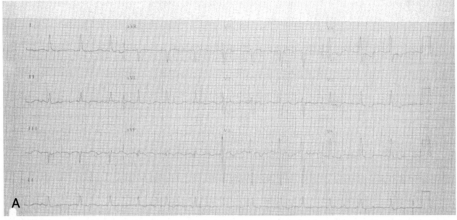

In 2004

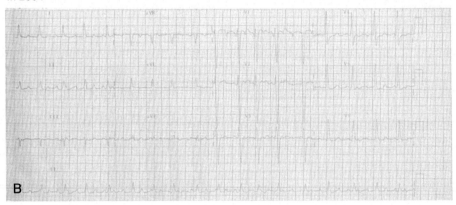

In 2005

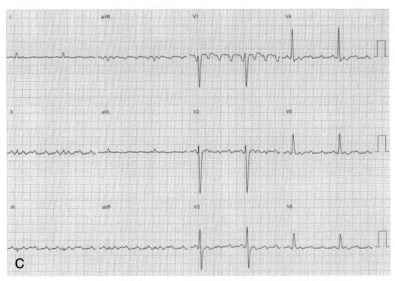

FIG. 10.1 Atrial tachycardia, **(A)** In 2002, **(B)** In 2004, **(C)** In 2005.

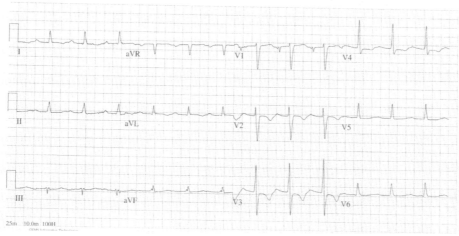

FIG. 10.2 First-degree atrioventricular block post AT ablation (PR ~ 300 ms).

Following his third catheter ablation, it was felt that the clinical priority was to reduce his cyanosis rather than pursue further attempts at electrophysiology (EP) intervention, regardless of arrhythmia recurrence. He remained on long-term anticoagulation with warfarin and a maintenance dose of 100 mg amiodarone once daily, which reduced the burden of his symptoms. The fenestration was closed in 2006 with a 4 mm Amplatzer Septal Occluder device and afterward there was no residual flow into the right atrium. Post device placement baseline oxygen saturations were 97% on room air.

Subsequently he was well, in sinus rhythm with an unremarkable cardiorespiratory examination, normal blood pressure, and no signs of heart failure. In view of his age, the amiodarone was converted to dronedarone 400 mg twice daily, which he tolerated well. During this time he was in full-time employment with an active social life and regularly participated in light/moderate sporting activities. He smoked 10 cigarettes per day and drank a little alcohol socially.

In 2011 he again started to become more troubled with intermittent symptoms of palpitations. He also complained of occasional dizziness.

Ambulatory monitoring in February 2011 showed an atrial arrhythmia burden of 34% with frequent atrial ectopics as well as periods of atrial bigeminy and sustained atrial arrhythmia (Fig. 10.3). Heart rate histograms showed normal diurnal variation with a minimum heart rate of 47 bpm at night and a maximum heart rate of 105 bpm during the day. In view of the documented symptomatic atrial tachycardia, it was decided that more aggressive management of his arrhythmia was required and in 2012 he had two further attempts at catheter ablation. At the first in early 2012, he had evidence of two predominant circuits, one related to the scar on the posterolateral right atrium and the second to the isthmus between the IVC and AV valve. Ablation was successfully undertaken of both these circuits. By this time, venous cannulation was only possible via the left (not right) femoral route due to right femoral vein occlusion. Just over 6 months later, another procedure was undertaken; on this occasion there were three tachycardias ablated: one a macroreentrant tachycardia related to scarring on the lateral and septal aspects of the tunnel and also two focal/microreentrant tachycardias, arising from the high right atrium and also the lateral right atrium both within the tunnel. At the end of the procedure he had evidence of nonsustained atrial arrhythmia only.

2015

Despite an apparently successful procedure in 2012, by 2015 he had a further recurrence of atrial tachycardia. Having had multiple ablation procedures over the previous decade, however, a consensus decision was made after the fifth procedure, not to pursue an invasive approach and to continue with medical therapy. Functionally he had otherwise remained stable. Available serial ETT/CPEX data are shown in Table 10.1.

Atrial bigeminy

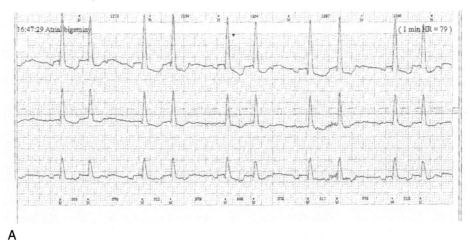

A

Atrial tachycardia

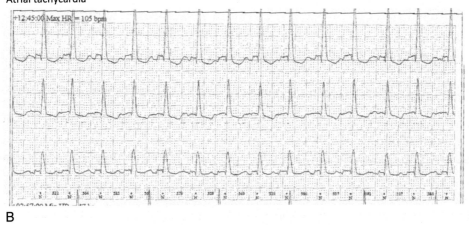

B

FIG. 10.3 **(A)** Atrial bigeminy; **(B)** Atrial tachycardia.

Transthoracic echocardiography in February 2015 showed no LV outflow obstruction, a dilated left ventricular cavity with mildly reduced systolic function, moderate left-sided AV valve regurgitation (longstanding), no spontaneous echo contrast within the TCPC or residual fenestration detected. The patient remained in a persistent atrial tachycardia; however, the ventricular rate was well controlled (Fig. 10.4), and there was no hemodynamic compromise or intrusive symptoms.

In 2015, the patient had worsening palpitations and was started on bisoprolol 2.5 mg once daily. These symptoms considerably improved; however, he began to experience infrequent but severe presyncope. 12

lead ECG showed a junctional rhythm at 36 bpm (Fig. 10.5). The bisoprolol was reduced to 1.25 mg once daily and ambulatory ECG was undertaken which showed sinus pauses (up to 9 s—Fig. 10.6), paroxysms of rapidly conducted atrial tachycardia, and frequent periods of junctional rhythm.

His case was reviewed at a multidisciplinary team meeting and a decision was made to implant a surgical pacing system. This was initially attempted via a subxiphoid incision; however, it was not possible to obtain acceptable ventricular lead pacing parameters through this approach, therefore a further lateral thoracotomy was performed. It was noted that the epicardium was extremely fragile, however, and it was still not possible

TABLE 10.1
Serial functional (exercise) assessments

	2001	2006	2010	2011
Study	Modified Bruce	Bruce	CPEX	CPEX
Time (mins)	18	13:24	7:35	
RER	—	—	1.15	
METS		15		
Vo2 max (% predicted)	—	—	20.3 mL/kg/min (51)	21.2 mL/kg/min (54)
Resting HR			78	
Max HR (% predicted)	140	96	102 (68)	117 (61)
Resting BP (mmHg)		120/70	110/80	
Peak BP		150/80	150/80	
Rhythm/arrhythmia		Intermittent Wenckebach and atrial flutter	SR, first-degree AV Block, LBBB (QRS 116 ms)	Sinus rhythm with frequent atrial ectopy
Test terminated due to		Leg fatigue	SOB	

BP, blood pressure; *HR*, heart rate; *LBBB*, left bundle branch block; *METS*, Metabolic Equivalents; *RER*, respiratory exchange ratio; *SOB*, shortness of breath; *SR*, sinus rhythm.

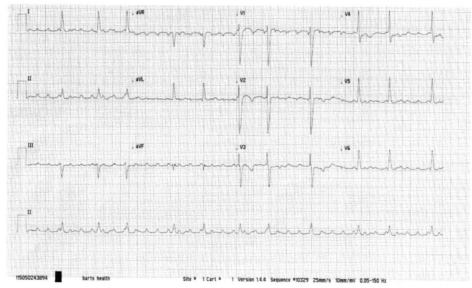

FIG. 10.4 Persistent atrial tachycardia in 2015 with controlled ventricular response.

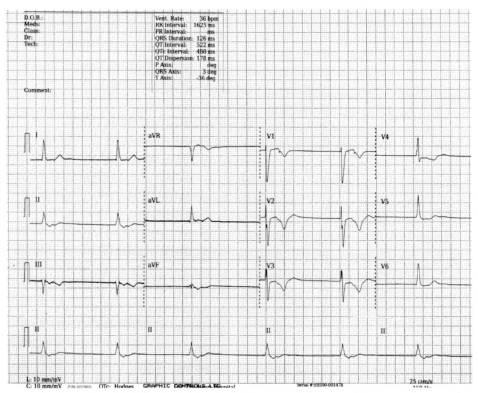

FIG. 10.5 Junctional bradycardia in 2015.

to anchor a pacing lead adequately here and the patient was closed without pacemaker insertion.

In view of the necessity for pacing and the failed surgery, a decision was made to attempt placement of an endocardial system percutaneously via a transbaffle puncture. The procedure was performed during therapeutic anticoagulation with warfarin. This was a long and complex procedure and the transbaffle puncture was difficult as the baffle was heavily calcified. Although the baffle was eventually successfully punctured, it was only possible to pass a single guide wire and not a sheath via an anterograde approach. The guide wire was then snared via a retrograde (transfemoral) route, allowing eventual passage of a guide sheath and placement of a single pacing lead at the ventricular apex with satisfactory parameters. A single chamber device was implanted as it was felt that there was insufficient space in the transbaffle puncture to implant a second lead and that this would also be too high risk. On balance, although there was no evidence of AV conduction disease, it was decided that a ventricular lead should be

placed rather than an atrial lead, in the event of developing more advanced AV conduction disease in the future, and in the hope that in the meantime, ventricular pacing would rarely be needed. Postprocedural chest X-ray is shown in Fig. 10.7. The generator was placed prepectorally and the wound closed without complications. However, femoral arterial access was unintentionally lost during the terminal part of the case, resulting in a significant retroperitoneal hematoma which required vascular surgery. Despite this, the patient made a good recovery and was successfully discharged home. At review in outpatient clinic in early 2016 the patient confirmed that he was no longer having presyncope, and pacing check showed 3% ventricular pacing. He remains in a regular atrial tachycardia with a ventricular rate of 74 bpm on dronedarone 400 mg bd. He complains of occasional palpitations; however, there have been no high rate episodes detected on device check. His main complaint is of generalized mild tiredness. Saturations are reduced from 97% preprocedurally to 91% at latest follow-up. At the current time, there is

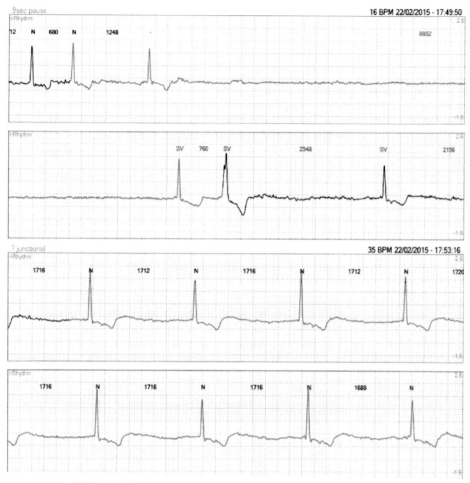

FIG. 10.6 Nine second sinus pause followed by junctional bradycardia.

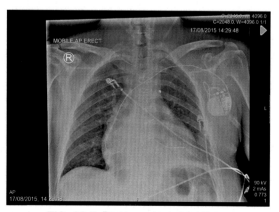

FIG. 10.7 Postprocedural chest X-ray.

no intention for him to undergo any further catheter ablations.

Questions

1. Should a further attempt at catheter ablation be considered/have been considered either now or prior to permanent pacemaker implantation?
2. Should a dual chamber system or atrial lead only have been implanted?
3. Should a leadless pacemaker have been considered an option?
4. Should the patient be given amiodarone again?
5. Should a further closure device be considered in view of his hypoxia (with obligate jailing of the pacing lead)?

Consultant Opinion #1

AKASH R. PATEL, MD • RONN E. TANEL, MD

This patient has a complicated history that includes an atriopulmonary Fontan operation for complex congenital heart disease that was subsequently revised to a lateral tunnel Fontan modification. As occurs in some patients, the atrial arrhythmia burden increased and became more difficult to treat. In addition, lateral tunnel pressures increased significantly from 2001 to 2005. This was coincident with the first mention that the single left ventricle systolic function was compromised. In addition, there was new dilation of the pulmonary venous atrium, coronary veins, and lateral tunnel. Although, ventricular dysfunction is multifactorial in this population, it is possible that persistent tachycardia resulted in a tachycardia-mediated cardiomyopathy. It is a reasonable goal to decrease or eliminate chronic cyanosis in a complex congenital heart patient, but addressing this problem alone is unlikely to result in overall clinical improvement if the arrhythmia is not addressed. This case clearly illustrates the problems often encountered in patients with complex congenital heart disease who develop late arrhythmias. There should always be a concerted effort to care for all aspects of the patient's cardiac issues since they are closely interrelated.

1. **Should a further attempt at catheter ablation be considered/have been considered either now or prior to pacemaker implantation?**

Another attempt at catheter ablation may seem futile after so many prior procedures. However, there are several additional modalities to consider that could potentially result in an improved outcome. As demonstrated by this case, the use of electroanatomic mapping systems have greatly advanced the field of catheter ablation by more rapidly and definitively identifying arrhythmia substrates through incorporation of anatomic and electrical activation data on a single system. However, the advent of newer high-density mapping systems (Rhythmia, Boston Scientific; Ensite Precision, St. Jude Medical) may allow for improved resolution and identification of more complex circuits present in this type of patient who tends to have significant scars. In addition, these systems register regions of electrical interest and sites where previous ablation was performed. In subsequent procedures, this may assist in

determining if substrates are new, different, or recurrent. The use of image integration with magnetic resonance imaging and computed tomography has proven to be helpful in delineating complex and unusual anatomic structures. Especially in patients with Fontan physiology, atrial thickness may be underestimated.[1] In this situation, ablation catheter specifications are important, including open-irrigated radiofrequency ablation catheters to increase lesion depth. Finally, intracardiac electrical signals in these patients may be low amplitude and attenuated, and thus misrepresent a sense of endocardial contact. The use of contact force-sensing systems may further provide for improved lesion delivery.

Based on the case description, it appears that some of the arrhythmias identified in the electrophysiologic (EP) laboratory represented recurrence of sites that were previously addressed with catheter ablation, while others were novel. It is also possible that some of the same substrates appeared different if they were modified by prior ablation attempts. Finally, it is possible that linear applications of radiofrequency energy might be incomplete and could result in new zones of slow conduction that could become new critical isthmuses for the development of new macroreentrant circuits. Many of these issues could potentially be addressed to some extent by the use of more recently developed catheters, both the irrigated tip catheter and the contact force-sensing catheter. Therefore, there are new technologies that may make another attempt at catheter ablation worthwhile, but these new tools do not necessarily ensure a better outcome. Finally, it should be recognized that further attempts at catheter ablation may be limited by the history of transient atrioventricular block during a previous ablation procedure. This should be taken into consideration before scheduling another procedure and atrioventricular block should be avoided at all costs in this population since they may fare poorly in a ventricular paced rhythm.[2]

Whether or not another catheter ablation procedure is performed, it should be mentioned that outcomes for catheter ablation in the complex congenital heart disease patient (Fontan patient) should not be measured by the same metrics that are used for ablation outcomes in less complex populations. Triedman et al. clearly showed that complete elimination of arrhythmia is often not achievable and that improving symptom burden is an acceptable goal.[3] Triedman, et al. measured outcome in these patients by using a symptom severity score and showed significant subjective and objective improvement.[4]

2. **Should a dual chamber system or atrial lead only have been implanted?**

Late sinus node dysfunction (SND) is commonly observed in patients who have had a Fontan operation. With periods of sinus bradycardia, sinus pauses, and junctional rhythm associated with paroxysms of rapidly conducted atrial tachycardia (tachy-brady syndrome), it is unlikely that this patient can be managed without a pacemaker. Pacing would be effective in managing sinus bradycardia and the atrioventricular dyssynchrony that occurs during junctional rhythm. However, in addition, pacing at physiologic rates may be sufficient to prevent atrial arrhythmias that are bradycardia- or pause-dependent and often observed in patients with complex congenital heart disease who have had multiple prior surgeries. Discontinuation of the β-blocker therapy is potentially helpful, but the SND will probably persist and progress with time, requiring pacing at some point in the future.

Epicardial pacing systems can be challenging to implant due to difficulty accessing the heart following prior sternotomies and due to epicardial scar. A left lateral thoracotomy approach to the back of the left atrium is an alternative option, since this area should be relatively preserved. This patient did have a prior left Blalock-Taussig shunt, so this approach may not be as straightforward as in those without a prior left lateral thoracotomy. The left atrium, generally via a left lateral thoracotomy, has been shown to be an effective approach to pacing in the patient with complex congenital heart disease.[5] In addition, since the problem is SND and there did not appear to be any residual atrioventricular block since the ablation in 2011, it seems that a transvenous atrial pacemaker may have been all that is necessary. Although much of the lateral tunnel is graft material, there is often some viable atrial tissue accessible for pacing.[6] It is true that the ventricular pacing lead might be used very little if it was only programmed to pace during sinus pauses, but this patient also has junctional rhythm, which is a suboptimal rhythm for the long term in a single ventricle patient. In addition, the transbaffle lead that was advanced to the left ventricular apex is potentially a much higher risk lead than a transvenous atrial lead

that stays within the lateral tunnel in a patient who had a right-to-left shunt previously closed with an occluder device. It is expected that the SND will continue to advance. Therefore, the argument that the patient will not use the ventricular lead for pacing may not be true in the future. An increasing percentage of ventricular pacing in a single ventricle patient could have significant deleterious effects.[2] The anatomy of this patient is not known in enough detail, but pacing the left ventricle from a coronary sinus branch has been described in a patient with tricuspid atresia who underwent a Fontan operation.[6] Therefore, a single chamber transvenous atrial pacemaker might have been a more optimal choice. Finally, the concern that more advanced atrioventricular conduction disease might develop is an important concern, but may not be relevant in this patient. With his progressive and cumulative hemodynamic and EP issues, it is concerning that this heart may not maintain an adequate cardiac output over the long term. Therefore, one could argue that an important strategy to consider is optimizing the current situation so that if transplantation is considered, the patient will be in his best possible state of health.

3. **Should a leadless pacemaker have been considered an option?**

A leadless pacemaker is certainly an option, but currently, it still has the limitations of being a single chamber device and being implanted in the systemic ventricle, with the significant risk of systemic thromboemboli and stroke. There is currently one report of successful implantation of a leadless pacemaker in a systemic ventricle.[7] In addition to the possibility of thromboemboli from the device, a more concerning event would be embolization of the device itself, which could result in systemic ventricle outflow obstruction. Finally, another more subtle concern is that currently the leadless pacemaker is implanted through an 18 Fr (St. Jude Medical) or 27 Fr (Medtronic) delivery sheath. This is not a trivial concern in a patient receiving anticoagulation therapy. In addition, the sheath would need to cross either a heavily calcified lateral tunnel baffle or the aortic valve in a retrograde manner for the device to be implanted in the left ventricle.

4. **Should the patient be given amiodarone again?**

The medical management of this patient, following numerous successful, partially successful, and unsuccessful ablation procedures is certainly a challenge. It is important to examine the risk:benefit profile of amiodarone, especially in the young patient who has potentially many years to develop side effects. Amiodarone is a reasonable option for medical therapy, especially if there is an expected endpoint to treatment with this agent. Unfortunately, this patient will likely need antiarrhythmic medication therapy for the rest of his life or for as long as he has this heart. Not only do the side effects cause problems in their own right, but side effects that involve the lung, liver, and other organs can certainly indirectly adversely affect cardiac function. Alternatively, it may be possible to attempt treatment with low-dose amiodarone, as this may pose a lower risk of some of the side effects.[8] A strategy with low-dose amiodarone, frequent monitoring for side effects, and discontinuing the amiodarone at the first sign of the development of an unacceptable side effect is a reasonable approach. In addition to amiodarone, dronedarone and dofetilide may be considered.[9] The question remains "Which is the lesser of two evils? Rate control, but not rhythm control, accepting that rate control may not be sufficient in a patient with complex congenital heart disease. Finally, surgical options should also be considered in patients with complex congenital heart disease who have both hemodynamic and EP abnormalities. In this case, Fontan revision to an extracardiac conduit with atrial reduction and surgical Maze procedure may be considered.

5. **Should a further closure device be considered in view of his hypoxia (with obligate jailing of the pacing lead)?**

This question assumes that the desaturation to 91% compared to the previous saturation of 97% is based on the transbaffle puncture that was performed in order to place the transvenous ventricular pacing lead. In order to consider this question, it is important to first determine if this is, in fact, the cause of the desaturation. There are many other causes of desaturation in Fontan patients, and these other etiologies should be considered. For example, a closure device would do nothing for pulmonary arteriovenous malformations or venovenous collaterals, both being significant causes of desaturation in this patient population. Once the mechanism of the desaturation is determined, the extent of desaturation should be assessed. Is this the new baseline oxygen saturation? Does the oxygen saturation worsen with exercise? Is the patient's hematocrit elevated, indicating chronic hypoxemia? Finally, if there is truly a significant right-to-left shunt where the pacing leads cross the lateral tunnel baffle, it is important to determine if the current hemodynamic status may actually need that pressure "pop-off." In other words, it is possible that the hemodynamic status has deteriorated to a degree that the right-to-left shunt now provides an adequate cardiac output that might not be possible if the lateral

tunnel baffle was intact. An obvious intervention that may be beneficial, but more difficult than implanting another occluder device, is getting the patient to stop smoking cigarettes and modifying any other relevant lifestyle behaviors that might adversely affect cardiopulmonary physiology. If this is not possible, and all of the other issues raised have been adequately addressed, it may be worth considering another closure device despite trapping the ventricular pacing lead.

It is important to consider the current clinical status of the patient and whether the medical and interventional management of this patient is acceptable or whether Fontan revision or conversion is an option. Orthotopic heart transplant may be an option if all else fails and if there is continued clinical deterioration. It is not clear from the data provided whether this patient is a candidate. However, among the complicated issues that providers address in adult patients with congenital heart disease complicated by hemodynamic issues and arrhythmias, it is important to remember that transplantation should be considered and discussed before the patient is so sick that he is a poor candidate. In other words, consideration of this option should start early since there may be a better outcome if a patient is transplanted when he or she are in a better state of health. The patient may turn down this option or he or she may be an obvious contraindication, but this is best addressed before the patient is so sick that there are no other options.

REFERENCES

1. Wolf CM, Seslar SP, den Boer K, et al. Atrial remodeling after the Fontan operation. *Am J Cardiol.* 2009;104: 1737–1742.
2. Fishberger SB, Wernovsky G, Gentles TL, et al. Long-term outcome in patients with pacemakers following the Fontan operation. *Am J Cardiol.* 1996;77:887–889.
3. Triedman JK, Bergau DM, Saul JP, Epstein MR, Walsh EP. Efficacy of radiofrequency ablation for control of intraatrial reentrant tachycardia in patients with congenital heart disease. *J Am Coll Cardiol.* 1997;30:1032–1038.
4. Triedman JK, Alexander ME, Love BA, et al. Influence of patient factors and ablative technologies on outcomes of radiofrequency ablation of intra-atrial re-entrant tachycardia in patients with congenital heart disease. *J Am Coll Cardiol.* 2002;39:1827–1835.
5. Ramesh V, Gaynor JW, Shah MJ, et al. Comparison of left and right atrial epicardial pacing in patients with congenital heart disease. *Ann Thorac Surg.* 1999;68:2314–2319.
6. Lopez JA. Transvenous right atrial and left ventricular pacing after the Fontan operation: long-term hemodynamic and electrophysiologic benefit of early atrioventricular resynchronization. *Tex Heart Inst J.* 2007;34(1):98–101.

7. Ferrero P, Yeong M, D'Elia E, Duncan E, Graham Stuart A. Leadless pacemaker implantation in a patient with complex congenital heart disease and limited vascular access. *Indian Pacing Electrophysiol J*. 2016;16:201−204.
8. Harris L, McKenna WJ, Rowland E, Holt DW, Storey GCA, Krikler DM. Side effects of long-term amiodarone therapy. *Circulation*. 1983;67:45−51.
9. El-Assaad I, Al-Kindi SG, Abraham J, et al. Use of dofetilide in adult patients with atrial arrhythmias and congenital heart disease: a PACES collaborative study. *Heart Rhythm*. 2016;13:2034−2039.

Consultant Opinion #2

REINA BIANCA TAN, MD • MAULLY SHAH, MBBS

This case highlights several important points in the management of adult congenital patients after Fontan palliation. Intraatrial reentrant tachycardia (IART) is the most common form of supraventricular tachycardia in ACHD.[1−4] The Fontan operation predisposes to atrial arrhythmias due to extensive sutures lines and long-standing hemodynamic stress which lead to thickened and enlarged atrial myocardium with multiple IART circuits. Up to 50% of atriopulmonary Fontan patients develop atrial tachycardia within a decade of surgery.[5] The Fontan modifications (lateral tunnel and extracardiac conduit) bypass most of the right atrium with resultant decrease in incidence of IART to 2%−7%.[4] IART and sinus node dysfunction (SND) are both common post-Fontan operation with SND typically presenting as tachy-brady syndrome. SND can be further exacerbated by antiarrhythmic drugs needed for control of atrial arrhythmias. Conversion of Fontan from an atriopulmonary anastomosis to a total cavopulmonary anastomosis may lead to reduction of right atrial pressure with concomitant decrease in atrial tachycardia burden.[6]

The first issue to be addressed is whether further attempts at catheter ablation should be undertaken or should have been done prior to pacemaker implantation.

Catheter ablation for IART has advanced since the introduction of 3D mapping and irrigated-tip or large-tip ablation catheters with short-term success rates of up to approximately 90%. However, long-term recurrence risk remains significant in the Fontan population (up to 53%).[1,7] In general, ablation is the curative treatment modality of choice over long-term antiarrhythmic management.[3] Typical approach for catheter ablation of IART is identification of an isolated diastolic atrial potential or critical isthmus using entrainment pacing maneuvers during tachycardia and/or with the assistance of 3D electroanatomic mapping and creating a fixed line of conduction block by placing linear radiofrequency lesions between atrial scars or an atrial scar and an anatomic barrier. This results in successful ablation in ~70−90% of patients, however with 30%−55% recurrence. Another approach is substrate-based ablation in which electroanatomic voltage maps are created to identify channels of conduction between dense scars and ablation of all identified channels is performed with the intent of eliminating all potential reentrant circuits.[8] Also, focal atrial tachycardia is common, often emanating from atrial suture lines. Frequently, the arrhythmia substrate is complex with multiple reentrant circuits, all of which must be addressed in order to achieve long-term control.[7,8] Ablation is generally considered acutely successful if there is arrhythmia termination during the application of energy in the absence of atrial ectopy and subsequent failure to reinduce the previously identified tachycardia or noninducibility alone if ablation was performed during sinus rhythm. Whenever possible, bidirectional conduction block across the lesion line should also be established.

This case demonstrates the familiar scenario of a patient s/p Fontan in the third decade of life with both hemodynamic and EP challenges. The patient had multiple arrhythmia circuits including macroreentrant tachycardia and focal atrial tachycardia. From the case description, it is unclear how many of the ablation procedures were actually successful. 3D mapping was used for all ablations but again it is not known whether the ablation was performed with irrigated tip catheters which are likely to provide more effective lesions. The patient was maintained on antiarrhythmic medication (amiodarone and then dronedarone) following the ablations but periodically had recurrent arrhythmias and a total of five catheter ablations were performed after which the patient continued to have symptomatic arrhythmias. Whether there were recurrences of previously ablated arrhythmia circuits or new arrhythmias due to ongoing atrial remodeling is unclear. There probably is not a consensus on the maximum number of catheter ablations that should be attempted to eliminate atrial tachyarrhythmias in a Fontan. However, if multiple catheter ablations are unsuccessful despite performance by experienced operators, reliable 3D electroanatomic maps and utilization of irrigated tip catheters, we would have considered a surgical maze procedure and conversion to an extracardiac Fontan.

In recalcitrant atrial arrhythmias, surgical atrial maze operation is performed at the time of Fontan conversion.[3,9–12] In this case, the patient had a Fontan conversion to a total cavopulmonary connection (TCPC) in 1995 with excision of the right atrial wall but without a maze procedure. Given that the arrhythmia substrate was mapped in both the lateral tunnel and systemic venous atrium as well as the pulmonary venous atrium, a surgical maze with conversion to an extracardiac Fontan and implantation of an epicardial pacemaker would have been our approach.

The next issue is considering the most appropriate pacemaker system for this patient.

Pacemaker implantation is the most common procedure after Fontan surgery and is estimated to be implanted in 0%–9.2% of patients.[13,14] The incidence of SND after Fontan procedure is between 15% and 45% likely due to scarring in the right atrium, interruption of the sinus node artery during surgery, right atrial hypertension, and manipulation of the RA-SVC junction during cannulation.[15] Current recommendations for permanent pacing in adults with congenital heart disease include symptomatic SND with chronotropic incompetence that is intrinsic or secondary to required drug therapy (Class I) and sinus or junctional bradycardia for the prevention of recurrent IART (Class IIA).[3]

At the time of pacemaker implantation, the patient demonstrated only SND and therefore our opinion is that only an atrial lead was necessary. The advantages of atrial pacing in this patient are (1) appropriate management of atrial arrhythmias with antiarrhythmic drugs via antibradycardia atrial pacing; (2) decreased episodes of IART via rate-adaptive pacemaker ability, thus preventing episodes of sinus bradycardia; (3) improve

ventricular function by maintaining AV synchrony; and (4) treatment of episodes of IART with programmed automatic atrial antitachycardia pacing (ATP).[16–18] Conventionally, the latter requires implantation of a dual chamber pacemaker because ventricular events to generate V–V intervals are required for the manufacturer specific atrial tachycardia (AT) detection algorithm to be operative. However, this can also be accomplished using a dual chamber device that can provide automatic atrial ATP with implantation of an atrial lead but with the ventricular port plugged. The pacemaker paces/senses in the atrium but is unable to sense the 1:1 conducted rhythm in the ventricle and is still able to deliver ATP as the AT algorithm criteria are fulfilled.[19]

Given that this patient had a TCPC, a transvenous lead could be placed on the atrial tissue within the lateral tunnel. In the absence of a residual right-to-left shunt, transvenous atrial lead placement has been shown to have lower procedural morbidity compared to epicardial placement with no significant difference in lead performance and longevity.[13,15] Based on published literature and on our own experience, we do not recommend implantation of an endocardial pacemaker lead in a systemic ventricle due to significant risk of thromboembolism despite anticoagulation. In this patient ventricular pacing could possibly be detrimental as it may cause ventricular dyssynchrony in an already compromised systemic ventricle and possibly worsen ventricular function. Furthermore, lack of AV synchrony with VVI pacing can lead to elevated atrial pressure and thus elevated Fontan pressure.[20]

Recently, leadless cardiac pacemakers (LCPs) have been developed for single chamber use (VVIR) with few reports of use in ACHD.[22,23] The LCP is a self-contained intracardiac device with a screw-in helix that attaches it to the endocardium. Several advantages include use for patients with limited vascular access, obviating the need for pacemaker pocket creation, and avoidance of venous occlusion by pacing leads. In this patient, a leadless system will allow for closure of Fontan fenestration without jailing of pacemaker lead. As the system is designed for use as a single ventricular chamber pacemaker, this limits the utility in a patient that would ultimately benefit from atrial pacing. Also, implanting a device in the endocardial surface of a systemic ventricle may be a nidus for thromboembolism with potentially serious consequences.

The next issue that needs to be addressed is whether the fenestration created by the transvenous lead should be closed.

Intracardiac shunts can lead to embolic strokes particularly with right-to-left shunts and in the presence of a transvenous lead in the systemic circulation. In this case, the patient has a significant right-to-left shunt across the Fontan fenestration with a transvenous lead in the systemic ventricle. Device closure of the fenestration will risk jailing the transvenous lead. As mentioned earlier, the patient will have a greater benefit from atrial pacing rather than ventricular pacing. In our opinion, extraction of ventricular lead with device closure of fenestration and placement of an atrial lead within the tunnel should be considered. While there remains a risk for thrombus formation with a transvenous atrial lead, closure of the fenestration will likely decrease the risk of stroke. In this patient with recurrent atrial arrhythmias and the added risk of a fenestration, long-term anticoagulation should be considered and is a class I indication based on the presence of complex congenital heart disease and sustained/recurrent IART.[3]

The last issue is whether the antiarrhythmic agent can be optimized to gain rhythm control.

The reason for switching to dronedarone was not clarified. It is possible the authors made the switch because of thyroid toxicity from amiodarone. Randomized controlled trials in the non-CHD adult population have failed to show significant difference in all-cause and cardiovascular mortality, heart failure—related hospitalizations, thromboembolic events, and quality of life.[3] Generally, in patients with complex congenital lesions particularly in univentricular hearts and heart failure, rhythm controlled is preferred over rate control. Amiodarone is a class III antiarrhythmic with potent antiatrial fibrillatory effects but has serious potential side effects.[24] The incidence of thyroid dysfunction in CHD is estimated to be 36% with increased risk for thyrotoxicosis in Fontan patients.[25] Therefore, amiodarone is probably not a good long-term medication. Dronedarone is a derivative of amiodarone made by removal of iodine group and addition of a methanesulfonyl group. These changes intend to decrease the lipophilicity of the drug, thus decreasing the side effect profile; however, there have been several reports of severe liver failure after dronedarone use. Studies comparing both drugs for atrial fibrillation and atrial flutter have shown dronedarone is superior to placebo, however is less effective than amiodarone in maintaining sinus rhythm.[26] Based on current recommendations, dronedarone is not recommended is patients with moderate or complex CHD due to concerns of worsening heart failure over time and increased mortality.[3,27] While amiodarone is considered a first-line agent for long-term maintenance of sinus rhythm in adults

with CHD and IART, the presence of cyanosis and risk of developing hepatic disease from Fontan physiology makes this a less favorable choice as well as risk for thyroid dysfunction.[28]

Our recommendation would be to consider using either dofetilide or sotalol. Both are class III antiarrhythmic drugs that block the rapidly acting delayed rectifier potassium channel (I_{Kr}) and prolong the effective refractory period of atrial and ventricular myocardium. Sotalol also has β-blocking effects. Both have been shown to be effective in restoration of sinus rhythm in patients with atrial tachycardia and atrial fibrillation. Currently, use of dofetilide is a class IIa indication as first-line antiarrhythmic adults with CHD and ventricular dysfunction.[3] This is based on adult studies that have showed no associated increase in mortality in high-risk patients with recent myocardial infarction or heart failure.[29] In two studies, 47%—55% of patients remain on the drug after initiation with complete or partial control.[30,31] Sotalol use is currently a class IIb indication for the maintenance of sinus rhythm in adults with CHD, IART, or atrial fibrillation with preserved ventricular function.

Recommendations

1. Lead extraction of transvenous ventricular pacing lead with device closure of Fontan fenestration with implantation of atrial lead within lateral tunnel of the Fontan. We would also recommend discontinuation of dronedarone and instituting dofetilide with proper precautions at the time of drug initiation.
2. If the patient continues to have symptomatic atrial arrhythmias with the aforementioned strategy, then we would recommend surgical revision of Fontan to an extracardiac conduit with a Maze procedure and placement of epicardial dual chamber pacemaker.
3. Anticoagulation with warfarin is recommended in the presence of an endocardial lead even in the absence of a right-to-left shunt.

TAKE-HOME POINTS (EDITORS)

1. While there is no limit to the number of ablations that can be performed in patients with complex atrial arrhythmias in the setting of a Fontan circulation, repeated recurrence after multiple ablations should warrant evaluation for surgical Fontan conversion with Maze operation.
2. SND is common in Fontan patients.

3. In general, patients with Fontan circulation and SND only need an atrial pacemaker. Ventricular pacing should be avoided if at all possible in such patients.
4. Leadless pacemakers have no role in patients with SND since they can currently only be used for ventricular pacing.
5. The presence of an endocardial pacing (or defibrillation) lead should be considered an indication for anticoagulation in Fontan patients.
6. Amiodarone is an excellent short-term option. In patients who need long-term antiarrhythmic therapy, it is important to consider an exit strategy (such as surgical Maze or catheter ablation) in order to stop amiodarone.

REFERENCES

1. Walsh EP, Cecchin F. Arrhythmias in adult patients with congenital heart disease. *Circulation.* 2007;115:534−545.
2. Janson CM, Shah MJ. Supraventricular tachycardia in adult congenital heart disease: mechanisms, diagnosis, and clinical aspects. *Card Electrophysiol Clin.* 2017;9:189−211.
3. Khairy P, Van Hare GF, BALAJI S, et al. PACES/HRS expert consensus statement on the recognition and management of arrhythmias in adult congenital heart disease. *Heart Rhythm.* 2014;11:e102−e165.
4. Balaji S, Daga A, Bradley DJ, et al. An international multicenter study comparing arrhythmia prevalence between the intracardiac lateral tunnel and the extracardiac conduit type of Fontan operations. *J Thorac Cardiovasc Surg.* 2014; 148(2):576−581.
5. Walsh EP. Interventional electrophysiology in patients with congenital heart disease. *Circulation.* 2007;115: 3224−3234.
6. Marcelletti CF, Hanley FL, Mavroudis C, et al. Revision of previous Fontan connections to total extracardiac cavopulmonary anastomosis: a multicenter experience. *J Thorac Cardiovasc Surg.* 2000;119:340−346.
7. Triedman JK, Bergau DM, Saul JP, Epstein MR, Walsh EP. Efficacy of radiofrequency ablation for control of intraatrial reentrant tachycardia in patients with congenital heart disease. *J Am Coll Cardiol.* 1997;30:1032−1038.
8. Nakagawa H, Shah N, Matsudaira K, et al. Characterization of reentrant circuit in macroreentrant right atrial tachycardia after surgical repair of congenital heart disease: isolated channels between scars allow "focal" ablation. *Circulation.* 2001;103:699−709.
9. Backer CL. Rescuing the late failing Fontan: focus on surgical treatment of dysrhythmias. *Semin Thorac Cardiovasc Surg Pediatr Card Surg Annu.* 2017;20:33−37.
10. Mavroudis C, Backer CL, Deal BJ, et al. Evolving anatomic and electrophysiologic considerations associated with Fontan conversion. *Semin Thorac Cardiovasc Surg Pediatr Card Surg Annu.* 2007:136−145.
11. Backer CL, Tsao S, Deal BJ, Mavroudis C. Maze procedure in single ventricle patients. *Semin Thorac Cardiovasc Surg Pediatr Card Surg Annu.* 2008:44−48.
12. Mavroudis C, Deal BJ, Backer CL, et al. J. Maxwell Chamberlain Memorial Paper for congenital heart surgery. 111 Fontan conversions with arrhythmia surgery: surgical lessons and outcomes. *Ann Thorac Surg.* 2007;84: 1457−1465. discussion 1465−6.
13. Takahashi K, Cecchin F, Fortescue E, et al. Permanent atrial pacing lead implant route after Fontan operation. *Pacing Clin Electrophysiol.* 2009;32:779−785.
14. Lasa JJ, Glatz AC, Daga A, Shah M. Prevalence of arrhythmias late after the Fontan operation. *Am J Cardiol.* 2014; 113:1184−1188.
15. Shah MJ, Nehgme R, Carboni M, Murphy JD. Endocardial atrial pacing lead implantation and midterm follow-up in young patients with sinus node dysfunction after the Fontan procedure. *Pacing Clin Electrophysiol.* 2004;27: 949−954.
16. Gillis AM, Koehler J, Morck M, Mehra R, Hettrick DA. High atrial antitachycardia pacing therapy efficacy is associated with a reduction in atrial tachyarrhythmia burden in a subset of patients with sinus node dysfunction and paroxysmal atrial fibrillation. *Heart Rhythm.* 2005;2: 791−796.
17. Stephenson EA, Batra AS, Knilans TK, et al. A multicenter experience with novel implantable cardioverter defibrillator configurations in the pediatric and congenital heart disease population. *J Cardiovasc Electrophysiol.* 2006;17: 41−46.
18. Kamp AN, LaPage MJ, Serwer GA, Dick M, Bradley DJ. Antitachycardia pacemakers in congenital heart disease. *Congenit Heart Dis.* 2015;10:180−184.
19. Noheria A, Friedman PA, Asirvatham SJ, McLeod CJ. Dual chamber pacing mode in an atrial antitachycardia pacing device without a ventricular lead - a necessary evil. *Indian Pacing Electrophysiol J.* 2015;15:133−137.
20. Fishberger SB, Wernovsky G, Gentles TL, et al. Long-term outcome in patients with pacemakers following the Fontan operation. *Am J Cardiol.* 1996;77:887−889.
21. Tsao S, Deal BJ, Backer CL, Ward K, Franklin WH, Mavroudis C. Device management of arrhythmias after Fontan conversion. *J Thorac Cardiovasc Surg.* 2009;138: 937−940.
22. Ferrero P, Yeong M, D'Elia E, Duncan E. Graham Stuart A: leadless pacemaker implantation in a patient with complex congenital heart disease and limited vascular access. *Indian Pacing Electrophysiol J.* 2016;16:201−204.

23. Reddy VY, Exner DV, Cantillon DJ, et al. Percutaneous implantation of an entirely intracardiac leadless pacemaker. *N Engl J Med.* 2015;373:1125−1135.

24. Singh BN, Connolly SJ, Crijns HJGM, et al. EURIDIS and ADONIS Investigators: dronedarone for maintenance of sinus rhythm in atrial fibrillation or flutter. *N Engl J Med.* 2007;357:987−999.

25. Thorne SA, Barnes I, Cullinan P, Somerville J. Amiodarone-associated thyroid dysfunction: risk factors in adults with congenital heart disease. *Circulation.* 1999; 100:149−154.

26. Christiansen CB, Torp-Pedersen C, Køber L. Efficacy and safety of dronedarone: a review of randomized trials. *Expert Opin Drug Saf.* 2010;9:189−199.

27. Køber L, Torp-Pedersen C, McMurray JJV, et al. Dronedarone Study Group: increased mortality after dronedarone therapy for severe heart failure. *N Engl J Med.* 2008;358: 2678−2687.

28. Martino E, Bartalena L, Bogazzi F, Braverman LE. The effects of amiodarone on the thyroid. *Endocr Rev.* 2001; 22:240−254.

29. Pedersen OD, Bagger H, Keller N, Marchant B, Køber L, Torp-Pedersen C. Efficacy of dofetilide in the treatment of atrial fibrillation-flutter in patients with reduced left ventricular function: a Danish investigations of arrhythmia and mortality on dofetilide (diamond) substudy. *Circulation.* 2001;104:292−296.

30. Wells R, Khairy P, Harris L, Anderson C, Balaji S. Dofetilide for atrial arrhythmias in congenital heart disease: a multicenter study. *Pacing Clin Electrophysiol.* 2009;32: 1313−1318.

31. El-Assaad I, Al-Kindi SG, Abraham J, et al. Use of dofetilide in adult patients with atrial arrhythmias and congenital heart disease: a PACES collaborative study. *Heart Rhythm.* 2016;13:2034−2039.

CHAPTER 11

Transposition With Mustard Operation Patient With Risk of Sudden Death

Case submitted by Jim T. Vehmeijer, MD, Barbara J.M. Mulder, MD, PhD, Joris R. de Groot, MD, PhD

CASE SYNOPSIS

A 37-year-old man with transposition of the great arteries (TGA), ventricular septal defect (VSD), and pulmonary valve stenosis presented with a history of Mustard repair, surgical VSD closure, and pulmonary valvulotomy. Because of sick sinus syndrome and intermittent complete atrioventricular (AV) block he underwent permanent pacemaker implantation in 2006. Atrial and ventricular leads were routed via the systemic venous baffle to the left atrium and—subpulmonary—left ventricle, respectively. Fig. 11.1 displays an electrocardiogram showing left atrial and left ventricular pacing.

Over the years, his systemic right ventricle deteriorated (ejection fraction 20%), partly due to an inferior wall myocardial infarction with right ventricular (RV) involvement. This infarction was ascribed to embolization of a thrombus in the systemic right ventricle. In addition, moderate to severe tricuspid regurgitation was present, but surgical intervention was deemed to be too great of a risk. In 2009 he was diagnosed with atrial tachycardia, which converted to sinus rhythm with atrial antitachycardia pacing. Sotalol was started, but resulted in heart failure symptoms necessitating intravenous diuretic treatment, and was thus discontinued.

After a period of relative stability, he presented in 2014 with dyspnea, fever, and leukocytosis. The diagnosis was pneumonia, for which antibiotic therapy was started. During this period he also experienced syncope, which was attributed to a ventricular arrhythmia, particularly because of observed nonsustained ventricular tachycardia in the presence of poor systemic RV function. Therefore, an implantable cardioverter-

defibrillator (ICD) implantation was considered. However, the addition of ICD leads through the systemic venous baffle was thought to be a risk for the development of baffle obstruction. After the signs of infection had dissipated, he underwent implantation of a subcutaneous implantable cardioverter-defibrillator (S-ICD), which was placed under the left serratus muscle (Fig. 11.2). S-ICD sensing was accurate, during both normally conducted rhythm and during ventricular pacing, and there were no signs of pocket infection.

One week after discharge, the patient was readmitted with fever and chills. Again, there were no signs of S-ICD pocket infection. Transthoracic and transesophageal ultrasound revealed a long vegetation on one of the intracardiac pacemaker leads (Fig. 11.3). After treatment for endocarditis was started with broad-spectrum antibiotics, blood cultures showed *Propionibacterium acnes*, and the antibiotic treatment was narrowed to penicillin, 2 million international units, 6 times daily, which was continued for 6 weeks. The anticipated high risk of intra- and periprocedural complications precluded lead extraction. As the PET-CT showed no signs of inflammation afterward, the patient was discharged in relatively good clinical condition. However, 1 week later he presented with chest pain, dyspnea, and general discomfort. Multiple pulmonary emboli were visible on CT scan, ascribed to a flare-up of the lead endocarditis. The patient's condition deteriorated due to a combination of endocarditis, pulmonary emboli, and therapy-resistant systemic RV failure. Eventually, the ICD was turned off, and together with the patient and his family, a choice was made to provide comfort care without further medical intervention. The patient passed away in his sleep.

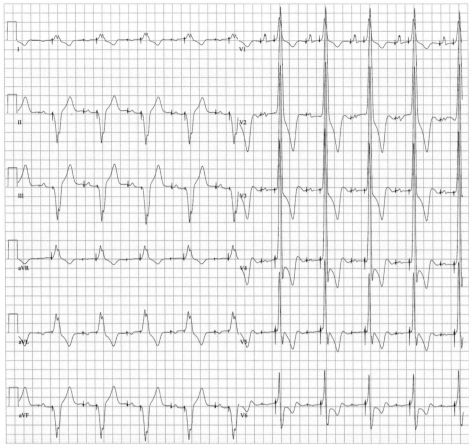

FIG. 11.1 Electrocardiogram after pacemaker implantation showing (left) atrial and ventricular pacing.

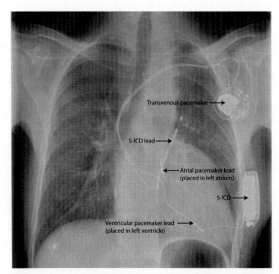

FIG. 11.2 Lead configuration of subcutaneous implantable cardioverter-defibrillator (S-ICD) and transvenous dual-chamber pacemaker on chest X-ray.

Questions

1. What is the role of biventricular pacing for a patient of this nature when they present with systemic RV failure?
2. In cases of supraventricular tachycardia (SVT) or atrial tachycardia, what are the first-line therapies? Is antitachycardia pacing a first-line therapy or should he have been tried on other treatment modalities such as medications or ablation first?
3. What are the ways to deal with systemic baffle obstruction prior to placing leads? Does the concern for baffle obstruction preclude lead placement?
4. What is the place of SICD therapy in patients with a Mustard operation? Should presence of prior devices be considered a potential problem in patients being evaluated for SICD?

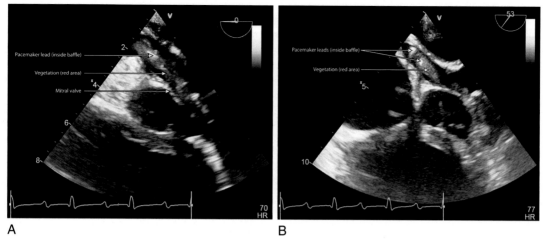

FIG. 11.3 (A) and (B): Vegetation on transesophageal ultrasound.

Consultant Opinion #1

RONALD KANTER, MD

I will attempt to address the questions in the order provided. Following atrial switch operation, the incidence of RV dysfunction leading to heart transplantation is 20% at 20 years,[1] and this seems to apply to both simple transposition and those having associated lesions.[1] Although the etiologies may include chronic atrial tachyarrhythmias or, as in this patient, myocardial infarction, more often, the cause is not known. Tricuspid valve regurgitation with secondary volume overload is often contributory. Although occasionally there are structural abnormalities of the valve or papillary muscle infarction, improvement in valve function can be expected as ventricular function improves.

1. What is the role of biventricular pacing for a patient of this nature when they present with systemic RV failure?

The contribution of intraventricular dyssynchrony of the systemic right ventricle to systolic dysfunction in this patient group has recently been demonstrated. Dyssynchrony and electromechanical delay, especially of the free wall, has been shown to correlate with myocardial fibrosis of the systemic right ventricle.[2] Speckle tracking of the right ventricle has identified the "classic pattern" of dyssynchrony in a handful of Mustard patients who subsequently clinically benefitted from cardiac resynchronization therapy (CRT).[3] This approach seems especially applicable in the presence of severe intraventricular conduction delay with a QRS duration >140 ms, either due to intrinsic delay, or—as in this case—related to left ventricular pacing.

The technique for CRT in these patients nearly always requires a limited right thoracotomy or sternotomy for access to the epicardial surface of the systemic right ventricle. The lead should be placed near the acute angle, just anterior to the tricuspid valve. We prefer a hybrid approach with a transvenous lead to the left ventricle. This eliminates the need for extensive surgical dissection to place a left ventricular lead. As is true in patients having structurally normal hearts, lead placement as close to the base of the heart is desirable so as to accomplish maximal lead separation. Because this patient had had a myocardial infarction, identification of a nonviable ventricular wall is necessary in order to avoid ventricular lead placement onto electrically inactive tissue. This may be accomplished by either radionuclide or electromechanical techniques.

2. In cases of SVT or atrial tachycardia, what are the first-line therapies? Is antitachycardia pacing a first-line therapy or should he have been tried on other treatment modalities such as medications or ablation first?

First-line therapy for intraatrial reentry tachycardia (IART) should be guided by the clinical context, although, in general, a recently published consensus statement favors ablative therapy over antiarrhythmic drugs (Class IIa).[4]

Because this patient required bradycardia pacing for both sinoatrial node dysfunction and impaired AV conduction, a pacing system having atrial antitachycardia pacing capability was a reasonable—and safe—first approach. However, antitachycardia pacing has the potential for conversion of the index tachycardia into a different one. In atrial switch patients having normal AV conduction, this could result in an unpredictable and potentially faster ventricular response, even leading to ventricular tachycardia and death. Whenever possible, we only program atrial antitachycardia pacing in patients whose system also has ventricular defibrillation capability.

Antiarrhythmic drugs have limited efficacy (e.g., AV nodal blocking agents), dangerous proarrhythmic potential (e.g., class IC, III agents), or undesirable long-term noncardiac side-effects (amiodarone). That said, sotalol is a reasonable first therapeutic option, followed by dofetilide, although amiodarone is also considered a reasonable second-line drug (Class IIa recommendation).[4]

Catheter ablation for IART may be successfully accomplished in over 85% of patients.[5-7] Although the recurrence rate is greater than that seen following IART ablation in patients who are postrepair of tetralogy of Fallot or atrial septal defects, it is not as high as in patients who have undergone Fontan-style operations. AV nodal reentrant tachycardia and focal atrial tachycardia are also encountered in these patients and are also highly responsive to catheter ablation.[6] The majority of tachycardia substrates requiring ablation are located in the pulmonary venous atrial side of the circulation. Catheter courses requiring both retroaortic valve/retrotricuspid valve and transbaffle techniques have been well described.[6,8]

3. What are the ways to deal with systemic baffle obstruction prior to placing leads? Does the concern for baffle obstruction preclude lead placement?

In general, whenever a patient who has undergone surgery for congenital heart disease (CHD) is determined to require transvenous placement of conduction hardware to treat bradycardias or tachycardias, meticulous evaluation of postsurgical intracardiac anatomy is required in advance. In no circumstance is this more relevant than in post-Senning and (especially) post-Mustard patients. Atrial baffle obstruction and/or residual baffle leaks exist in as many as half of these patients,[9] particularly in the Mustard group. These residual problems should always be addressed prior to placement of transvenous leads. We have seen patients in whom leads were placed across stenotic baffles with resultant SVC syndrome or new onset of cyanosis due to right-to-left shunting across unappreciated proximal baffle leaks. Superior systemic venous baffle obstruction is more common than either inferior systemic or pulmonary venous baffle obstruction, making this issue especially pertinent to the implanting electrophysiologist. Total obstruction may be present in asymptomatic patients due to decompression of upper body venous return down the azygos vein. In general, we recommend dilatation and (usually) stent placement if the narrowest cross-sectional area (as determined by careful MRI-, echocardiography-, or venography-guided measurements) is less than twice that of the combined cross-sectional area of the leads to be used. Even total obstruction over a short segment can be recanalized and stented by the interventionalist, so that leads may be placed. Residual baffle leaks result in left-to-right shunts and may not be evident by transthoracic echocardiography. Cardiac MRI or transesophageal echocardiography is usually required for detection and precise localization. Placement of leads, especially atrial, in the presence of such a defect places the patient at risk for paradoxical embolization. Once identified, the interventionalist can occlude the defect using occluder devices or covered stents. Two additional caveats are as follows: (1) Before the interventionalist places a stent in an atrial baffle in these patients, evaluation for IART should be performed. Although most IART substrates are in the inferior portion of the atrial mass and most obstructions and baffle leaks are in the superior portion, once a stent is placed—especially a covered stent—catheter access to the IART substrate may be rendered impossible. (2) Coordination between the electrophysiologist and the interventionalist is crucial in these cases. Anatomic details should be discussed in advance. For example, although the interventionalist may wish to implant a superior baffle stent quite inferiorly into the systemic venous atrium, this may impede the ability to place an atrial lead. Liberal flaring of the inferior portion of that stent will help avoid chronic lead damage. The interventionalist and electrophysiologist together should be able to rehabilitate the anatomy and place device hardware in nearly all of these patients.

Also, pertinent to the patient presented, baffle obstruction may be observed in the presence of chronically implanted leads. Balloon dilatation may be attempted in these patients, so long as lead functionality is assessed immediately afterward. However, stents should never be placed in such situations. That is, jailing of chronic leads is poor practice because it is then impossible to extract those leads, should the patient develop endocarditis. Open heart surgery would be the only way to remove potentially infected hardware. If baffle stenosis has become a clinical problem in a patient having transvenous leads, the better practice is lead extraction, treatment of obstruction, and lead replacement.

4. What is the place of S-ICD therapy in patients with a Mustard operation? Should the presence of prior devices be considered a potential problem in patients being evaluated for S-ICD?

There is increasing experience with implantation of the S-ICD in patients with CHD. Patient eligibility for S-ICD requires that their surface QRS-T complex conforms to one of several predetermined templates in at least one of three lead configurations and in lying and standing positions. In patients having CHD, the eligibility failure rate is higher (21%) than in those having a normal heart, but eligibility may be improved (from 79% to 88%) by placing right (compared with left) parasternal surface leads (and, hence, a right parasternal subcutaneous lead).[10] Once placed, S-ICD systems appear to be as effective in congenital heart patients as in those with normal hearts.[11] In Moore's report of 21 patients, two had undergone the Mustard operation. The compatibility of an S-ICD with a preexisting transvenous bradycardia system, as in the patient presented, is established in patients having a normal cardiac anatomy.[12] Eligibility in those having normal heart anatomy seems to be influenced by permanent RV lead placement, with apical lead placement having a lower eligibility rate than septal or biventricular sites.[13] In the presence of CHD and ventricular pacing, eligibility seems to be reduced, although again, placement of a right parasternal lead may improve the eligibility rate.[10] In Okamura's report, eligibility was negatively impacted by inverted T waves in leads V2–V6 or a long QTc interval.[10] In a small series of four patients having CHD and bradycardia pacing systems, successful implantation, defibrillation threshold testing, and device function were demonstrated.[14] This experience even included a patient having a unipolar lead. Those

authors recommended programming the upper tracking rate to less than one half the S-ICD's tachycardia detection zone in order to prevent inappropriate therapy due to double sensing (pacing spike and QRS). We would be very wary of placing an S-ICD in the presence of any unipolar pacing system.

CONCLUSION

This case is a tragic illustration of the complex issues facing patients with complex CHD and arrhythmias. As a rule, there are no perfect solutions, and, one has to do one's best in trying circumstances.

REFERENCES

1. Cuypers JA, Eindhoven JA, Slager MA, et al. The natural and unnatural history of the Mustard procedure: long-term outcome up to 40 years. *Eur Heart J.* 2014;35:1666–1674.
2. Babu-Narayan SV, Prati D, Rydman R, et al. Dyssynchrony and electromechanical delay are associated with focal fibrosis in the systemic right ventricle – insights from echocardiography. *Int J Cardiol.* 2016;220:382–388.
3. Forsha D, Risum N, Smith PB, et al. Frequent activation delay-induced mechanical dyssynchrony and dysfunction in the systemic right ventricle. *J Am Soc Echocardiogr.* 2016;29:1074–1089.
4. Khairy P, Van Hare GF, Balaji S, et al. PACES/HRS expert consensus statement on the recognition and management of arrhythmias in adult congenital heart disease. *Heart Rhythm.* 2014;11:e102–e165.
5. Wu J, Deisenhofer I, Ammar S, et al. Acute and long-term outcome after catheter ablation of supraventricular tachycardia in patients after the Mustard or Senning operation for D-transposition of the great arteries. *Europace.* 2013;15:886–891.
6. Kanter RJ, Papagiannis J, Carboni MP, Ungerleider RM, Sanders WE, Wharton JM. Radiofrequency catheter ablation of supraventricular tachycardia substrates after mustard and senning operations for d-transposition of the great arteries. *J Am Coll Cardiol.* 2000;35:428–441.
7. Khairy P, Van Hare GF. Catheter ablation in transposition of the great arteries with Mustard or Senning baffles. *Heart Rhythm.* 2009;6:283–289.
8. Perry JC, Boramanand NK, Ing FF. "Transseptal" technique through atrial baffles for 3-dimensional mapping and ablation of atrial tachycardia in patients with d-transposition of the great arteries. *J Interv Card Electrophysiol.* 2003;9:365–369.
9. Patel S, Shah D, Chintala K, Karpawich PP. Atrial baffle problems following the Mustard operation in children and young adults with dextrotransposition of the great arteries: the need for improved clinical detection in the current era. *Cong Heart Dis.* 2011;6:466–474.

10. Okamura H, McLeod CJ, DeSimone CV, et al. Right parasternal lead placement increases eligibility for subcutaneous implantable cardioverter defibrillator therapy in adults with congenital heart disease. *Circ J.* 2016;80:1328–1335.

11. Moore JP, Mondesert B, Lloyd MS, et al. Clinical experience with the subcutaneous implantable cardioverter-defibrillator in adults with congenital heart disease. *Circ Arrhythm Electrophysiol.* 2016;9:e004338.

12. Kuschyk J, Stach K, Tulumen E, et al. Subcutaneous implantable cardioverter-defibrillator: first single-center

experience with other cardiac implantable devices. *Heart Rhythm.* 2015;12:2230–2238.

13. Ip JE, Wu MS, Kennel PJ, et al. Eligibility of pacemaker patients for subcutaneous implantable cardioverter defibrillators. *J Cardiovasc Electrophysiol.* 2017;28: 544–548.

14. Huang J, Patton KK, Prutkin JM. Concomitant use of the subcutaneous implantable cardioverter defibrillator and a permanent pacemaker. *Pacing Clin Electrophysiol.* 2016; 39:1240–1245.

Consultant Opinion #2

EDWARD P. WALSH, MD

This case demonstrates the difficult clinical judgments that often must be made in older patients with CHD in the absence of firm outcome data to guide our decisions. In a complex patient such as this, multiple options exist for treatment of atrial tachycardia, pacemaker implant, ICD implant, and management of infectious complications, none of which can be said to be truly superior to another. Whenever the outcome is poor, we are always left second-guessing ourselves, but the fact remains that we still lack the data necessary to move beyond ad hoc decisions that, to our best reckoning, seem to be in the best interest of the individual patient. Several specific questions were attached to this case for my opinion, and these will be addressed with my own bias on the matter, but broadly speaking, I can only say that each decision made for this patient was entirely reasonable within the current state of the art. The unfortunate outcome did not result from any one specific approach or intervention, but rather was a function of a long-standing compromised hemodynamic substrate with associated electrophysiologic challenges and ultimately, infectious complications. The only thing I can state with confidence is that a similar patient would have a better outcome nowadays with the benefit of an arterial switch procedure rather than struggling in early adulthood with the known late complications of the Mustard operation, most all of which seemed to be present in this case.

1. What is the role of Biventricular pacing for a patient of this nature when they present with systemic RV failure?

The first question posed to me was whether biventricular pacing would have been beneficial in this case to address RV dysfunction. Outcome data on the benefits of CRT pacing in the population with a systemic RV are, to say the least, inconclusive. The consensus guidelines for adult CHD[1] would have considered this patient to have a Class IIa indication for CRT, but the level of evidence to support that recommendation is still only C. Keeping in mind that addition of an RV lead would almost certainly necessitate an epicardial approach in this anatomic arrangement, I have usually not been a strong advocate in similar patients of my own. This particular case is further complicated by myocardial infarction with RV involvement, as well as advanced tricuspid regurgitation, neither of would have been likely to reverse even if a CRT system was implanted successfully. I would have been considering a patient like this for transplant evaluation rather than CRT.

2. In cases of SVT or atrial tachycardia, what are the first-line therapies? Is antitachycardia pacing a first-line therapy or should he have been tried on other treatment modalities such as medications or ablation first?

The therapy chosen for atrial tachycardia management in this case was antitachycardia pacing. No information was provided regarding how successful this was for the patient, but I assume it proved efficacious. My own experience/concern with atrial antitachycardia pacing is that it can sometimes cause a shift in atrial reentry circuits to one with a different cycle length (or precipitate atrial fibrillation) with a faster ventricular response,[2] but assuming that was never an issue in this patient, it was certainly a reasonable approach as a pacemaker was already needed for bradycardia indications. Some patients can be managed successfully long term with this approach, but I have found them to be in the minority of Mustard and Senning patients. My own preference is catheter ablation as location of the atrial reentrant circuit(s) is fairly predictable in this condition, and the outcomes have been quite favorable,[3] but I would not take issue with antitachycardia pacing if it was working in an individual case. Regarding medical therapy, I believe drugs for rate control are reasonable to consider, but have little or no confidence in their ability to prevent atrial tachycardia itself.[4]

3. What are the ways to deal with systemic baffle obstruction prior to placing leads? Does the concern for baffle obstruction preclude lead placement?

The issue of SVC baffle narrowing in relation to pacemaker leads and addition of an ICD lead is likewise a judgment call. One could consider elective extraction of chronic pacing leads with dilation and stenting of narrowed portions of the SVC baffle[5] followed by reimplantation of new pacing leads (or a transvenous ICD lead if needed). This assumes availability of a skilled and experienced interventionalist to address the baffle narrowing, which is not a trivial undertaking. In a hemodynamically compromised patient, the risks involved must be balanced carefully against potential benefit.

4. What is the place of S-ICD therapy in patients with a Mustard operation? Should the presence of prior devices be considered a potential problem in patients being evaluated for S-ICD?

The clinicians managing this patient chose instead to implant an S-ICD system, which seems a reasonable decision as QRS sensing proved accurate. My own experience with the S-ICD in Mustard patients is that most do not qualify based on inadequate QRS discrimination (particularly if they have bundle branch block from VSD closure or intermittent ventricular pacing), but we continue to check individual patients to see if it would be an option in selected cases such as this.

The subacute problem leading to this patient's demise was endocarditis involving the transvenous pacemaker leads. Infectious disease consultants I have worked with always advocate hardware removal in this setting, although we do not always follow that advice in tenuous patients. Would the outcome have differed if the infected leads been extracted? Perhaps, but we have certainly had anecdotal success sterilizing similar infections in our own patients with prolonged antibiotic therapy, and I do not think it was unreasonable to try in a hemodynamically compromised patient such as this.

We are fortunate that there are multiple effective therapeutic options to address the complex presentation of late complications in CHD patients, although it is always unsettling to be responsible for major therapy decisions in the absence of data. Now that more patients with CHD are reaching adulthood, the population is fast approaching the size where a more organized appraisal of the many options through multicenter study will be possible.

TAKE-HOME POINTS (EDITORS)

1. Patients with atrial switch (Mustard's and Senning's operations for transposition) and a combination of arrhythmias and systemic RV failure present extremely difficult management conundrums in adult congenital heart disease.
2. Ablation therapy for atrial arrhythmias is encouraging in this group and should be considered early.
3. The frequent presence of baffle stenosis and or baffle leaks should be considered in such patients prior to any interventional and/or device procedures.
4. In general, transplantation should be considered early in the course of patients with complex CHD and systemic ventricular failure.

REFERENCES

1. Khairy PC, et al. PACES/HRS expert consensus statement on the recognition and management of arrhythmias in adult congenital heart disease. *Heart Rhythm*. 2014;11: e102−e165.
2. Rhodes LA, Walsh EP, Gamble WJ, Triedman JK, Saul JP. Benefits and potential risks of atrial antitachycardia pacing after repair of congenital heart disease. *PACE*. 1995;18: 1005−1016.
3. Sherwin ED, Triedman JK, Walsh EP. Update on interventional electrophysiology in patients with congenital heart disease: evolving solutions for complex hearts. *Circ Arrhythm Electrophysiol*. 2013;6:1032−1040.
4. Walsh EP. Interventional electrophysiology in patients with congenital heart disease. *Circulation*. 2007;115:3224−3234.
5. Walsh EP, Cecchin F. Arrhythmias in adult patients with congenital heart disease. *Circulation*. 2007;115:534−545.

CHAPTER 12

Complex Congenital Heart Disease With Brady-Tachy Syndrome and Antitachycardia Pacing

TABITHA G. MOE, MD • VICTOR A. ABRICH, MD • EDWARD K. RHEE, MD

CASE SYNOPSIS

This case involves a 33-year-old woman with complex congenital heart disease consisting of heterotaxy with a single systemic right ventricle, pulmonary artery atresia, and an interrupted inferior vena cava (IVC) with hemiazygous continuation to a persistent left superior vena cava (SVC) (Fig. 12.1). She is status postpulmonary artery banding, creation of bilateral bidirectional cavopulmonary anastomoses (Kawashima procedure), creation of a lateral tunnel Fontan, right atrial plication, and tricuspid valve repair. She presented to the emergency room multiple times for recurrent episodes of tachycardia (Fig. 12.2 EKG). She was started on amiodarone but continued to have recurrent episodes. She then had an electrophysiologic study where three distinct atrial flutters and a focal atrial tachycardia were induced (Fig. 12.3 EGM). Subsequently, she underwent a biatrial maze procedure and implantation of a dual chamber antitachycardia pacemaker (Medtronic EnRhythm model P1501DR) with epicardial lead placement and an abdominal generator (Fig. 12.4); however, the initial generator was faulty and required replacement.

During normal operation, the pacemaker delivers ATP if the atrial rate is above the atrial detection rate. However, the device also assesses the atrioventricular (AV) relationship and can only deliver ATP if the atrial rate is faster than the ventricular rate. Therefore ATP would not be delivered for atrial arrhythmias with a 1:1 AV relationship. Because of this software limitation, the pacemaker was loaded with custom software from Medtronic (TPARx) under compassionate use allowing patient-activated ATP. At the onset of symptoms, the patient presses a button on a wireless transmitter that starts a timer (typically 30 min). During this period, the pacemaker suspends the AV relationship criteria

and delivers ATP for atrial rhythms above the atrial detection limit. The pacemaker returns to normal operation once the atrial arrhythmia ends or the timer expires. Placing a magnet over the device will also stop delivery of therapy by TPARx.

Following pacemaker implantation, atrial arrhythmias with a 1:1 AV relationship were documented during pacemaker interrogation (Fig. 12.5). The pacemaker did

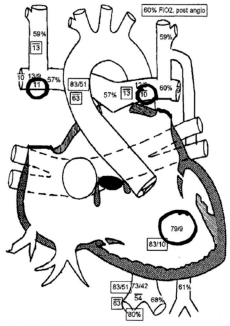

FIG. 12.1 A right heart catheterization report depicting the patient's anatomy along with chamber pressures and oxygen saturations. There is an interrupted inferior vena cava with hemiazygos continuation to a persistent left superior vena cava.

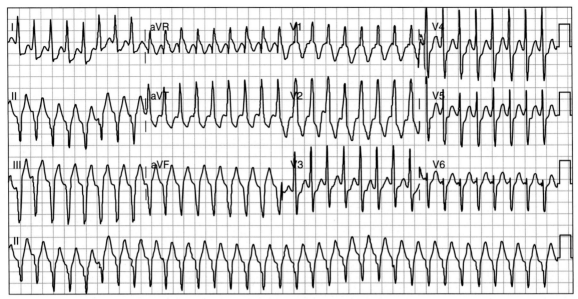

FIG. 12.2 ECG revealing a wide complex tachycardia.

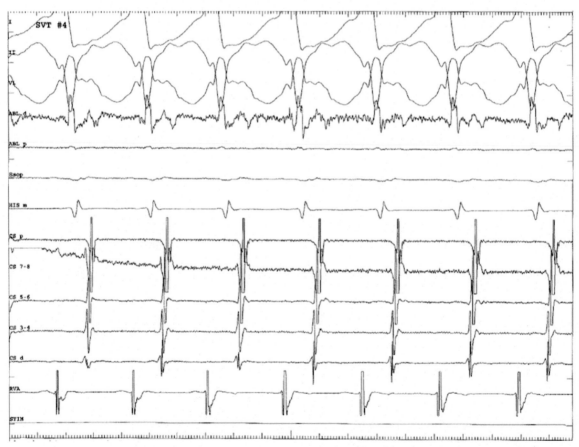

FIG. 12.3 Intracardiac electrogram of one of the inducible tachycardias. CS activation is distal to proximal, suggestive of a counterclockwise atrial flutter.

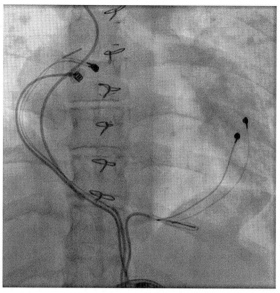

FIG. 12.4 Fluoroscopic view of epicardial pacemaker leads and abdominal pacemaker generator.

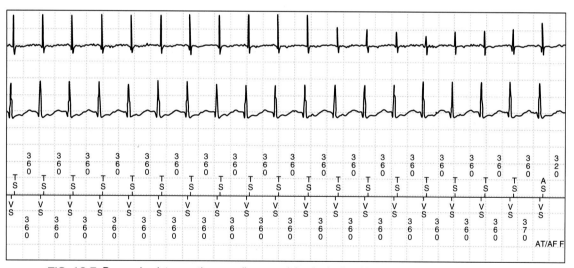

FIG. 12.5 Pacemaker interrogation revealing an atrial arrhythmia with a 1:1 atrioventricular relationship.

not initially deliver ATP after patient activation because the heart rates were below the atrial detection limit. Once the atrial detection limit was lowered, ATP was able to be delivered with patient activation. The TPARx software has successfully terminated the patient's subsequent atrial arrhythmias (Figs. 12.6 and 12.7).

Questions

1. Is there a role for repeat ablation in this patient?

2. What would be the challenges to another ablation attempt and how to go about ensuring success?
3. Would you continue amiodarone? If yes, why? If no, why not?
4. Is there a different drug that you would try?
5. Is it acceptable to leave the patient with current ATP management?
6. Are there any downsides to ATP management and how can we minimize those?

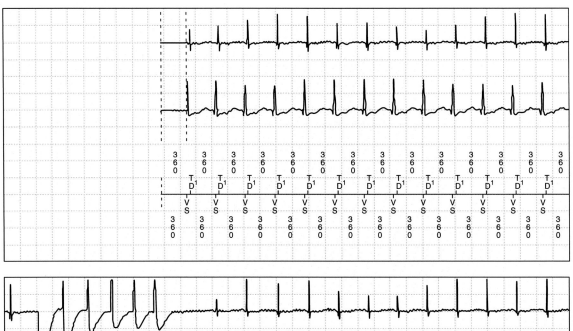

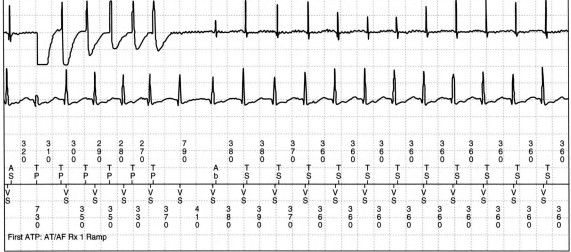

FIG. 12.6 Rhythm strip showing atrial arrhythmia that does not terminate with first ATP sequence.

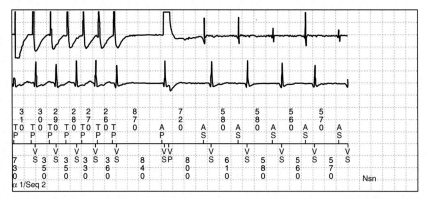

FIG. 12.7 Rhythm strip showing termination of atrial arrhythmia during second ATP sequence.

Consultant Opinion #1

CHARLOTTE A. HOUCK, MD • NATASJA M.S. DE GROOT, MD, PHD

This case represents a patient with complex congenital heart disease who underwent multiple palliative surgical procedures and who presented with symptomatic postoperative atrial tachyarrhythmias. Several attempts were made to treat these atrial tachyarrhythmias, including antiarrhythmic drug therapy with amiodarone, a biatrial Maze procedure, and finally, implantation of a dual chamber antitachycardia pacemaker. Antitachycardia pacing with patient activation successfully terminated atrial tachyarrhythmias in this patient.

Multiple treatment modalities for postoperative atrial tachyarrhythmias have been described in patients after Fontan-type surgery, including antiarrhythmic drug therapy, antitachycardia pacing, conversion surgery, arrhythmia surgery, and catheter ablation.

POSTOPERATIVE ATRIAL TACHYARRHYTHMIAS IN FONTAN PATIENTS

Atrial tachyarrhythmias are the most commonly observed postoperative arrhythmias after Fontan-type surgery, occurring in up to 50% of patients by 20 years of follow-up.[1] Risk factors for development of atrial tachyarrhythmias in Fontan patients include right atrial enlargement, elevated atrial pressure, dispersion of atrial refractoriness, sinus node dysfunction, older age at the time of cardiac surgery, elevation of pulmonary pressure, low oxygen saturation, preoperative arrhythmias, prior palliation with an atrial septectomy, AV valve replacement, and aging.[2–4]

Macroreentrant circuits involving the right atrium are most often observed (Fig. 12.1). However, in lateral tunnel-type repairs, a part of the anatomic right atrium (and thus the reentrant circuit) may end up in the pulmonary venous (left) atrium after surgery.[5] Slowed conduction with reentry is facilitated by both anatomic and surgical barriers. Anatomic barriers include the orifices of the inferior and SVC, the ostium of the coronary sinus, and an atrial septal defect. Scar tissue, suture lines, and prosthetic materials form surgically induced barriers. Patients with a Fontan circulation often have multiple reentry circuits because of the extensiveness of areas of scar tissue that are scattered throughout the

dilated atria.[6] Follow-up of patients with lateral tunnel and extracardiac Fontan modifications show that patients with lateral tunnel repair experience more atrial tachyarrhythmias, consistent with the increased placement of suture lines in this procedure.[7]

Focal atrial tachycardias have also been described in Fontan patients, although infrequently. A focal atrial tachycardia is defined as an atrial tachycardia originating from a circumscribed region from where it expands centrifugally to the remainder of the atrium, as

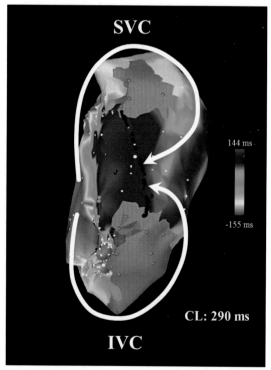

FIG. 12.1 Three-dimensional electroanatomic activation map of a macroreentrant tachycardia (CL 290 ms) involving the right atrial free wall of a patient after the Fontan procedure. The tachycardia was caused by a figure of eight type reentry around two scars (gray areas) as indicated by the *arrows*. The *dark red dots* indicate the line of ablation that was made between the two scars. *IVC*, inferior vena cava; *SVC*, superior vena cava.

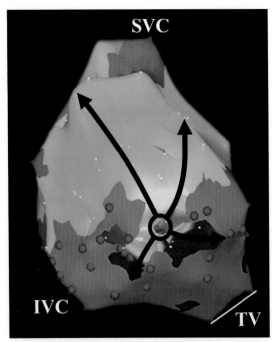

FIG. 12.2 Three-dimensional electroanatomic activation map of the right atrium obtained from a patient with a Fontan circulation revealing a focal atrial tachycardia originating from the lower part of the anterior wall. The tachycardia emerges from a small circumscribed region nearby an area of scar tissue (gray areas). The *arrows* indicate main propagation directions. *IVC*, inferior vena cava; *SVC*, superior vena cava; *TV*, tricuspid valve.

demonstrated in Fig. 12.2. Whether these tachycardias are caused by ectopic activity or microreentry remains questionable.[6] Atrial fibrillation also occurs in patients with a Fontan circulation and this arrhythmia tends to occur at a much younger age (28 ± 9 years) in Fontan patients than in the normal population.[8]

1. **Is there a role for repeat ablation in this patient?**
2. **What would be the challenges to another ablation attempt and how to go about ensuring success?**

CATHETER ABLATION

Catheter ablation is a good alternative in case of failure or adverse effects of medical therapy. Although numerous studies have reported ablation outcomes in patients with a variety of congenital heart diseases, only a few studies assessed results of catheter ablation in Fontan patients specifically. Outcomes of these studies are summarized in Table 12.1. Acute success rates of ablative therapy for atrial tachyarrhythmias

are variable and follow-up after catheter ablation is complicated by many recurrences. Successive atrial tachyarrhythmias developing over time may be caused by different mechanisms. It is most likely that recurrences of atrial tachyarrhythmias are caused by a progressive atrial cardiomyopathy instead of an unsuccessful ablation procedure or arrhythmogenicity of prior ablative lesions.[6,9]

Difficulties in catheter ablation in patients after Fontan-type surgery include the frequent existence of multiple tachycardia circuits, restricted catheter access, distorted anatomy, hemodynamic instability, and the inability to deliver lesions of sufficient depth. Moreover, extensive ablation results in focal wall thinning, which in itself may produce an additional area of slowed conduction, facilitating tachycardia development.[5] Catheter access is limited due to difficulties in accessing the pulmonary venous atrium from the systemic veins. Several approaches have been described, including transbaffle puncture, retrograde access via the systemic artery, direct via sternotomy, or transthoracic via percutaneous access. Disadvantages of retrograde aortic access include poor stability and flexibility of the ablation catheter, hemodynamic instability, and risk of valve dysfunction or injury by manipulation of the catheter past the systemic semilunar and the AV valve.[10] Outcomes might improve by using remote-controlled magnetic navigation, but this technology is not widely available.[11] Transthoracic or trans-sternotomy access is associated with a high incidence of complications and technical limitations.[12,13] Another method to reach the pulmonary venous atrium is transbaffle puncture, which was first described in 1959.[14] Several studies showed that puncture through intra-atrial baffles or patches is a safe and simple technique, without residual shunts during follow-up.[10,15] Performance of transbaffle puncture can be guided by angiogram or by transesophageal or intracardiac echocardiography. Transbaffle access can be achieved by puncture with a transseptal needle or with the use of radiofrequency energy. In order to avoid unnecessary transbaffle puncture, preprocedural echocardiography can be considered to investigate the presence of residual baffle leaks or fenestrations.

After access is obtained, electroanatomic activation and/or voltage mapping in addition to entrainment techniques contribute to the identification of arrhythmogenic substrates and the selection of suitable target sites for ablation. Three-dimensional electroanatomic contact or noncontact mapping visualizes the activation wavefront throughout the atria, which is especially useful in the presence of areas of scar tissue, prior incision

TABLE 12.1

Results of Ablation of Atrial Tachyarrhythmias in Patients With Fontan Circulation

Reference	Patients (N)	At Circuits (N)	Acute Success	Follow-Up	Recurrence
Betts et al.[33]	5	11	60%	6.4 mo	67%
Weipert et al.[1]	30	—	83%	1.7 y	—[a]
De Groot et al.[15]	19	41	78%	53 mo	60%
Yap et al.[34]	11	—	45%	2.3 y	47%

[a] Arrhythmia recurrence not specifically stated: Kaplan-Meier estimate for freedom from tachycardia after initially successful ablation was 81% ± 10% at 3 years' follow-up.

AT, atrial tachyarrhythmia; *mo*, months; *y*, years.

sites, and prosthetic material, as is generally always the case in Fontan patients. As most atrial tachyarrhythmias in Fontan patients are caused by macroreentrant tachycardias related to scar tissue, accurate identification of areas of scar tissue is crucial. Prior endovascular voltage mapping studies have demonstrated that successful ablative therapy of atrial tachyarrhythmias was often targeted at arrhythmogenic areas from which atrial potentials with small peak-to-peak amplitudes were recorded. In a cohort of patients with and without congenital heart disease, bipolar voltages of 0.1 mV or less were never recorded in the latter group.[16] Based on these observations, a cut-off value of 0.1 mV was used to discriminate between healthy and diseased (e.g., scarred) myocardium. It was suggested that scar tissue mapping using a cut-off value of 0.1 mV in combination with activation and propagation mapping facilitated ablation outcomes in patients with congenital heart disease.[16]

In the electrophysiology study prior to the biatrial maze procedure in our patient, there were multiple, different atrial tachyarrhythmias inducible by programmed electrical stimulation. It is very likely that after this surgical procedure there are still multiple tachyarrhythmias inducible due to the presence of an extensive arrhythmogenic substrate. In patients such as this, while attempting to perform wavefront analysis, a different wavefront arising from an ectopic beat (for instance) may alter the course of the initial wavefront and give rise to another clinically relevant tachycardia. The first decision when scheduling a second ablation procedure would thus be either to target only the clinical tachyarrhythmia or to target all inducible tachyarrhythmias. In the first case, when the patient is in sinus rhythm at the onset of the ablation procedure, inducing the clinical tachyarrhythmia can be challenging. In the second case, noninducibility of all atrial tachyarrhythmias as a procedural endpoint could result

in an extensive ablation procedure of considerable duration and prolonged fluoroscopy times. Owing to limited atrial access and the distorted cardiovascular anatomy and particularly the interrupted IVC, creation of effective lesions at the desired target site can be difficult but may be overcome by using a remote magnetic navigation system. Because of all these complexities, ablative therapy should only be considered when all other therapies, including antitachycardia pacing and pharmacologic rhythm control, fail, and the patient has multiple, long symptomatic episodes.

ARRHYTHMIA SURGERY

Atrial tachyarrhythmias can also be treated at the moment of Fontan conversion. Recurrence rate of atrial tachyarrhythmias after Fontan conversion without arrhythmia surgery is reported to be around 76%.[5] Intraoperative ablation consists of a right-sided Maze operation for right atrial reentry tachycardias and a Cox-Maze III procedure for atrial fibrillation or left atrial reentry tachycardias.[6] Several studies have shown that Fontan conversion with concomitant arrhythmia surgery is safe and effective, improves clinical outcome, and has an acceptable recurrence rate (9%–25%).[17–21] The success rate of arrhythmia surgery in Fontan patients can be limited by several factors, including the type of atrial fibrillation [paroxysmal vs. (longstanding) persistent], the size of the (remaining) left and right atria or single atrium, the anatomy and function of the systemic ventricle, the technique and procedure applied, and the presence of clots in the left atrial appendage.[6]

In case of the heterotaxy syndrome, additional ablative lesions will be necessary to connect the left-sided SVC to the confluence of the pulmonary veins in order to improve outcomes.[19] It is of note that focal atrial tachycardia is not addressed by the right-sided Maze procedure and requires direct elimination of the tachycardia focus.[5]

3. **Would you continue amiodarone? If yes, why? If no, why not?**
4. **Is there a different drug that you would try?**

Drug Therapy

Persistent atrial tachyarrhythmias can be treated with chemical or electrical cardioversion and, if tachyarrhythmias are recurrent, with antiarrhythmic drug therapy. Unfortunately, medical management of atrial tachyarrhythmias in patients with congenital heart disease is often difficult, achieving low success rates.[22] Moreover, antiarrhythmic drugs may be proarrhythmic, negative inotropic, and may aggravate sinus and AV node dysfunction.[6] In turn, sinus node dysfunction might contribute to development of atrial tachyarrhythmias.[23] Amiodarone is the most effective antiarrhythmic drug available, but severe side effects such as thyroid dysfunction and liver or pulmonary toxicity—which are dose- and time dependent—occur particularly in young adults.[24] Hence, it is not a preferable therapy for a patient like this who is only 33 years old.

Sotalol may be an alternative, yet meta-analysis has shown that sotalol usage is associated with an increased mortality and it has therefore become a class IIb indication for patients with congenital heart defects and intraatrial reentrant tachycardias or atrial fibrillation.[25-27]

5. **Is it acceptable to leave the patient with current ATP management?**
6. **Are there any downsides to ATP management and how can we minimize those?**

Antitachycardia Pacing

Antitachycardia pacing is another treatment modality for atrial tachyarrhythmias. The value of antitachycardia pacing is based on the principle of entrainment with termination. Termination is only likely to occur if the pacing cycle length is <80% of the tachycardia cycle length.[28] Results of antitachycardia pacing in the treatment of atrial tachyarrhythmias in patients with congenital heart disease are questionable, especially in the presence of multiple clinical atrial tachycardia types.[28, 29] In addition, antitachycardia pacing may increase the risk of acceleration of atrial tachycardia and degeneration into atrial fibrillation. It has been suggested that antitachycardia pacing might be more efficacious when combined with antiarrhythmic drugs or after radiofrequency ablation of some of the reentry circuits.[28,30]

For appropriate therapy, the pacing algorithm requires that the atrial tachyarrhythmia has ≥2:1 AV

relation. This algorithm acts as a safety measure to ensure that rapid antitachycardia pacing is not conducted 1:1 to the ventricle and to assist in arrhythmia identification. However, patients with congenital heart disease often have slower atrial tachyarrhythmias that conduct 1:1 to the ventricle. In these cases, the algorithm does not recognize the rhythm as atrial tachyarrhythmia.

With TPARx software, the device uses the usual algorithm until the patient feels symptomatic and activates antitachycardia pacing. Patients with congenital heart disease are often very well able to recognize an atrial tachyarrhythmia. However, several disadvantages of the patient-activated device include 1) the need for the patient to be conscious or in the presence of someone familiar with the device and 2) the potential risk of inducing a ventricular tachyarrhythmia by manipulation of a 1:1 atrial tachyarrhythmia. For the latter limitation, concomitant administration of an AV node-blocking drug has been suggested when activating the device.[31]

In addition to the aforementioned case, two other cases of congenital heart disease and patient-activated antitachycardia pacing have been described in the literature. One report described an 18-year-old woman with complex congenital heart disease and a Fontan circulation with frequent episodes of atrial tachyarrhythmias with 1:1 AV conduction.[31] The other case concerned a 28-year-old woman after surgical repair of total anomalous pulmonary venous return with a long history of paroxysmal atrial tachyarrhythmias and also 1:1 AV conduction of the tachycardia.[32] TPARx software was installed to allow use of patient-activated antitachycardia pacing. In both cases, subsequent atrial tachyarrhythmias with 1:1 AV conduction could be terminated successfully. No proarrhythmic effect regarding acceleration of atrial tachycardia or induction of ventricular tachycardia was documented.

Hence, there is no objection to continue patient-activated antitachycardia pacing in our patient.

REFERENCES

1. Weipert J, Noebauer C, Schreiber C, et al. Occurrence and management of atrial arrhythmia after long-term Fontan circulation. *J Thorac Cardiovasc Surg.* 2004;127:457–464.
2. Agnoletti G, Borghi A, Vignati G, Crupi GC. Fontan conversion to total cavopulmonary connection and arrhythmia ablation: clinical and functional results. *Heart.* 2003;89:193–198.
3. Cecchin F, Johnsrude CL, Perry JC, Friedman RA. Effect of age and surgical technique on symptomatic arrhythmias after the Fontan procedure. *Am J Cardiol.* 1995;76:386–391.

4. Gelatt M, Hamilton RM, McCrindle BW, et al. Risk factors for atrial tachyarrhythmias after the Fontan operation. *J Am Coll Cardiol.* 1994;24:1735–1741.

5. Deal BJ, Mavroudis C, Backer CL. Arrhythmia management in the Fontan patient. *Pediatr Cardiol.* 2007;28:448–456.

6. de Groot NMS, Bogers A. Development of tachyarrhythmias late after the Fontan procedure: the role of ablative therapy. *Card Electrophysiol Clin.* 2017;9:273–284.

7. Nurnberg JH, Ovroutski S, Alexi-Meskishvili V, Ewert P, Hetzer R, Lange PE. New onset arrhythmias after the extracardiac conduit Fontan operation compared with the intraatrial lateral tunnel procedure: early and midterm results. *Ann Thorac Surg.* 2004;78:1979–1988;discussion 1988.

8. Teuwen CP, Ramdjan TT, Gotte M, et al. Time course of atrial fibrillation in patients with congenital heart defects. *Circ Arrhythm Electrophysiol.* 2015;8:1065–1072.

9. de Groot NM, Lukac P, Blom NA, et al. Long-term outcome of ablative therapy of postoperative supraventricular tachycardias in patients with univentricular heart: a European multicenter study. *Circ Arrhythm Electrophysiol.* 2009;2:242–248.

10. Correa R, Walsh EP, Alexander ME, et al. Transbaffle mapping and ablation for atrial tachycardias after Mustard, Senning, or Fontan operations. *J Am Heart Assoc.* 2013;2: e000325.

11. Ernst S, Babu-Narayan SV, Keegan J, et al. Remote-controlled magnetic navigation and ablation with 3D image integration as an alternative approach in patients with intra-atrial baffle anatomy. *Circ Arrhythm Electrophysiol.* 2012;5:131–139.

12. Khairy P, Fournier A, Ruest P, Vobecky SJ. Transcatheter ablation via a sternotomy approach as a hybrid procedure in a univentricular heart. *Pacing Clin Electrophysiol.* 2008; 31:639–640.

13. Nehgme RA, Carboni MP, Care J, Murphy JD. Transthoracic percutaneous access for electroanatomic mapping and catheter ablation of atrial tachycardia in patients with a lateral tunnel Fontan. *Heart Rhythm.* 2006;3:37–43.

14. Ross Jr J, Braunwald E, Morrow AG. Transseptal left atrial puncture; new technique for the measurement of left atrial pressure in man. *Am J Cardiol.* 1959;3:653–655.

15. El-Said HG, Ing FF, Grifka RG, et al. 18-year experience with transseptal procedures through baffles, conduits, and other intra-atrial patches. *Catheter Cardiovasc Interv.* 2000;50:434–439;discussion 440.

16. De Groot NM, Kuijper AF, Blom NA, Bootsma M, Schalij MJ. Three-dimensional distribution of bipolar atrial electrogram voltages in patients with congenital heart disease. *Pacing Clin Electrophysiol.* 2001;24: 1334–1342.

17. Aboulhosn J, Williams R, Shivkumar K, et al. Arrhythmia recurrence in adult patients with single ventricle physiology following surgical Fontan conversion. *Congenit Heart Dis.* 2010;5:430–434.

18. Jang WS, Kim WH, Choi K, et al. The mid-term surgical results of Fontan conversion with antiarrhythmia surgery. *Eur J Cardiothorac Surg.* 2014;45:922–927.

19. Mavroudis C, Deal BJ, Backer CL, et al. J. Maxwell Chamberlain Memorial Paper for congenital heart surgery. 111 Fontan conversions with arrhythmia surgery: surgical lessons and outcomes. *Ann Thorac Surg.* 2007;84: 1457–1465;discussion 1465–1466.

20. Sridhar A, Giamberti A, Foresti S, et al. Fontan conversion with concomitant arrhythmia surgery for the failing atriopulmonary connections: mid-term results from a single centre. *Cardiol Young.* 2011;21:665–669.

21. Terada T, Sakurai H, Nonaka T, et al. Surgical outcome of Fontan conversion and arrhythmia surgery: need a pacemaker? *Asian Cardiovasc Thorac Ann.* 2014;22: 682–686.

22. Garson Jr A, Bink-Boelkens M, Hesslein PS, et al. Atrial flutter in the young: a collaborative study of 380 cases. *J Am Coll Cardiol.* 1985;6:871–878.

23. de Groot NM, Schalij MJ. The relationship between sinus node dysfunction, bradycardia-mediated atrial remodelling, and post-operative atrial flutter in patients with congenital heart defects. *Eur Heart J.* 2006;27: 2036–2037.

24. Thorne SA, Barnes I, Cullinan P, Somerville J. Amiodarone-associated thyroid dysfunction: risk factors in adults with congenital heart disease. *Circulation.* 1999;100: 149–154.

25. Freemantle N, Lafuente-Lafuente C, Mitchell S, Eckert L, Reynolds M. Mixed treatment comparison of dronedarone, amiodarone, sotalol, flecainide, and propafenone, for the management of atrial fibrillation. *Europace.* 2011; 13:329–345.

26. Khairy P, Van Hare GF, Balaji S, et al. PACES/HRS Expert Consensus Statement on the Recognition and Management of arrhythmias in adult congenital heart disease: developed in partnership between the pediatric and congenital Electrophysiology Society (PACES) and the Heart Rhythm Society (HRS). Endorsed by the governing bodies of PACES, HRS, the American College of Cardiology (ACC), the American Heart Association (AHA), the European Heart Rhythm Association (EHRA), the Canadian Heart Rhythm Society (CHRS), and the International Society for Adult Congenital Heart Disease (ISACHD). *Heart Rhythm.* 2014;11:e102–e165.

27. Lafuente-Lafuente C, Longas-Tejero MA, Bergmann JF, Belmin J. Antiarrhythmics for maintaining sinus rhythm after cardioversion of atrial fibrillation. *Cochrane Database Syst Rev.* 2012:CD005049.

28. Kanter RJ, Garson Jr A. Atrial arrhythmias during chronic follow-up of surgery for complex congenital heart disease. *Pacing Clin Electrophysiol.* 1997;20:502–511.

29. Rhodes LA, Walsh EP, Gamble WJ, Triedman JK, Saul JP. Benefits and potential risks of atrial antitachycardia pacing after repair of congenital heart disease. *Pacing Clin Electrophysiol.* 1995;18:1005–1016.

30. Fukushige J, Porter CB, Hayes DL, McGoon MD, Osborn MJ, Vlietstra RE. Antitachycardia pacemaker treatment of postoperative arrhythmias in pediatric patients. *Pacing Clin Electrophysiol.* 1991;14:546–556.

31. Batra AS. Patient-activated antitachycardia pacing to terminate atrial tachycardias with 1:1 atrioventricular conduction in congenital heart disease. *Pediatr Cardiol*. 2008;29: 851–854.
32. Weber S, Jeron A, Schneider HJ, Muders F. Efficacy of patient activated antitachycardia pacing therapy using the Medtronic AT500 pacemaker. *Europace*. 2006;8: 413–415.
33. Betts TR, Roberts PR, Allen SA, et al. Electrophysiological mapping and ablation of intra-atrial reentry tachycardia after Fontan surgery with the use of a noncontact mapping system. *Circulation*. 2000;102:419–425.
34. Yap SC, Harris L, Downar E, Nanthakumar K, Silversides CK, Chauhan VS. Evolving electroanatomic substrate and intra-atrial reentrant tachycardia late after Fontan surgery. *J Cardiovasc Electrophysiol*. 2012;23:339–345.

Consultant Opinion #2

KEVIN SHANNON, MD

1. **Is there a role for repeat ablation in this patient?** In general, the answer to this question would be yes, even though the success rates for ablation of multiple atrial arrhythmias in patients after a Fontan procedure are low,[1] arrhythmia burden is often diminished, and the intervening biatrial maze may alter the tachycardia substrate enough that it will be more amenable to ablation. The risk of both transbaffle and transconduit access is low,[2] and so even a slight reduction in arrhythmia burden is worthwhile.

2. **What would be the challenges to another ablation attempt and how to go about ensuring success?** The biggest challenge to repeated ablation in this population is the frequent finding of multiple tachycardias. The use of multipolar mapping catheters can shorten the time it takes to create high-density electroanatomic maps and increase success rates.[3] The use of irrigated ablation catheters or large tip catheters has also improved the efficacy of ablation for atrial flutter and would be useful in this situation, as would force sensing technology.[4]

3. **Would you continue amiodarone? If yes, why? If no, why not?** In this situation, the amiodarone is likely playing an important role in slowing the tachycardia and making it amenable to ATP. Stopping the amiodarone may lead to a higher atrial tachycardia rate, necessitating higher ATP rates and raising the risk of the current tachycardia treatment strategy. Hence it would be important to continue amiodarone.

4. **Is there a different drug that you would try?** Amiodarone has the best safety and efficacy profile of all the available antiarrhythmic agents, and so I would not be in favor of attempting therapy with alternative medications in the current situation. I would consider additional AV nodal blocking agents to minimize the risk of rapid conduction of ATP and or more rapid atrial tachycardia induced by ATP. I would also consider flecainide if ventricular function is normal and arrhythmia burden remains unacceptable. Dofetilide is another alternative to amiodarone and flecainide.

5. **Is it acceptable to leave the patient with current ATP management?** If the patient's symptoms are adequately controlled with the current management and the patient has an acceptable quality of life, then continuing the current ATP management would be reasonable.

6. **Are there any downsides to ATP management and how can we minimize those?** There are several downsides to ATP management.
   a. Battery longevity can be significantly reduced by frequent ATP, particularly when it becomes less effective. In this situation, the ATP only occurs after the patient uses a manual activation device, thus the patient can be instructed to stop attempting ATP if it has not been effective during the 30-min window.
   b. 1:1 conduction of antitachycardia pacing and or induction of more rapid atrial tachycardia with 1:1 conduction are a known cause of fatal outcomes from this approach.[5] This can be minimized with the continued use of amiodarone and may be further minimized by the addition of AV nodal blocking agents, including digoxin. Another strategy that I would seriously consider

would be upgrading the current device to an ICD. A subcutaneous shocking lead can be tunneled posteriorly or placed in the pericardium and the existing bipolar leads used as pace-sense leads.[6,7]

c. The risk of thromboembolic events may be elevated in this situation where the patient may not activate the ATP in a timely fashion of arrhythmia episodes may be frequent. This can be minimized with anticoagulation as appropriate.

TAKE-HOME POINTS (EDITORS)

1. Antitachycardia pacemakers can be an important adjunct therapy in select patients with atrial arrhythmias unresponsive to medications, ablation, and surgery. It can reduce arrhythmia duration, arrhythmia burden, the number of emergency room visits and hospitalizations.

2. In patients with antitachycardia pacemakers, amiodarone (and other antiarrhythmic therapy) can slow the atrial arrhythmia sufficiently to make the antitachycardia pacing effective.

3. In general, repeat ablation procedure should be attempted in such patients except in situations such as interrupted IVC.

REFERENCES

1. Moore JP, Shannon KM, Fish FA, et al. Catheter ablation of supraventricular tachyarrhythmia after extracardiac Fontan surgery. *Heart Rhythm.* 2016;13(9):1891−1897.
2. Correa R, Walsh EP, Alexander ME, et al. Transbaffle mapping and ablation for atrial tachycardias after Mustard, Senning, or Fontan Operations. *J Am Heart Assoc.* 2013;2(5):e000325.
3. Bun SS, Delassi T, Latcu DG, et al. A comparison between multipolar mapping and conventional mapping of atrial tachycardias in the context of atrial fibrillation ablation. *Arch Cardiovasc Dis.* 2017. S1875-2136(17) 30151−1.
4. Reddy VY, Shah D, Kautzner J, et al. The relationship between contact force and clinical outcome during radiofrequency catheter ablation of atrial fibrillation in the TOCCATA study. *Heart Rhythm.* 2012;9(11):1789−1795.
5. Lau CP, Cornu E, Camm AJ. Fatal and nonfatal cardiac arrest in patients with an implanted antitachycardia device for the treatment of supraventricular tachycardia. *Am J Cardiol.* 1988;61(11):919−921.
6. Gupta N, Moore JP, Shannon K. A novel approach to eliminate intraventricular lead placement in patients with congenital heart disease. *J Interv Card Electrophysiol.* 2012; 35(1):115−118. https://doi.org/10.1007/s10840-012-9682-5. Epub 2012 May 4.
7. Cannon BC, Friedman RA, Fenrich AL, Fraser CD, McKenzie ED, Kertesz NJ. Innovative techniques for placement of implantable cardioverter-defibrillator leads in patients with limited venous access to the heart. *Pacing Clin Electrophysiol.* 2006;29(2):181−187.

CHAPTER 13

Tetralogy of Fallot and Biventricular Heart Failure

Submitted by Adam J. Small, MD and Jeremy Moore, MD

CASE SYNOPSIS

AGE: 18 years
GENDER: Male
PERSONAL INFORMATION: High school senior
WORKING DIAGNOSIS: Repaired Tetralogy of Fallot with progressive severe biventricular dysfunction in the setting of sinus node dysfunction and refractory atrial arrhythmias.

HISTORY

The patient was born with tetralogy of Fallot and underwent complete repair with transannular patch and ventricular septal defect closure in infancy. By age 16 he had developed progressive right heart dilation and severe tricuspid regurgitation. He underwent pulmonary valve placement, tricuspid valvuloplasty, and right atrial plication.

Six months later, at age 17, he presented with supraventricular tachycardia. He was taken to the electrophysiology laboratory for evaluation. The tachycardia cycle length was 340 ms with 2:1 atrioventricular conduction. The P wave morphology was thought to be consistent with either an atrial tachycardia or atypical atrial flutter. Radiofrequency lesions were delivered to create a line of block from the superior vena cava to the midposterior free wall of the right atrium, as well as from the tricuspid valve to the inferior vena cava. After lesion delivery, the tachycardia could still be induced with isoproterenol administration. The area of earliest atrial activation was then located at the coronary sinus ostium, and ablation was

undertaken there. The tachycardia was terminated and was not inducible thereafter.

Four months later, the patient presented to the emergency room with a heart rate of 160 beats/min. Cardioversion was performed with a 50 J synchronized shock, with conversion to sinus rhythm. Unfortunately, the tachyarrhythmia recurred 2 h later. Repeat electrophysiology study and catheter ablation were then performed. An intraatrial reentrant tachycardia circuit was found to involve the isthmus between the right atriotomy and tricuspid valve. It was successfully ablated, along with two other tachycardia foci.

Over the next 2 months, the patient was admitted twice for symptomatic tachyarrhythmia. For both, direct current cardioversion was attempted but was unsuccessful. A 12 lead electrocardiogram from that time revealed atrial flutter with a ventricular rate of 120 beats/min, complete right bundle branch block, and QRS duration of 170 milliseconds. An echocardiogram demonstrated mildly to moderately diminished left ventricular systolic function, which had worsened since the previous month.

Soon after, at age 18, he was taken back to the operating room for a redo sternotomy, tricuspid valve replacement with 29 mm Mosaic porcine valve, modified Maze procedure, and biventricular implantable cardioverter-defibrillator (ICD) (St Jude Unify Assura CRT-D; St Jude Medical, St Paul, MN, USA). Eight cryolesions were delivered within the right atrium during the Maze procedure. A right atrial pacemaker lead implant was then attempted in numerous endocardial and epicardial locations. Reliable atrial sensing and pacing could not be achieved, a difficulty attributed to the MAZE procedure, but a bipolar lead was placed transmurally into the atrial myocardium (St Jude Tendril STS, 46 cm; St Jude Medical, St Paul, MN, USA). Likewise, an epicardial bipolar lead (Enpath Myopore Sutureless Myocardial Pacing Lead, 35 cm; Enpath Medical, Minneapolis, MN, USA) was placed with one electrode on the right ventricular free wall and the other electrode on the left ventricle for biventricular pacing. A subcutaneous defibrillation coil (Medtronic Subcutaneous Lead System, 41 cm; Medtronic, Minneapolis, MN) was then implanted along the posterior pericardium. After the operation, the patient was in junctional rhythm. Transesophageal echocardiogram demonstrated severely diminished biventricular function and moderate-to-severe tricuspid insufficiency.

The atrial tachyarrhythmia quickly recurred and his condition worsened over the next month. He re-presented to the hospital with lightheadedness, nausea, and chest pain. Cardioversion was unsuccessful with 100, 150, and 200 J synchronized energy. He was started on amiodarone and milrinone infusions. His tachyarrhythmia improved with amiodarone, but the left ventricular ejection fraction had deteriorated to 20%.

He was transferred to our facility for consideration of orthotopic heart transplantation. Device interrogation revealed a nonfunctioning atrial lead but otherwise normal device function and lead characteristics. The pacing mode was set to VVI with a lower rate of 70 beats/min. The underlying rhythm was junctional and poorly tolerated.

CURRENT SYMPTOMS

The patient experienced palpitations during episodes of supraventricular tachycardia, which were recurrent upon transfer. He also had chest pain at the site of his sternotomy incision. He had no dyspnea, diaphoresis, cough, fevers, chills, nausea, vomiting, or diarrhea.

CURRENT MEDICATIONS

Milrinone infusion 0.5 mcg/kg/min
Amiodarone 200 mg oral daily
Enalapril 2.5 mg oral twice daily
Furosemide 20 mg intravenous every 12 h
Enoxaparin 60 mg subcutaneous every 12 h

PHYSICAL EXAMINATION

104 BP/65 mmHg, HR 81 bpm, oxygen saturation 97% on 2 L via nasal cannula.

Weight 65.5 kg

Appearance: The patient appeared comfortable with normal work of breathing.

Neck veins: Jugular veins were distended.

Lungs/chest: Crackles were appreciated at the left base. Otherwise aeration was normal.

Heart: The rhythm was irregular. S1 and S2 were appreciated. A grade II/VI systolic ejection murmur was appreciated at the left upper sternal border.

Abdomen: The abdomen was normal with no ascites or organomegaly.

Extremities: The extremities were warm without edema.

Skin: Midline sternotomy and left upper chest incisions were clean, dry, and intact.

Laboratory Data (Obtained Prior to Transfer)

Hemoglobin 10.3 g/dL
Hematocrit 31%
Middle cardiac vein 87 fL
Platelet count 304 × 10^9/L
Sodium 134 mmol/L
Potassium 3.5 mmol/L
Creatinine 0.7 mg/dL
Blood urea nitrogen 10 mmol/L
Brain natriuretic peptide 369 pg/mL
Troponin I 0.09 ng/mL
Lactate 0.7 mmol/L

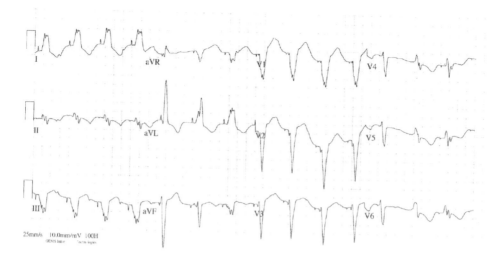

ELECTROCARDIOGRAM

Ventricular-paced rhythm with underlying sinus bradycardia and fusion complexes, paced QRS duration > 200 milliseconds. Ventricular rate at this time is 85 beats/min.

CHEST RADIOGRAPH

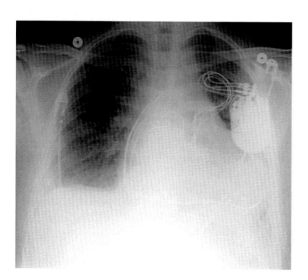

There is an ICD generator in the left chest wall. A right peripherally inserted central catheter (PICC) line extends to the right brachiocephalic vein. A prosthetic pulmonic valve is noted. The patient is status post-midline sternotomy. The heart is enlarged. There is no pneumothorax or pleural effusion. Opacity at the left lung base is noted, probably atelectasis.

CT SCOUT FILM

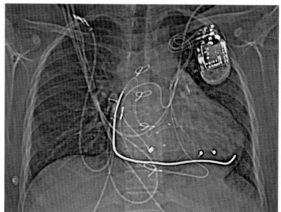

A bipolar transvenous lead is seen attached to the atrial myocardium in a transmural configuration. A bipolar epicardial pacing lead is seen with one electrode on the right ventricular free wall and the other electrode on the left ventricle near the anterior interventricular septum. A subcutaneous defibrillation coil is seen along the posterior pericardium.

Questions

1. What are the possible causes of the patient's ventricular dysfunction?
2. What are the therapeutic options? Does he require orthotropic heart transplantation?

Consultant Opinion #1

FRANK FISH, MD

1. **What are the possible causes of the patient's ventricular dysfunction?**
   - This patient may have multiple factors contributing to his ventricular dysfunction. First and foremost is the likelihood of chronic tachycardia leading to a tachycardia-induced myopathy.
   - Additionally, despite the presence of a biventricular pacing system, the paced QRS complex is quite prolonged, suggesting suboptimal electromechanical resynchronization. Fusion complexes during VVI pacing are further compromising resynchronization efforts
   - The patient has also developed severe tricuspid valve insufficiency. Thus, despite appropriate intervention in the past, there is significant right ventricular volume load which may contribute to adverse RV-LV interaction and decreased LV preload.
   - Finally, late diastolic and systolic dysfunction may be observed following repair of Tetralogy of Fallot. Whether the posterior epicardial placement of the ICD lead is further contributing to his left ventricular diastolic dysfunction is unclear.
2. **What are the therapeutic options? Does he require orthotopic heart transplantation?**
   - Of the multiple contributors to the patient's ventricular dysfunction and hemodynamic compromise, the two factors most amenable to therapy are his tachycardia and his ventricular dyssynchrony.
   - Medical control of this patient's tachycardia has proven ineffective and further effort should be made to eliminate the patient's tachycardia with repeat catheter ablation. Ideally, with detailed mapping and use of advanced high-density mapping and saline-irrigated catheters,

successful ablation could be achieved in a center experienced in this situation. Owing to his hemodynamic compromise, mechanical circulatory support with an Impella device or extracorporeal membrane oxygenation (ECMO) might be necessary. If this proved unsuccessful, AV node ablation to gain control of his ventricular rate would be appropriate. Although less ideal than rhythm control, control of the ventricular rate may allow recovery of ventricular function.
   - It is unclear whether the transmural atrial pacing lead is functional; if not, a left atrial lead might be considered.
   - More optimal cardiac resynchronization should also be attempted and may warrant placement of a new LV lead via the coronary sinus, if favorable resynchronization cannot be achieved with the existing unipolar epicardial pacing leads.
   - The patient may well have unrecoverable ventricular failure. However, the lengthy time course for recovery of ventricular function if rhythm control may be two or more months. If rhythm control and adequate resynchronization could be achieved, it would be reasonable to support by means other than transplant, possibly including advanced heart failure therapies such as a ventricular assist device for a period of several months before resorting to transplantation.
   - The tricuspid valve insufficiency is a concern and may ultimately prove to be the limiting factor in achieving recovery of ventricular function. Until and unless substantial recovery of ventricular function could be achieved, he would be a poor candidate for tricuspid valve replacement, unless a transcatheter approach could be utilized.

REFERENCES

1. Gopinathannair R, Etheridge SP, Marchlinski FE, Spinale FG, Lakkireddy D, Olshansky B. Arrhythmia-induced cardiomyopathies: mechanisms, recognition, and management. *J Am Coll Cardiol.* 2015;66:1714−1728.
2. Moore JP, Patel PA, Shannon KM, et al. Predictors of myocardial recovery in pediatric tachycardia-induced cardiomyopathy. *Heart Rhythm.* 2014;11:1163−1169.
3. Kempny A, Diller GP, Orwat S, et al. Right ventricular-left ventricular interaction in adults with Tetralogy of Fallot: a combined cardiac magnetic resonance and echocardiographic speckle tracking study. *Int J Cardiol.* 2012;154(3):259−264.
4. Praz F, George I, Kodali S, et al. Transcatheter tricuspid valvein-valve intervention for degenerative bioprosthetic tricuspid valve disease. *J Am Soc Echocardiogr.* 2018;31(4): 491−504.

Consultant Opinion #2

DAVID J. BRADLEY, MD

This is a challenging case of rhythm and hemodynamic management in the setting of two-ventricle congenital heart disease (CHD): a young adult patient with tetralogy of Fallot (TOF) has valvular lesions and recurrent atrial arrhythmias for which treatments have serially failed. This is followed by a decline in underlying hemodynamic status.

The case also highlights a number of clinical decisions. Preservation of this patient's clinical condition is a compelling priority; he is referred for consideration of transplantation given an observed decline in left ventricular function, which is a late sequela and poor prognostic indicator in TOF.

KEY CLINICAL EVENTS

Age	Event	Achievement	Detriment
Infancy	Tetralogy repair	Physiologic circulation	Ventriculotomy, conduction delay, PV insufficiency
16 years	PV replacement, TV repair, R atrial plication	Competent PV, improved TV	None
16 years	Atrial tachycardia ablation	Reduction in atrial arrhythmia substrates	None
16 years	Cardioversion	Sinus rhythm, transient	None
17 years	Cardioversion × 2	None	None
18 years	Tricuspid replacement, RA maze, epicardial CRT-D	Competent TV, possible reduction in A tachycardia	Nonfunctioning A lead, sinus node dysfunction

A, atrial; *PV*, pulmonary valve; *TV*, tricuspid valve; *CRT-D*, cardiac resynchronization defibrillator.

What are the possible causes of the patient's ventricular dysfunction?

The table summarizes the interventions and provides this young man's cardiologic timeline. Like many with TOF, he had an infant surgery followed by a "honeymoon" of nearly 2 decades, until a series of unfortunate medical events, comprising the majority of this case narrative, in his late teens.

There is no obvious solution to his predicament. Much could be said about the approach to his atrial arrhythmias, but these are not the topic at hand. An examination of his course identifies several contributors to his functional decline:

1. **Loss of sinus rhythm** is a serious one. Maintenance of sinus rhythm in repaired CHD is both a requirement for stable long-term cardiac status and an indicator of it; the adequacy of rate control in the setting of atrial tachyarrhythmia is debated in the normal heart but is clearly inferior in the repaired heart where AV synchrony and appropriate rate appear necessary. This patient follows a well-worn path from sinus, to increasingly frequent atrial tachycardia episodes, to atrial slowing due to both medication and surgery, to predominant ventricular pacing: more on pacing below.

2. **Ventricular dyssynchrony** was likely present from his first postoperative day as an infant. Yet his course was less favorable than many patients after TOF repair. Why? A history of transannular patch can mean anything from a small incursion on the ventricle by the surgeon to a large ventriculotomy with a long outflow patch. His QRS duration of 170 ms, right ventricular dysfunction and dilation, and tricuspid valve regurgitation suggest that he was of the latter type. Chronic volume overload results in slowed impulse propagation due to fibrosis, compounding the prolongation of ventricular activation; this degree of conduction delay is not a simple matter of right bundle branch block and a large area of ventricular wall.

The implantation of a resynchronization defibrillator/pacemaker was intended to address this but has not; the atrial lead does not capture or sense; and the ECG would suggest that only the right ventricular lead is capturing. The QRS duration on paced beats appears to exceed 200 ms. The M-mode echo shows paradoxical septal motion with a markedly reduced shortening fraction. As expected, the BNP is elevated.

A few comments on this cardiac resynchronization therapy (CRT) system are important:

Atrial lead implant failure: The maze operation, a long operation on cardiopulmonary bypass and redo sternotomy are a setup for a challenging epicardial implant. Even when available pacing sites can be found, this portion of the procedure is often literally the last priority for the surgical team. It comes after the case has been arduous and is nearly finished; patience for a lengthy device procedure may be gone. But the patient's intact AV conduction and atrial arrhythmias make this a major shortcoming. The transatrial approach used in this case is successful when routinely placed, but may be easily dislodged during chest closure.

Hardware choices: The screw-in Myopore bipolar lead is not steroid eluting. While this is a convenient lead in certain situations and can be precisely positioned, it should be a second choice due to its poor long-term performance. The sew-on Medtronic model 4968 bipolar electrode, with steroid-eluting contacts, has a higher impedance and thus requires lower pacing current. It is a superior long-term choice whenever possible. Finally, high-quality ICDs are available from several manufacturers, but only one, Medtronic, still offers atrial antitachycardia pacing. In a CHD patient with a history of atrial arrhythmias this device should be chosen.

Ventricular pacing sites: The paced QRS of >200 ms with the vector of forces propagating away from the RV represents a failure of this CRT implant. A slow but steady trickle of data on RV synchronization suggests that directly resynchronizing the RV conduction delay may be beneficial in TOF patients with ventricular dysfunction. And in the absence of AV synchrony, due to absence of the atrial lead, VV synchrony is paramount. This patient's system appears not to have a true LV lead. It is an understatement to say that the RV-LV electrical delay has not been optimized.

3. **What are the therapeutic options? Does he require orthotopic heart transplantation?**

This young man may have unrecoverable biventricular dysfunction, so a transplant workup is reasonable. But a concerted effort toward improving his immediate situation is also in order, and has a chance of a forestalling transplant.

A stepwise approach of the following should be considered:

1. Attempted placement of a transvenous atrial and coronary sinus (LV) lead

   A functioning atrial lead would allow for A-V synchrony and a functioning, properly located LV lead would provide V-V synchrony. If a substantial shortening of the QRS were achieved, it would be possible that remodeling of the ventricle would occur, with reduction in ventricular volumes and recovery of their function. The BNP trend would likely be downward.

2. Failing #1, open reattempt at epicardial LV and RA pacing sites

   It would be a difficult decision to return to the operating room for revision of this pacing system, but with the alternative of transplant, this could be considered. Confirmation of a late-activated site during RV paced rhythm would be essential in placing the LV lead.

A number of configurations could improve on the current system, all likely to recover the left ventricular function somewhat. Whether this would suffice to spare the patient transplant cannot be predicted. Even RV-only resynchronization could be considered. Should atrial arrhythmias resurface as a clinical problem, a Medtronic device with atrial antitachycardia features should be placed.

REFERENCES

1. Ait Ali L, Trocchio GL, Crepaz R, et al. Left ventricular dysfunction in repaired tetralogy of Fallot: incidence and impact on atrial arrhythmias at long term-follow up. *Int J Cardiovasc Imaging.* 2016;32(9):1441−1449. https://doi.org/10.1007/s10554-016-0928-7.
2. Janoušek J, Kovanda J, Ložek M, et al. Pulmonary right ventricular resynchronization in congenital heart disease: acute improvement in right ventricular mechanics and contraction efficiency. *Circ Cardiovasc Imaging.* 2017;10(9). https://doi.org/10.1161/CIRCIMAGING.117.006424.
3. Janoušek J, Tomek V, Chaloupecký VA, et al. Cardiac resynchronization therapy: a novel adjunct to the treatment and prevention of systemic right ventricular failure. *J Am Coll Cardiol.* 2004;44(9):1927−1931. https://doi.org/10.1016/j.jacc.2004.08.044.
4. Khairy P, van Hare GF, Balaji S, et al. PACES/HRS expert consensus statement on the recognition and management of arrhythmias in adult congenital heart disease. *Can J Cardiol.* 2014;30(10):e1−e63. https://doi.org/10.1016/j.cjca.2014.09.002.

TAKE-HOME POINTS (EDITORS)

1. Electrical causes of cardiac dysfunction include absence of AV synchrony, dyssynchronous ventricular activation, and tachycardia-induced cardiomyopathy.
2. Each of these three factors should be considered in any patient with severe ventricular dysfunction and every effort undertaken to eliminate them. Elimination or reduction of tachyarrhythmia burden (using drugs, ablation, surgery, and or anti-tachycardia pacing), reducing dyssynchrony (by elimination of ventricular pacing or appropriate resynchronization therapy), and providing AV synchrony by placement of appropriate leads are all important in the management.
3. Transplant can be delayed, or even avoided, by the abovementioned measures in select patients.

CHAPTER 14

Transposition Patient With Mustard's Operation and Brady-Tachy Issues

Case submitted by Vivienne Ezzat, MBChB

CASE SYNOPSIS

A 30-year-old female was referred to the congenital heart disease arrhythmia service in 2016. Diagnoses were transposition of the great arteries (TGA), bilateral superior vena cavae [with a left superior vena cava (SVC) draining into the systemic venous atrium (SVA) with no bridging vein], and Crohn's disease. She underwent atrial septostomy soon after birth and again at 5 months (balloon and blade, respectively), followed by a Mustard operation with a bovine pericardial patch aged 11 months. Postoperatively she developed persistent complete heart block with a narrow escape of ~60 bpm; however, there was no hemodynamic compromise, and a permanent pacemaker (PPM) was not implanted. Subsequent ambulatory monitoring and exercise testing demonstrated adequate heart rate variability; a 24 h ECG in 1995 (aged 9) showed complete heart block throughout, with a minimum heart rate of 38 bpm and maximum of 133 bpm, the daytime rate being consistently between 70 and 80 bpm. On exercise testing, also in 1995, a maximum heart rate of 145 bpm was reached.

Other than infrequent but severe migraines, she remained well until ~2004–05 when she started to experience shortness of breath on exertion with a suggestion of some mild systemic venous baffle stenosis on transthoracic echocardiogram (Vmax 2 m/s). This was felt to be dynamic, however, and possibly due to the mitral valve motion. Resting ECG at this time is shown in Fig. 14.1. She underwent an exercise test (2005) during which she exercised for 9 min of the Bruce protocol, achieving a maximum heart rate of 141 bpm (70% predicted); resting blood pressure was 100/70 mmHg, with no significant rise (peak blood pressure 105/70 mmHg), and maximum workload was 10 METS. The test was stopped due to fatigue, neck pain, and dizziness. There were also multiple ventricular ectopics. At this time her echocardiogram showed the systemic right ventricle (SRV) was mildly dilated with mild systolic dysfunction. A pacemaker was considered but not implanted.

By 2007 her symptoms of breathlessness had worsened such that she was easily short of breath on minimal exertion and also complained of tiredness and occasional light-headedness. A decision was made to go ahead with dual-chamber PPM implantation, prior to which she underwent cardiac magnetic resonance imaging and catheterization in order to fully assess her anatomy, particularly that of her baffle pathways. These investigations identified that there was in fact a stenosis of the superior systemic venous pathway at its entrance to the systemic venous atrium, as well as a significant communication/leak immediately adjacent to the stenotic area between the systemic and pulmonary venous atriums (PVAs). As the leak was proximal to the obstruction, flow was predominantly right to left (Qp:Qs 0.84), and the expected flow acceleration at the site of the SVC narrowing was, therefore, not observed. The pulmonary venous pathway was unobstructed. Systemic right ventricular function was good, and its indexed end diastolic volume was 120 mL/m^2 [indexed left ventricular (LV) end diastolic volume = 78 mL/m^2]. The right femoral vein was found to be occluded. It was noted in retrospect that saturations on room air had previously been documented as low as 92%.

She underwent successful stenting of the SVC/SVA junction stenosis with exclusion also of the SVA to PVA baffle leak with a covered stent. There was an excellent angiographic result, although it was noted that the right SVC was of a relatively small caliber. Postprocedure oxygen saturations were 98%–99% on room air. After the procedure she complained of some chest discomfort and developed new T wave inversion on 12-lead ECG (Fig. 14.3A) accompanied by a small troponin rise (Troponin T 0.17 ng/mL) but she was otherwise well. Echocardiography repeated the day after the procedure (before pacemaker implantation) demonstrated a moderately

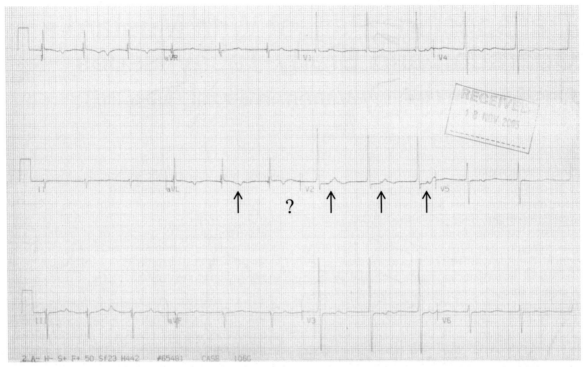

FIG. 14.1 Baseline ECG in 2005, showing sinus rhythm with mild sinus arrhythmia, complete heart block/AV dissociation with almost identical atrial and ventricular rates (~65 bpm)—the atrial rate is marginally faster. The QRS duration is 85 ms. The *arrows* show tiny dissociated p waves visible on occasions, most easily seen in this example in V2. The p wave is too small to be seen easily in aVL.

dilated SRV with moderate-severe systolic dysfunction, which appeared to be a new finding. There was mild systemic atrioventricular (AV) valve regurgitation. It was unclear as to why the SRV had deteriorated, although it was postulated that it may be as a result of the increased preload; however, a thromboembolic phenomenon could not be excluded. A right-sided dual-chamber pacemaker was implanted uneventfully a few days later. Both leads were active fixation and had satisfactory parameters at implant. The (subpulmonary, left) LV lead was placed apically. Chest X-ray and CT imaging illustrating her stent and pacing leads in situ are shown in Fig. 14.2. Pre- and postprocedural 12-lead ECGs are shown in Fig. 14.3. After pacemaker implantation, she was 100% ventricularly paced with ~30% atrial pacing, with a base rate set at 50 bpm. An exercise test was performed (2008) (bike 5–10W ramp) during which she exercised for over 9 minutes 5 seconds, reaching a maximum heart rate of 163 bpm (82% predicted)—and was atrially sensed, ventricularly paced throughout; VO_2 max was 16.5 mL/min/kg (45% predicted); peak watts 60; VE/VCO_2 slope 33.4 (predicted 23.5); RER 1.04. Blood pressure at rest was 110/70 mmHg, rising maximally to 130/70 mmHg. Height at this time was noted to be 163 cm and weight 48 kg. The test was stopped due to tired legs and shortness of breath.

Although she reported only NYHA class II symptoms, her history appeared to be somewhat unreliable, her lifestyle relatively inactive, and objectively her systemic ventricular systolic function had clearly deteriorated; transthoracic echocardiography in 2008 demonstrated the right ventricle to be moderate-severely dilated and impaired. Serial echocardiographic qualitative data on her SRV available from the reports are shown in Table 14.1. The precise cause of this deterioration was unclear. Subpulmonary ventricular function was preserved. She was started on ramipril 5 mg once daily; however, this caused a cough and was changed to losartan. On subsequent pacing checks there were no tachyarrhythmias detected and good heart rate histograms.

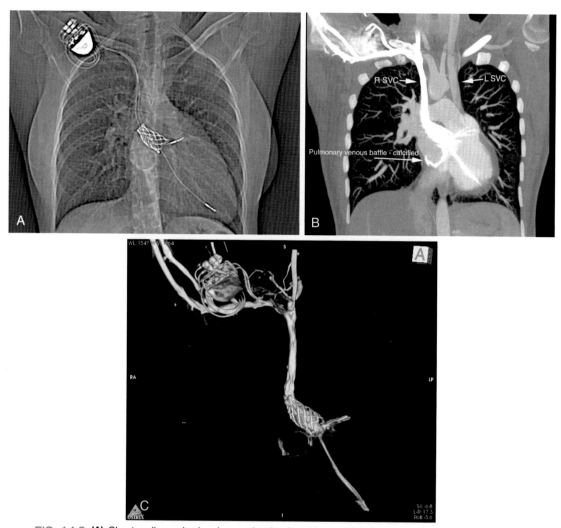

FIG. 14.2 **(A)** Chest radiograph showing pacing leads and stent. **(B)** Coronal cross-sectional CT (2016) showing calcified pulmonary venous baffle as well as bilateral superior vena cavae (SVCs). **(C)** CT 3D reconstruction of stent and ventricular pacing lead.

A generator change was required in 2012. A transvenous biventricular device was considered at this time; however, it was understood that there was no access to the coronary sinus (CS) via the systemic venous circulation (although interpretation of the CT images of her coronary/left SVC anatomy was felt to be difficult). By 2013, her symptoms had progressed and she was in functional class III. Her echocardiogram demonstrated a severely dilated and moderate-severely impaired systemic ventricle. At this time, her heart failure medications titrated up to the maximally tolerated doses, which subjectively did appear to improve her functional status. During a repeat exercise test in 2013 (bike

5–10 W ramp) she managed only 6 min 52 s of exercise, but the test was stopped due to heart rate limitation as a result of the programmed max tracking rate of the pacemaker (heart rate dropped from 153 to 130 bpm with 2:1 AV block and accompanying shortness of breath). Because of this, interpretation of the data was limited. Heart rate at rest was 84 bpm. The rhythm was atrially sensed, ventricularly paced throughout; VO_2 max was 16.3 mL/min/kg (49% predicted); peak watts 45; VE/VCO_2 slope 43.5 (predicted 24); RER 1.03. Blood pressure at rest was 120/80 mmHg, rising maximally to 130/80 mmHg. Height at this time was noted to be 163 cm and weight 52 kg.

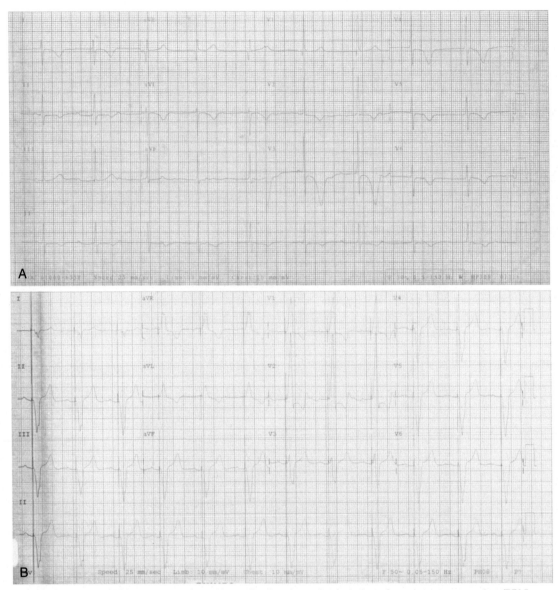

FIG. 14.3 **(A)** ECG post stenting and immediately prior to implantation of permanent pacemaker (PPM) (2007)—the T wave inversion was new and occurred after the stenting procedure. **(B)** ECG immediately after PPM implantation.

She underwent cardiac catheterization in 2014. Results were as follows:

Saturations (%): IVC 78.3, SVC 63.0, LV 70.2, PA 68.0, RV 98.3

Pressures (mmHg): RA 6, LV 35/7, PA mean 16, PCWP 6, RV 113/9, Ao 123/61

Calculations: TPG 9, CO (Fick) 2.49 L/min, CI 1.62 L/min/m², PVRI 5.6WU

CT scan showed at least moderate obstruction within the SVC stent. An epicardial (surgical) attempt at cardiac resynchronization therapy (CRT) was considered, but it was felt that this may be difficult without any certainty of benefit and instead she was referred to the regional transplant center for assessment. There, however, it was felt that she did not fulfill the criteria for transplant at the time based on symptomatology and functional

TABLE 14.1
Serial Systemic Right Ventricular Size and Function

	16/11/05	21/2/07	6/7/07	14/4/08	18/7/11	10/9/12	25/2/13	5/6/15
SRV size	Mildly dilated	Mildly dilated	Moderately dilated	Moderate-severely dilated	Severely dilated	Severely dilated	Severely dilated	Severely dilated
SRV function	Good	Mild dysfunction	Moderate-severe dysfunction	Moderate-severe dysfunction	Moderate dysfunction	Moderate dysfunction	Moderate-severe dysfunction	Severe dysfunction

The SVA was stented shortly prior to the scan performed in July 2007.
SVA, systemic venous atrium; SRV, systemic right ventricle.

status. Clinical observations were weight 48 kg, BP 112/76 mmHg, sats 98% on air, JVP +2 cm, no peripheral edema detectable, a 2/6 pansystolic murmur was heard, her chest was clear, and there was a 2 cm hepatomegaly with no ascites. Medications were spironolactone 25 mg daily, carvedilol 25 mg twice a day, losartan 150 mg daily, furosemide 20 mg daily, and digoxin 125 mcg daily. Her renal function was normal.

Between 2013 and 2015, the patient also suffered significant flare-ups of her Crohn's disease, which required treatment and subjectively became her predominant problem. When seen again after an interval for follow-up in the congenital heart disease clinic in 2015, she reported that her cardiac symptoms had improved significantly with medical therapy. A single reported syncopal episode did not correspond to any arrhythmia detected on device interrogation but sounded more likely to be vasovagal in nature, although the exact cause was unclear. Her resting ECG at this time is shown in Fig. 14.4. In 2015 she also presented to her local hospital with a left-sided hemiparesis which resolved after 2 days and was felt to be consistent with a transient ischemic attack. She was commenced on apixaban. Subsequent device check did not show any arrhythmia.

2016

The patient was referred to the congenital heart disease arrhythmia service in early 2016 following another syncopal episode. This event occurred unprovoked while out walking and was precipitated by chest pain and palpitations. By the time of paramedic arrival, the patient had regained consciousness and was not tachycardic. Pacemaker interrogation showed 10 atrial mode switch episodes due to atrial tachycardia (AT), all occurring for <1 min with CLs 280–400 ms

(mainly regular, but some faster episodes irregular) and ventricular pacing up to the maximum tracking rate of 160 bpm. An example is shown in Fig. 14.5. Ambulatory ECG monitoring was subsequently arranged and also showed frequent brief episodes of max tracking (HR 156 bpm) and periods of bigeminy (junctional/paced rhythm), both of which resulted in symptoms. Transthoracic echocardiographic observations were unchanged.

The patient's digoxin was stopped and carvedilol increased to 25 mg three times a day. The max tracking rate of the device was reduced to 140 bpm in the interim period while the patient awaited a catheter ablation of her AT. This was performed uneventfully in September 2016; however, under general anesthesia, despite aggressive pacing and the administration of isoprenaline, it was not possible to induce any sustained tachycardia and, therefore, an empirical cavotricuspid isthmus line was ablated with radiofrequency on either side of the baffle using a retrograde aortic approach to ablate the PVA aspect. Following a definitive review of imaging and a repeat CT in 2016, it was clear that the CS os was accessible from the inferior aspect of the SVA (effectively the IVC); however, it appeared to drain the apical LV and was difficult therefore to conceive any theoretical benefit to pacing here. The left-sided SVC entrance to the SVA was noted to be jailed by the stent and did not appear to drain any suitable veins in any case. The patient has been further reviewed at a multidisciplinary team meeting and a consensus decision made not to 'upgrade' the PPM to an implantable cardioverter defibrillator (ICD), given the lack of strong data to support implantation in the primary prevention setting and the not insignificant possibility of inappropriate shocks. On most recent exercise testing, the patient managed 6 minutes of a standard CPEX protocol with a VO_2 max of 19.2 mL/min/kg

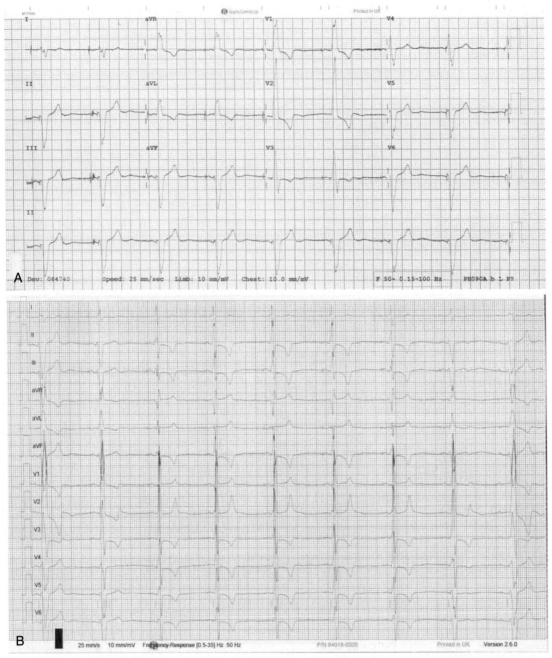

FIG. 14.4 **(A)** ECG in 2015 showing full ventricular pacing with a QRS duration ≥140 ms. **(B)** ECG showing fusion of ventricular pacing with isorhythmic junctional escape (i.e., junctional, sinus, and backup pacing rates all very similar). Note the differences in QRS morphology between beats. It is unlikely that the narrow QRS complexes represent atrioventricular (AV) conduction given the complete absence of any AV conduction prior to this.

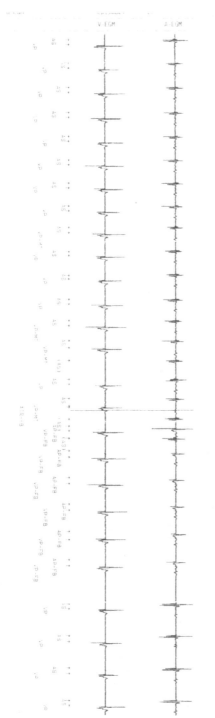

FIG. 14.5 Intracardiac electrograms showing atrial channel (top) and ventricular channel (bottom) with a 1:1 conducted atrial tachycardia (AT) until the max tracking rate is reached (VP-MT). The rate is initially regular and ~ 145 bpm. As the

(57% predicted) and a peak heart rate of 112 beats per minute. She has been referred once again back to the regional center for reconsideration of cardiac transplantation.

Questions

1. Should pacemaker implantation have been considered prior to 2005?
2. Should a biventricular pacemaker implantation have been considered in 2007 and what was the cause of her SRV deterioration at the time? Should further investigations have been considered at that time or now?
3. Should no pacemaker have been implanted at all?
4. Was an empiric catheter ablation (under GA) appropriate given the low burden of atrial arrhythmia or should she have been treated with device reprogramming +/− amiodarone with a view to bridging to transplant?
5. Is the decision not to implant an ICD correct? If an ICD were implanted, what would be the strategy with regard to redundant leads and where should it be placed?
6. Is there any rationale for considering a surgical epicardial lead in an attempt to resynchronize her ventricles while awaiting transplant? What are the potential risks/benefits/difficulties of this and what is the likelihood of being able to place a lead in a meaningful position with respect to resynchronization?

Consultant's Opinion #1

ANICA BULIC, MD • ANNE M. DUBIN, MD

This patient illustrates the numerous long-term sequelae that can arise following a Mustard procedure. Systemic and less commonly pulmonary venous baffle obstruction, baffle leaks, arrhythmias including sinus

AT becomes slightly faster, the subsequent atrially sensed beats fall into the post ventricular atrial refractory period [designated (AS)], resulting in atrial pacing which fortuitously results in termination of the tachycardia into an initial Ap,Vp rhythm followed by sinus rhythm (AsVp) at the end of the strip.

node dysfunction and atrial tachyarrhythmias, systemic right ventricular dysfunction, and sudden cardiac death are among the most common complications following a Mustard repair.

When reviewing this case, **the first question to be discussed is the indication and timing of pacemaker implantation in a patient with congenital heart disease and surgical heart block.** Postoperative advanced second- or third-degree AV block that is not expected to resolve or that persists at least 7 days after cardiac surgery has routinely been considered a class I indication for PPM implantation.[1,2] This is based on natural history data suggesting chronic postsurgical complete heart block is associated with an increased risk of sudden cardiac death of up to 40% over the longer term.[3,4] One could make the argument that pacemaker placement following this patient's Mustard procedure would have been warranted to both improve exercise tolerance and to decrease her risk of sudden cardiac death in the long run. However, it is also important to consider the negative impact of ventricular pacing. Pacing in the ventricle induces dyssynchrony and significantly increases the risk of pacing-induced cardiomyopathy. One possible strategy in this situation is to place a pacemaker but to program it in a backup VVI mode. While this will not address issues of exercise intolerance, it will act as a safety net if the patient does not have a reliable escape rhythm.

Baffle obstruction is a relatively common complication of the Senning or Mustard procedure. In a meta-analysis of the long-term outcome of atrial switch procedures, Khairy and colleagues reported a prevalence of 36% of obstruction of the superior limb of the systemic venous baffle.[5] These obstructions can often be asymptomatic, and thus a comprehensive evaluation involving cardiac catheterization and/or cardiac MRI to fully delineate baffle anatomy and assess hemodynamics is imperative prior to any device implantation, as transvenous pacemaker implantation can significantly worsen baffle obstruction. Baffle leaks are particularly common in Mustard patients and can be quite problematic when considering a transvenous system.[6] In the EVENT multicenter retrospective study of 202 patients with intracardiac shunts, Khairy and colleagues showed that patients with transvenous leads had a 15.6% prevalence of thromboembolic events, compared with 8.9% of those with epicardial leads.[7] Transvenous leads were associated with a 2.6-fold increased risk of systemic thromboembolic events. Interestingly, anticoagulation with aspirin or warfarin was not protective and did not mitigate the increased

thromboembolic risk. Thus, these issues must be addressed prior to transvenous pacemaker placement.

Intravascular stent placement for baffle obstruction offers an alternative to surgical baffle revision. Poterucha and colleagues reported the largest series of intravascular and intraoperative hybrid stent placements in TGA patients following an atrial switch with excellent midterm results.[8] A total of 20 d-TGA patients corrected to either a Mustard- or Senning-type atrial switch underwent stent placement for either systemic or pulmonary venous baffle obstruction. At follow-up of approximately 2 years, there was significantly improved NYHA class, and only two patients had mild baffle stenosis with a mean gradient 2–3 mmHg and did not require reintervention. These procedures are now often performed in conjunction with placement of the transvenous pacing system.

Right ventricular systolic dysfunction developed in this patient following superior systemic baffle obstruction stenting and baffle leak closure. Patients with d-TGA corrected with a Mustard-type atrial switch are at a higher risk of systemic ventricular dysfunction compared with arterial switch patients, mainly due to the presence of a pressure-loaded SRV. In this case, right ventricular systolic dysfunction was temporally related to baffle leak closure; this raises the question of thrombus embolization during the closure. It is possible with manipulation across the baffle leak that a small thrombus embolized to the coronaries causing some transient ischemia and decreased function. The rise in troponin and ECG findings of T wave inversions would support this.

Atrial arrhythmias are a common long-term complication of a Mustard procedure, in part due to the numerous suture lines in the atria as well as atriotomy scars. Atrial arrhythmias are not only burdensome to the patient but also increase the risk of arrhythmia-induced cardiomyopathy and incur a risk of sudden cardiac death, which is not insignificant in this vulnerable patient population. A previously published report on long-term outcomes after Mustard palliation reported an incidence of sudden cardiac death of 7%, and an all-cause mortality of 20% at 15 years of follow-up.[9,10] Kammeraad and colleagues investigated the risk factors of sudden cardiac death in a retrospective, multicenter, case-controlled study and found that heart failure and/or arrhythmic symptoms, and documented atrial flutter or fibrillation were predictors of sudden cardiac death.[11] Unfortunately, noninvasive tests such as ECG, chest X-ray, and Holter findings (e.g., ventricular ectopy) were not predictive of sudden cardiac arrest. In contrast to patients with tetralogy of Fallot (TOF), the role of programmed ventricular stimulation for risk stratifying d-TGA patients has not been well studied and is somewhat controversial. Inducible ventricular tachycardia (VT) has not been shown to predict future events.[12] Patients who have received an ICD for primary prevention based on a positive ventricular stimulation study had no appropriate discharges compared with 28% of patients with an ICD for secondary prevention. The paucity of data available and low appropriate shock rates in this population is reflected in the recent PACES/HRS guidelines.[13] **This patient would be considered to have a class IIb indication for an ICD (an adult congenital heart disease (ACHD) patient with systemic RV ejection fraction <35%, especially with additional risk factors such as complex ventricular arrhythmias, unexplained syncope, NYHA functional class II–III symptoms, QRS >140 ms, or severe systemic AV valve regurgitation).**

The mechanism of sudden death in this group has recently been elucidated with the use of ICD therapy. In a multicenter study of 37 adult patients with d-TGA palliated to a Mustard/Senning, Khairy and colleagues found that supraventricular tachycardia preceded the VT and appropriate shocks in 50% of patients.[12] It is certainly reasonable to aggressively treat atrial arrhythmias with medical therapy or ablation, in light of the abovementioned data suggesting atrial tachyarrhythmias are associated with an increased risk of sudden cardiac death.

Ablation of intra-atrial reentry tachycardia (IART) or atrial flutter is an attractive management option for d-TGA patients with an atrial switch procedure with medically refractory arrhythmias. It is thought that the extensive atrial baffle construction creates areas of scar and acts as a barrier for electrical signal propagation and thus creates atrial reentry circuits. Mapping in concert with a solid understanding of the surgical anatomy can identify areas of slow conduction within the atrial reentry circuit that are necessary for maintenance of the tachycardia and serve as a target for radiofrequency ablation. Van Hare and colleagues described one of the earliest series of mapping and radiofrequency ablation of IART in d-TGA patients following Mustard/Senning procedures.[14] These investigators found that these patients most frequently presented with "typical" flutter, utilizing the cavo-tricuspid isthmus. However, in patients with atrial switch procedures, it was necessary to approach this anatomic area from both the right and left side of the heart. Radiofrequency ablation

was successful in 77% of cases with successful locations requiring ablation in both the right atrium as well as the PVA. Pulmonary venous baffle access may be obtained either by a transseptal puncture with a Brockenbrough needle, or radiofrequency transseptal perforation, which has been shown to be a safe alternative.[15]

The final issue that merits discussion is the appropriateness of biventricular pacing, or CRT, in a patient with repaired cyanotic congenital heart disease and an SRV. There are no randomized controlled trials in the pediatric or ACHD populations, and the criteria for CRT are extrapolated from adult literature. Pediatric and ACHD CRT studies are limited but do support the hemodynamic and functional benefits seen in the adult population. In the largest multicenter pediatric study including 103 patients who underwent CRT, Dubin and colleagues showed that CRT decreased QRS duration by approximately 38 ms from a baseline of 166 ms, and modestly improved ejection fraction from approximately 26%–40%.[16] Subsequent studies have suggested that the benefits of CRT in congenital heart disease may depend on the underlying anatomy of the systemic ventricle, presence and degree of systemic AV valvar regurgitation, ventricular myocardial scarring, and type of electrical dyssynchrony. Janousek and colleagues have reported that patients with an SRV, systemic AV valvar regurgitation, and a poor initial NYHA class responded less favorably to CRT.[17,18] According to published PACES/HRS expert consensus statement on the management of arrhythmias in ACHD patients, our symptomatic patient with systemic RV dilatation and systolic dysfunction but a narrow QRS would not meet criteria for CRT implantation.[13]

REFERENCES

1. Frye RL, Collins JJ, DeSanctis RW, et al. Guidelines for permanent cardiac pacemaker implantation, May 1984. A report of the Joint American College of Cardiology/American Heart Association Task Force on Assessment of Cardiovascular Procedures (Subcommittee on Pacemaker Implantation). *Circulation.* 1984;70:331A–339A.
2. Epstein AE, DiMarco JP, Ellenbogen KA, et al. 2012 ACCF/AHA/HRS focused update incorporated into the ACCF/AHA/HRS 2008 guidelines for device-based therapy of cardiac rhythm abnormalities: a report of the American College of Cardiology Foundation/American Heart Association Task Force on Practice Guidelines and the Heart Rhythm Society. *J Am Coll Cardiol.* 2013;61:e6–75.
3. Gross GJ, Chiu CC, Hamilton RM, Kirsh JA, Stephenson EA. Natural history of postoperative heart block in congenital heart disease: implications for pacing intervention. *Heart Rhythm.* 2006;3:601–604.

4. Lillehei CW, Sellers RD, Bonnabeau RC, Eliot RS. Chronic postsurgical complete heart Block. With particular reference to prognosis, management, and a new P-Wave pacemaker. *J Thorac Cardiovasc Surg.* 1963;46:436–456.

5. Khairy P, Landzberg MJ, Lambert J, O'Donnell CP. Long-term outcomes after the atrial switch for surgical correction of transposition: a meta-analysis comparing the Mustard and Senning procedures. *Cardiol Young.* 2004;14:284–292.

6. Patel S, Shah D, Chintala K, Karpawich PP. Atrial baffle problems following the Mustard operation in children and young adults with dextro-transposition of the great arteries: the need for improved clinical detection in the current era. *Congenit Heart Dis.* 2011;6:466–474.

7. Khairy P, Landzberg MJ, Gatzoulis MA, et al. Epicardial versus Ep and Thromboembolic events I. Transvenous pacing leads and systemic thromboemboli in patients with intracardiac shunts: a multicenter study. *Circulation.* 2006;113:2391–2397.

8. Poterucha JT, Taggart NW, Johnson JN, et al. Intravascular and hybrid intraoperative stent placement for baffle obstruction in transposition of the great arteries after atrial switch. *Catheter Cardiovasc Interv.* 2017;89:306–314.

9. Wilson NJ, Clarkson PM, Barratt-Boyes BG, et al. Long-term outcome after the mustard repair for simple transposition of the great arteries. 28-year follow-up. *J Am Coll Cardiol.* 1998;32:758–765.

10. Walsh EP. Sudden death in adult congenital heart disease: risk stratification in 2014. *Heart Rhythm.* 2014;11:1735–1742.

11. Kammeraad JA, van Deurzen CH, Sreeram N, et al. Predictors of sudden cardiac death after Mustard or Senning repair for transposition of the great arteries. *J Am Coll Cardiol.* 2004;44:1095–1102.

12. Khairy P, Harris L, Landzberg MJ, et al. Sudden death and defibrillators in transposition of the great arteries with intra-atrial baffles: a multicenter study. *Circ Arrhythm Electrophysiol.* 2008;1:250–257.

13. Khairy P, Van Hare GF, Balaji S, et al. PACES/HRS expert consensus statement on the recognition and management of arrhythmias in adult congenital heart disease: developed in partnership between the Pediatric and Congenital Electrophysiology Society (PACES) and the Heart Rhythm Society (HRS). Endorsed by the governing bodies of PACES, HRS, the American College of Cardiology (ACC), the American Heart Association (AHA), the European Heart Rhythm Association (EHRA), the Canadian Heart Rhythm Society (CHRS), and the International Society for Adult Congenital Heart Disease (ISACHD). *Heart Rhythm.* 2014;11:e102–e165.

14. Van Hare GF, Lesh MD, Ross BA, Perry JC, Dorostkar PC. Mapping and radiofrequency ablation of intraatrial reentrant tachycardia after the Senning or Mustard procedure for transposition ofthe great arteries. *Am J Cardiol.* 1996;77:985–991.

15. Esch JJ, Triedman JK, Cecchin F, Alexander ME, Walsh EP. Radiofrequency-assisted transseptal perforation for electrophysiology procedures in children and adults with repaired congenital heart disease. *Pacing Clin Electrophysiol.* 2013;36:607–611.

16. Dubin AM, Janousek J, Rhee E, et al. Resynchronization therapy in pediatric and congenital heart disease patients: an international multicenter study. *J Am Coll Cardiol.* 2005;46:2277–2283.

17. Janousek J, Gebauer RA, Abdul-Khaliq H, et al. Cardiac resynchronisation therapy in paediatric and congenital heart disease: differential effects in various anatomical and functional substrates. *Heart.* 2009;95:1165–1171.

18. Janousek J, Kubus P. Cardiac resynchronization therapy in congenital heart disease. *Herzschrittmacherther Elektrophysiol.* 2016;27:104–109.

Consultants Opinion #2

PETER P. KARPAWICH, MsC, MD, FAAP, FACC, FAHA, FHRS

1. **Should pacemaker implantation have been considered prior to 2005?**
This case is a great example of the need to stay "proactive" when dealing with congenital heart disease patients, especially those in whom a surgical intervention may result in potentially adverse problems even years later. D-TGA repair with the Mustard (or Senning) intra-atrial baffle is known to be associated with three important problems that commonly become more apparent as the patient ages: sinus node dysfunction, atrial arrhythmias, and early heart failure. In addition, a precise working knowledge of vascular anatomy is important when dealing with potential device implants, as in this case: an absent innominate vein with left SVC continuation. This may preclude subsequent left subclavicular device implants.

Heart block following the Mustard repair does occur, with a reported 12% incidence.[1] However, it may be argued that at 11 months of age, with no symptoms and a narrow QRS rhythm, ventricular pacing was not required. Also, in this situation, by 2004 (age 18 years) with fatigue, a dilated systemic ventricle, and systolic dysfunction, it is evident that the patient was exhibiting signs of early heart failure. Although chronotropic incompetence, per se, may not be an indication for pacing among repaired CHD patients, the associated clinical and ECHO findings do favor a device implant.[2] Ventricular ectopy during exercise can also be a marker for myocardial stress. For these reasons, a pacemaker should have been implanted. In addition, selective ventricular pacing lead implant, with the intent of improving contractility, may delay the onset of heart failure.[3] The finding of atrial baffle obstruction, especially the SVC, is not an uncommon finding following the Mustard procedure, due typically to patient growth and reangulation of the baffle. This obstruction is typically relieved by a transvenous stent. Pacing lead implant through the stent can then be readily performed.[4] Entrapment of the pacing lead outside the stent will preclude later lead extraction if required and may damage the lead. So, vascular stenting before lead implant is recommended.

2. **Should a biventricular pacemaker implantation have been considered in 2007 and what was the cause of her SRV deterioration at that time? Should further investigations have been considered at that time or now?**

   A systemic ventricle with "right" ventricular morphology is architecturally not designed for prolonged contractility against systemic pressures. It will fail earlier than one with "left" morphology. This patient had several factors which caused relatively early cardiac decompensation: heart block with loss of atrial synchronization, chronotropic incompetence, and ventricular anatomy. Obviously, any patient presenting with new-onset heart failure should be evaluated for other possible etiologies (e.g., myocarditis, etc). However, in this patient, the heart failure appears to have been progressive and not sudden. Biventricular or CRT is definitely applicable to patients with repaired CHD and can improve ventricular function to forestall heart failure, often for many years. Although there have been several publications indicating its efficacy,[5] application of published "guidelines" for older patients with

structurally normal hearts is not appropriate for CHD patients, especially those with altered systemic ventricular anatomy. In this particular patient, CRT pacing should have been considered in 2007 as an adjunct to heart failure therapies. In that regard, determination of which CHD patients might improve from CRT pacing, based on their respective paced-contractility response, has been shown to be an effective means of preselecting appropriate candidates.[6]

3. **Should no pacemaker have been implanted at all?**

   No, the patient met several criteria for pacemaker implant.[2]

4. **Was an empiric catheter ablation (under GA) appropriate given the low burden of atrial arrhythmia or should she have been treated with device reprogramming +/− amiodarone with a view to bridging to transplant?**

   Atrial arrhythmias are common following the intra-atrial baffle surgery with a reported incidence of 25%[7]. Although most are IART and do involve the cavo-tricuspid isthmus, atrial fibrillation can also occur.[8] The patient had a syncopal episode as well as a transient hemiparesis. In that regard, transient atrial fibrillation with rapid ventricular response could not be completely excluded. Although no arrhythmias could be induced during the electrophysiology study (EPS), it would be appropriate to at least attempt ablation along the cavo-tracuspid isthmus as a means to potentially prevent other arrhythmias. Device programming to attempt to overdrive IART is not always effective and would not be effective for atrial fibrillation.[9] Amiodarone does have negative inotropic qualities and should be used with caution in patients with heart failure.

5. **Is the decision not to implant an ICD correct? If an ICD were implanted, what would be the strategy with regard to redundant leads and where should it be placed?**

   There is no documentation of any ventricular arrhythmias or aborted sudden death in this patient. However, the patient does have a systemic "right" ventricle, is a clinical NYHA II-III classification, and did have an episode of syncope with associated palpitations. For these reasons, an ICD may be considered (Class IIa, Level of evidence C) appropriate therapy based on the recent PACES/HRS published statement.[2] The patient underwent an EPS in 2016 that was negative. At that time, the venous ventricular lead could have been explanted and exchanged for a transvenous ICD lead as a precaution against further potentially dangerous arrhythmias. Alternatively, the existing transvenous pacing lead could have been abandoned. If the existing lead was retained, a new ICD lead could have been implanted along the LV septum as a way of performing "bi-septal" ventricular pacing.

6. **Is there any rationale for considering a surgical epicardial lead in an attempt to resynchronize her ventricles while awaiting transplant? What are the potential risks/benefits/difficulties of this and what is the likelihood of being able to place a lead in a meaningful position with respect to resynchronization?**

Among patients following the atrial baffle repair, the CS is frequently not accessible from the venous SVC/IVC baffle. In this particular case, however, it was accessible. However, the CS is predominately a LV venous system. A transvenous pacing lead implanted via the SVC baffle would route to the venous "left" ventricle. In this regard, an additional lead placed in the CS would not constitute "biventricular" pacing as only the left ventricle would be electrically stimulated. The problem among repaired D-TGA patients with the Mustard/Senning procedures is that the "right" ventricle is the systemic ventricle and that is the one that requires stimulation. A combination "epi-endocardial" hybrid pacing effectively accomplishes that need. To perform this, a transvenous lead is placed in the venous LV septum via the SVC baffle, while an epicardial lead is implanted on the systemic "right" ventricle via a thoracotomy. The epicardial lead is then tunneled subcutaneously to connect to the usual subclavicular device implant site. In this manner, effective CRT pacing of the systemic ventricle can be achieved.[6]

The epicardial lead implant does carry typical risks associated with any surgical approach to epicardial lead implant. However, benefits of improving heart failure can outweigh those risks. By preselecting the proper RV implant site with temporary pacing, the cardiologist can effectively indicate to the surgeon if the epicardial lead should be placed at the free wall or apical regions. Often a "minithoracotomy" is all that is required for exposure. Due to typical postoperative epicardial fibrosis/fat, use of a helical electrode would be preferable. Alternatively, a small epicardial incision can be made to permit an intramyocardial lead implant.[10.]

TAKE-HOME POINTS (EDITORS)

1. Atrial switch (Mustard's and Senning's operation) patients can have complex plumbing and electrical issues. Proactive attention to both issues is important to reduce morbidity and mortality, to maintain quality of life, and to extend their longevity as much as possible.
2. The number and size of pacing leads traversing through the superior baffle should be minimized to reduce the risk of baffle stenosis/occlusion. Baffle stenosis should be addressed before lead implantation.
3. Most patients in this group do not need ventricular pacing. Ventricular pacing can increase the risk of dyssynchrony-induced ventricular dysfunction and should be avoided if possible.
4. If ventricular pacing is unavoidable (mostly due to the rare presence of complete heart block), biventricular pacing should be considered in order to minimize dyssynchrony.

REFERENCES

1. Gelatt M, Hamilton R, McCrindle B, et al. Arrhythmia and mortality after the Mustard procedure: a 30-year single center experience. *J Am Coll Cardiol.* 1997;29:194−201.
2. Khairy P, Van Hare G, Balaji S, et al. PACESZ/HRS expert consensus statement on the recognition and management of arrhythmias in adult congenital heart disease. *Heart Rhythm.* 2014;11(10):e102−e165.
3. Karpawich PP, Singh H, Zelin K. Optimizing paced ventricular function in patients with and without repaired congenital heart disease by contractility-guided lead pacing lead implant. *Pacing Clin Electrophysiol.* 2015;38(1):54−62.
4. Patel S, Shah D, Chintala K, Karpawich PP. Clinically unrecognized atrial baffle complications following the Mustard operation in young adults with d-transpopsition of the great arteries: improved detection is required. *Congenit Heart Dis.* 2011;6(5):466−467.
5. Montonga K, Dubin A. Cardaic resynchronization therapy for pediatric patients with heart failure and congenital heart disease: a reappraisal of results. *Circulation.* 2014; 129:1879−1891.
6. Karpawich PP, Bansal N, Samuel S, Sanil Y, Zelin Kathleen. 16 years of cardiac resynchronization pacing among congenital heart disease patients: direct contractility (dP/dt) screening when the guidelines do not apply. *J Am Coll Cardiol-EP.* 2017;3(No 8):830−841.
7. Khairy P, Landzberg M, Lambert J, O'Donnell C. Long-term outcomes after the atrial switch for surgical correction of transposition: a meta-analysis comparing the Mustard and Senning procedures. *Cardiol Young.* 2004;14:284−292.

8. Frankel D, Shah M, Aziz P, Hutchinson M. Catheter ablation of atrial fibrillation in transposition of the great arteries treated with mustard atrial baffle. *Circ Arrhythm Electrophysiol.* 2012;5:e41–e43.

9. Stephenson E, Casavant D, Tuzi J, et al. Efficacy of atrial antitachycardia pacing using the medtronic AT500

Pacemaker in patients with congenital heart disease. *Am J Cardiol.* 2003;92:871–876.

10. Karpawich PP, Walters H, Hakimi M. Chronic performance of a transvenous steroid pacing lead as an epi-intramyocardial electrode. *Pacing Clin Electrophysiol.* 1998;21:1486–1488.

CHAPTER 15

A Crisscross Heart With Brady-Tachy Issues

Case submitted by Vivienne Ezzat, MBChB

CASE SYNOPSIS

A 39-year-old man was referred to the congenital heart disease (CHD) arrhythmia service in 2015. He was known to have crisscross heart with situs solitus, atrioventricular (AV) concordance, ventriculoarterial (VA) discordance, a large unrestrictive inlet ventricular septal defect (VSD), and a dysplastic pulmonary valve with severe pulmonary valve stenosis. His only intervention was a right-sided Blalock-Taussig (BT) shunt performed when he was 4.5 months old. Cardiac catheterization performed in 2003 showed a dilated BT shunt with a distal stenosis at the anastomosis to the right pulmonary artery, normal pulmonary artery pressures, and a mean pullback gradient over the BT shunt of 43 mmHg. The branch pulmonary arteries were of good size. He also had significant cardiomegaly and the calculated Qp:Qs at the time of this scan being ~3:1.

The patient had a background history of paroxysmal palpitations that had started in childhood. They could sometimes be stopped by vagal maneuvers. An ECG in 1988 was reported to show "atypical atrial flutter"; however, no traces were available to review in 2015. He had initially been treated with digoxin, disopyramide, and propranolol, and subsequently from 1987 was given flecainide and digoxin. Following transition from the pediatric to the adult congenital heart disease (ACHD) service, and subsequent multidisciplinary team (MDT) discussion, his flecainide was stopped in 2009 in view of his structural heart disease. At this time he had been free of symptoms from arrhythmia since 2005 and had been physically stable, in full-time employment, with NYHA Class II symptoms (shortness of breath on stairs or uphill, no ankle edema, no orthopnea) and no major limitations in his daily life. He was a nonsmoker and consumed alcohol infrequently.

The patient remained well until 2007 when he experienced a transient episode of diplopia and abnormal eye movements, which spontaneously resolved after 9 h. He reported to the local ophthalmology service where his eyes were examined and no abnormalities detected. A head CT was not performed. He was seen 1 month later by the regional ACHD service.

On examination at this time he was clubbed; height and weight were 172 cm and 50.4 kg, respectively, oxygen saturations 89% on air, blood pressure 90/50 mmHg, heart rate 68 bpm and regular, jugular venous pressure was not raised, and first and single second heart sounds were normal. There was a left ventricular heave and a grade 4/6 continuous murmur.

Blood workup showed a Hb of 16.8 g/dL (MCV 94.3) and was otherwise normal.

His ECG at this time was described as showing sinus rhythm with very large P waves, marked first-degree AV block (PR interval 380 ms); QRS duration 150 ms with a right bundle branch block pattern.

A transthoracic echocardiogram was performed (2007). Peak velocity across the pulmonary valve was 5 m/s; there was very mild left- and right-sided AV valve regurgitation and good ventricular function. There was a high velocity flow in the BT shunt (maximum systolic gradient ~80 mmHg). No intracardiac thrombus was seen.

It was felt that the episode most likely represented a transient ischemic attack (TIA) and the patient was started on oral aspirin 75 mg once daily. A 24 h ambulatory ECG was performed, and this showed sinus rhythm throughout with first-degree heart block, occasional Wenckebach phenomenon (Fig. 15.1), episodes of aberrant conduction (Fig. 15.1B), and sinus bradycardia (Fig. 15.1C). There were no tachyarrhythmias observed. Heart rate histograms are shown in Fig. 15.3D. Similar findings were again recorded on ambulatory monitoring in 2008.

He remained under regular follow-up and was stable until 2011 when he started to have intermittent

135

palpitations again. There was no history of syncope or presyncope. A 12 lead ECG from 2010 is shown in Fig. 15.2. During a Bruce protocol exercise test performed in 2010, he exercised for 7.39 min with an increase in heart rate from 51 bpm to a peak of 146 bpm (78% of maximum predicted). His blood pressure rose from 104/45 mmHg to a peak of 136/66 mmHg. The test was stopped due to shortness of breath. There were no significant arrhythmias noted (occasional ventricular ectopics only) and no ST segment changes with exercise. His resting saturations were 88% and fell to 63% at peak exercise.

Repeat Holter monitoring was performed (2011), while he was taking digoxin only and showed no tachyarrhythmia, but bradyarrhythmia was noted. As previously observed, there was first-degree AV block and periods of AV Wenckebach; in addition there was evidence of more pronounced bradyarrhythmia on two separate recordings, including a daytime sinus

pause of 3.59s (Fig. 15.3A) and P wave asystole of 5.8 s, also in the daytime (Fig. 15.3B); however, it did appear that in all instances of AV block, the non-conducted beats were preceded by PR lengthening. He was asymptomatic on both occasions. When symptomatic with palpitations and breathlessness, ventricular ectopics, and periods of bigeminy/trigeminy were recorded, accounting for ~0.5% of the beat counts. Cross-sectional imaging at this time confirmed that ventricular function remained good. His digoxin was stopped and he was started on bisoprolol 1.25 mg.

Over the next 2 years, he reported a very slow deterioration in his functional status, becoming more easily short of breath and tired on exertion; however, he remained generally well and stable until 2014 when he started to experience "dizziness," the exact nature of which was unclear. A 48 h Holter monitoring demonstrated both sinus node and AV nodal conduction disease, with occasional sinus pauses of

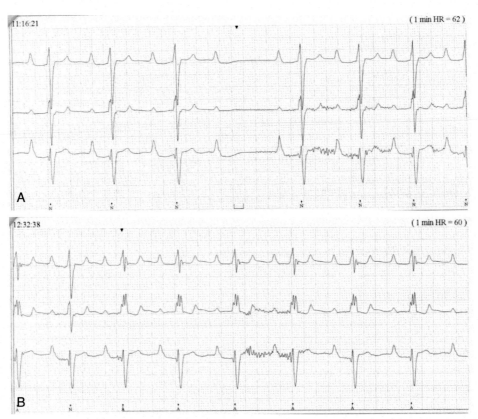

FIG. 15.1 24 h ambulatory monitoring (2007); a marker channel is shown at the bottom of each trace. **(A)** Lengthening of the PR interval followed by a nonconducted P wave. **(B)** An example of aberrant conduction with a change in the morphology of the QRS complex. **(C)** Sinus bradycardia. **(D)** Heart rate histograms over the 24-h period showing some diurnal variation.

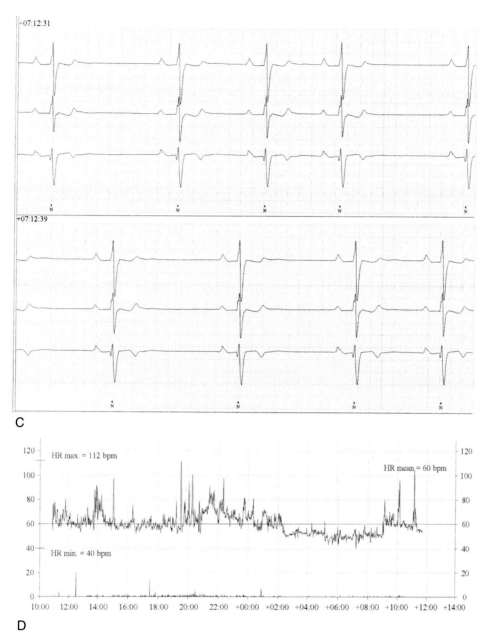

FIG. 15.1 cont'd.

up to 3 s and brief periods of 2:1 AV block during the daytime (traces unavailable). He continued to deny any syncope or presyncope, however, and given the potential challenges of implanting a permanent pacemaker, it was decided to continue to manage him conservatively with periodic repeat Holter monitoring.

In 2015, the patient was seen in the regional center for routine follow-up, during which he gave a history of two syncopal episodes. He was unconcerned about these episodes and had not presented himself to hospital at the time. He had been well in the interim period and his palpitations had become less intrusive. A

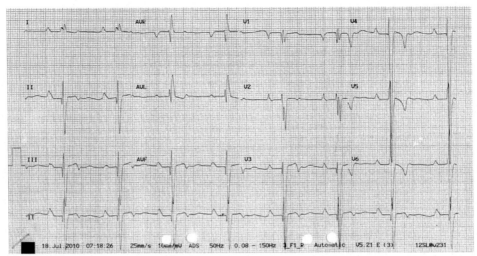

FIG. 15.2 12 lead ECG in 2010 showing sinus rhythm, first-degree atrioventricular block (PR interval 336 ms) and right bundle branch block (QRS duration 146 ms).

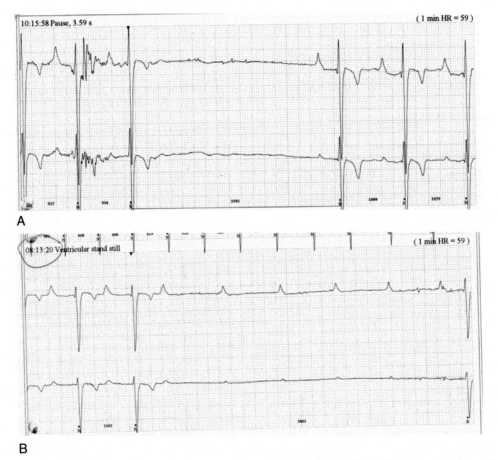

FIG. 15.3 **(A)** Ambulatory monitoring 2011—daytime sinus pause of 3.59 s (the patient was asymptomatic). **(B)** Daytime atrioventricular conduction block with P wave asystole of 5.8 s (the patient was asymptomatic).

detailed history revealed one episode of syncope was nocturnal, postmicturition, and sounded possibly vagal in etiology; however, the second occurred while supine in bed and at rest. The patient was witnessed by his partner to suddenly lose consciousness and this was accompanied by pallor and grunting/agonal breathing for ~30 s. He was unable to recall the event. This occurred while the patient was on bisoprolol 1.25 mg od. His baseline 12 lead ECG from 2015 is shown in Fig. 15.4.

He was seen in the CHD arrhythmia clinic, and in view of the clear history of cardiogenic syncope in the context of previously documented conduction abnormalities, permanent pacemaker (PPM) implantation was empirically discussed with the patient; however, he was reluctant to undergo invasive intervention. Ambulatory monitoring off β-blockers was therefore repeated which showed nocturnal bradycardia as well as brief periods of asymptomatic second-degree block/nonconducted P waves (Fig. 15.5). An MDT meeting was convened and all of the patient's data reviewed. It was concluded that the patient should undergo PPM implantation as soon as possible. At this time ventricular function was felt to be mildly impaired.

After discussion and consideration of the risks involved via different access routes, an endocardial/transvenous approach was considered, but shortly prior to the scheduled procedure, the patient experienced an episode of very transient left-sided weakness and numbness with mouth drooping and slurred speech. He was reviewed by his local neurology service who felt that his symptoms were consistent with a further TIA. The procedure was postponed while the potential thromboembolic risks were reconsidered and he was started on warfarin.

A further MDT meeting was convened and an epicardial (surgical) pacemaker was recommended. The patient was reluctant to undergo general anesthesia and enquired about the possibility of a leadless pacemaker implant. On balance it was felt that the risks of general anesthesia were outweighed by the unknown thromboembolic risk of a leadless device without the capacity for AV synchrony, therefore a dual chamber epicardial system was implanted via a median sternotomy. A single chamber system was considered (which could have been performed via a limited left anterior thoracotomy); however, it was agreed that the benefit of synchronous AV contraction outweighed the increased risk of a sternotomy versus a more limited approach. The surgery was carried out uneventfully, lead parameters were satisfactory, and an abdominal box was placed without complications.

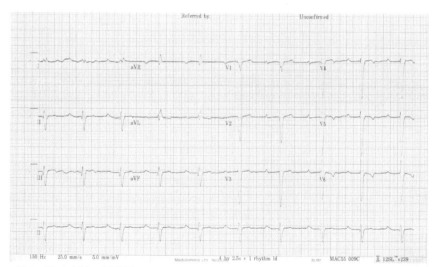

FIG. 15.4 12 lead ECG in 2015 showing pronounced first-degree atrioventricular block.

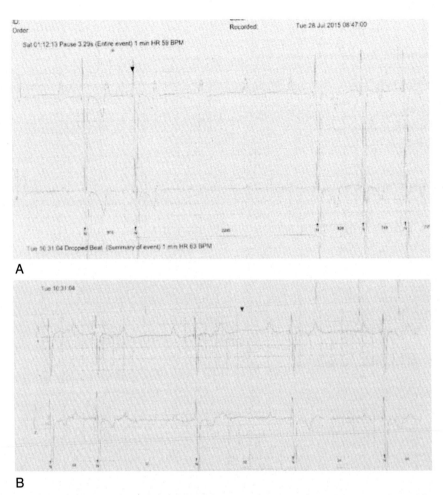

FIG. 15.5 **(A)** Ambulatory monitoring in 2015—PR lengthening followed by three nonconducted P waves, a sinus beat which is conduced, and then two junctional beats. **(B)** Sinus rhythm with 2:1 atrioventricular conduction.

The device was programmed to promote intrinsic conduction. The patient made a satisfactory recovery but developed persistent atrial tachyarrhythmia (both a relatively organized atrial tachycardia and atrial fibrillation, Fig. 15.6) in the early postoperative period. He declined DC cardioversion and was treated with oral amiodarone, which eventually cardioverted him to sinus rhythm which he has maintained since with very occasional episodes of paroxysmal nonsustained atrial arrhythmia detected on pacing check (Fig. 15.7). He remains well and recently became father to a healthy baby boy.

Questions

1. What would have been the optimal choice of antiarrhythmic agent in the early period?
2. Should he have been anticoagulated in 2007?
3. Was there any indication for PPM implantation prior to his syncopal episode?
4. Was the PPM definitely indicated at the time it was implanted?
5. What would be the preferred initial route for PPM implantation? And following the possible TIA?
6. Was there a role for a leadless device in this patient?
7. Should he undergo catheter ablation if he continues to experience atrial arrhythmia?

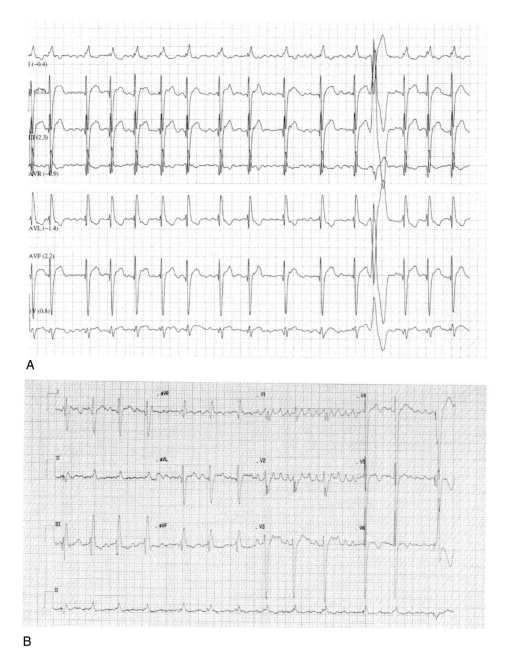

FIG. 15.6 **(A)** Postoperative atrial fibrillation. **(B)** Postoperative organized atrial tachycardia.

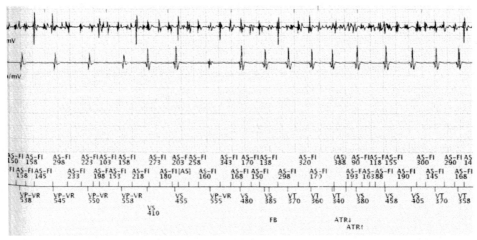

FIG. 15.7 Intracardiac electrograms from pacemaker check showing paroxysmal atrial fibrillation.

Consultant Opinion #1

ANNA KAMP, MD, MPH • NAOMI J. KERTESZ, MD

CASE SUMMARY

This patient has complex single ventricle anatomy and was palliated with a BT shunt in infancy, without further surgical interventions. As a consequence, he has both intracardiac shunting and chronic cyanosis. Bradyarrhythmias and tachyarrhythmias are known to be common in the adult congenital population, and this patient exemplifies the challenges that come with complex single ventricle physiology. Treatment of tachyarrhythmias is often limited by sinus and AV node disease. Treatment of bradycardia with permanent pacing can be delayed due to the subtlety of symptoms and the invasive approach required for epicardial lead placement. Furthermore, these adults have substantial comorbidity burdens, and the benefits of invasive procedures have to be repeatedly weighed against the risks; and symptom threshold for procedures are understandably higher. A multidisciplinary approach to these complex patients, including adult congenital cardiologists, congenital electrophysiologists, congenital surgeons, and congenital cardiac anesthesiologists are often needed to accurately weigh the risks and benefits of invasive procedures.

1. **What would have been the optimal choice of antiarrhythmic agent in the early period?**

In 1987, this patient was treated with digoxin and flecainide for symptoms of palpitations which responded to vagal maneuvers; however, there was also a reported history of atypical atrial flutter. Antiarrhythmic therapy was initiated without clear documentation of arrhythmia. In the current era, it would be uncommon to initiate antiarrhythmic therapy without documentation of arrhythmia, as it would certainly guide therapy. The use of flecainide has been variable in the last several decades, initially starting with the CAST trial in 1991, which demonstrated increased mortality in postmyocardial infarction patients who received flecainide.[1] Additionally, early analysis of flecainide use in young patients with supraventricular tachycardia or ventricular tachycardia demonstrated a similar finding of increased risk of proarrhythmias in patients with ventricular dysfunction or structural heart disease.[2] In more recent years, the use of flecainide in children with cardiomyopathy or structural heart disease was not found to be associated with mortality.[3] However, the use of flecainide or other Class I agents in adults with CHD has not been well studied and the risk of proarrhythmic events remains unclear. Therefore, it is now recommended to avoid Class I agents in adults with CHD.[4] Digoxin would not be considered first line as antiarrhythmic therapy in a single ventricular patient with atrial tachyarrhythmia largely due to lack of effectiveness. Additionally, its use in the setting of AV node disease could be problematic. With the concern for AV node disease in this patient, the combination of flecainide and digoxin would be avoided. The balance between effective treatment of tachyarrhythmias in adults with CHD and exacerbation of their sinus node disease or AV node disease with antiarrhythmic therapy is well demonstrated in this case.

With a history of palpitations which were amenable to vagal maneuvers, documentation of arrhythmia would guide therapy. β blocker therapy would likely be considered as first-line therapy unless there was significant sinus node disease. One could also consider calcium channel blocker use in this situation. However, with only rare symptoms and no known sustained arrhythmias, in addition to sinus node and AV node disease, consideration of no antiarrhythmic therapy would be quite reasonable.

2. **Should he have been anticoagulated in 2007?**

In this patient with cyanotic heart disease and complex single ventricle physiology, anticoagulation would be indicated after a TIA.[5] Evaluation with head CT or MRI to exclude brain abscess should also be considered. As was done in this case, it would be appropriate to evaluate for occult arrhythmias as an etiology for possible intracardiac clot and a cardiovascular accident. Unless there was a contraindication to do so, anticoagulation would be considered. Recent data in adults with single ventricle palliation demonstrated warfarin to be effective in resolving and decreasing thromboembolic complications.[6,7] While this patient has not undergone Fontan palliation, he has complex single ventricle physiology and many would consider treatment strategies for adults with Fontan palliation to be appropriate for this patient as well. Atrial arrhythmias are known to increase risk of thromboembolic events in adults with single ventricle palliation,[8] and, in the current era, stronger consideration for anticoagulation would be given in this patient.[9] Additionally, this patient has long-standing chronic cyanosis and secondary erythrocytosis with likely hypercoagulability; therefore, initiating anticoagulation with suspected atrial arrhythmia would be reasonable.

3. **Was there any indication for PPM implantation prior to his syncopal episode?**

This patient reported symptoms of shortness of breath with exertion and dizziness in 2014. At that time, he had symptoms of dizziness with known sinus node disease, brief 2:1 AV block, and sinus pauses of 3 s. By history, he had a slow decline in his functional status in the setting of good ventricular function, and it is possible that chronotropic incompetence contributed to this, but additional hemodynamic factors (i.e., high filling pressures, limited pulmonary blood flow; hyperviscocity, relative iron anemia) are also possible contributing factors. He does not have a Class I indication for pacing,[10,11] and permanent pacing in this patient with intracardiac shunt would require an epicardial pacing system to avoid potential systemic thromboembolism. Therefore, symptom thresholds are reasonably high in this patient, and pacemaker placement was not clearly indicated.

4. **Was the PPM definitely indicated at the time it was implanted?**

This patient had unexplained syncope in the setting of AV node disease with evidence of high-grade AV block on Holter monitoring off anti-arrhythmic medications. It is reasonable to ascribe his syncope to AV node disease. It is possible that his syncope could have been due to tachyarrhythmia given his symptoms of palpitations. However, with a history of palpitations for nearly 10 years and no history of documented tachyarrhythmia, this would seem less likely. Medical management of tachyarrhythmias would be limited by sinus node and AV node disease and would require permanent pacing for medical treatment. In this setting of unexplained syncope, one must consider the risk of ventricular dysrhythmias and sudden cardiac death. He has no documented ventricular arrhythmias in the past, his ventricular function is well preserved, and he does not have pulmonary hypertension; therefore, ventricular arrhythmias seem less likely.

5. **What would be the preferred initial route for PPM implantation? And following the possible TIA?**

This patient has unrepaired cyanotic heart disease with intracardiac shunt. Epicardial pacemaker is the preferred route with or without history of TIA. A transvenous system would only be considered as a palliative approach in a terminal patient for relief of symptoms. Consideration of permanent pacing must also consider optimal AV synchrony. A single chamber pacemaker in this patient could have been achieved through a less invasive route; however, the long-term benefits of AV synchrony in single ventricle physiology outweigh the less invasive approach that may be achieved with epicardial ventricular pacing only.

6. **Was there a role for a leadless device in this patient?**

In this patient with complex single ventricle anatomy, there is no clear role for a leadless pacemaker. The thromboembolic complication with leadless pacemaker in this patient who has already demonstrated thrombotic events is likely too high to consider it as a reasonable option. Additionally, at this time, leadless pacemakers are limited as a single chamber system. The benefits of AV synchrony in this patient far outweigh the risk of thromboembolic events with leadless pacemaker in this clinical presentation. However, it could be considered as a palliative option for symptom improvement in a terminal patient. A recent single case report of leadless pacing system in a Fontan patient has been reported but no long-term follow-up is known.[12]

7. **Should he undergo catheter ablation if he continues to experience atrial arrhythmia?**

Ablation therapy in adults with CHD is one arm of a multifaceted treatment approach. Certainly if he has sustained atrial tachycardia, consideration of ablation therapy is warranted.[4] For sustained atrial tachyarrhythmias, consideration of attempt at ablation therapy would be preferable to long-term amiodarone use. Current ablative technologies, including advanced electroanatomic mapping, integration of advanced imaging acquisition, multielectrode high-density mapping, and irrigated ablation catheters could potentially contribute to long-term success in this patient.

This patient had sustained postoperative atrial tachyarrhythmias, but no sustained arrhythmias since. If he remains on amiodarone therapy, it would be preferable to eliminate need for amiodarone and one would consider discontinuing amiodarone to assess for atrial tachyarrhythmias. Consideration of ablation for atrial tachycardia is different in comparison to atrial fibrillation as success rate of ablation of paroxysmal atrial fibrillation in this population is unknown. Additionally, careful consideration of the patient's anatomy is warranted in consideration of ablation therapy. Large atrial size is associated with lower success rates for ablation of atrial tachyarrhythmias.

This patient has demonstrated an avoidance of invasive procedures. Therefore, optimizing antiarrhythmic therapy and atrial pacing may be advantageous for minimizing atrial tachyarrhythmias. Adding back β blocker therapy now that he has permanent pacing may be quite effective in controlling the nonsustained atrial tachycardia.

REFERENCES

1. Echt DS, Liebson PR, Mitchell LB, et al. Mortality and morbidity in patients receiving encainide, flecainide, or placebo: the Cardiac Arrhythmia Suppression Trial. *N Engl J Med.* 1991;324(12):781–788.
2. Fish F, Gillette P, Benson D. Proarrhythmia, cardiac arrest and death in young patients receiving encainide and flecainide. *J Am Coll Cardiol.* 1991;18:356–365.
3. Moffett B, Valdes S, Lupo P, et al. Flecainide use in children with cardiomyopathy or structural heart disease. *Pediatr Cardiol.* 2015;36:146–150.
4. Khairy P, Van Hare G, Balaji S, et al. PACES/HRS expert consensus statement on the recognition and management of arrhythmias in adult congenital heart disease. *Heart Rhythm.* 2014;11:e102–e165.
5. Potter B, Leong-Sit P, Fernandes S, et al. Effect of aspirin and warfarin therapy on thromboembolic events in patients with univentricular hearts and Fontan palliation. *Int J Cardiol.* 2013;168:3940–3943.
6. Egbe A, Connolly H, Niaz T, et al. Prevalence and outcome of thrombotic and embolic complications in adults after Fontan operation. *Am Heart J.* 2017;183:10–17.
7. Pujol C, Niesert A, Engelhardt A, et al. Usefulness of direct oral anticoagulants in adult congenital heart disease. *Am J Cardiol.* 2016;117:450–455.
8. Egbe A, Connolly H, McLeod C, et al. Thrombotic and embolic complications associated with atrial arrhythmia after Fontan operation. *J Am Coll Cardiol.* 2016;68:1312–1319.
9. Contractor T, Levin V, Mandapati R. Drug therapy in adult congenital heart disease. *Card Electrophysiol Clin.* 2017;9:295–309.
10. Epstein A, DiMarco J, Ellenbogen K, et al. 2012 ACCF/AHA/HRS focused update incorporated into the ACCF/AHA/HRS 2008 guidelines for device-based therapy of cardiac rhythm abnormalities. *JACC.* 2013;5:e6–e75.
11. Epstein A, DiMarco J, Ellenbogen K, Estes N, Freedman, et al. ACC/AHA/HRS 2008 guidelines for device-based therapy of cardiac rhythm abnormalities. *Heart 1Rhythm.* 2008;5:e1–e62.
12. Ferrero P, Yeong M, D'Elia E, Duncan E, Graham Stuart A. Leadless pacemaker implantation in a patient with complex congenital heart disease and limited vascular access. *Indian Pacing Electrophysiol J.* 2016;16:201–204.

Consultant Opinion #2

BRYAN CANNON, MD

The patient presented in this scenario represents a complex congenital patient with both tachyarrhythmias and bradyarrhythmias as well as AV conduction disease. This is a relatively common scenario in patients with complex CHD. In considering the management of this patient, it is important to balance all factors of the patient's care. Several factors come into play. The first, and likely most important, is that the ventricular function is normal. The normal ventricular function gives some degree of flexibility when treating arrhythmias in AV block. In patients with poor ventricular function, a much more aggressive approach to treat both arrhythmias and AV block is warranted. The second factor that comes into play is that the patient is cyanotic and has right-to-left shunting. In addition to this, he has a history of a TIA. This may put him for a higher risk of clot formation from atrial arrhythmias and atrial fibrillation and markedly limits the ability to place any type of transvenous pacemaker.

1. **What would have been the optimal choice of antiarrhythmic agent in the early period?**

Therapy of arrhythmias in patients with underlying sinus and AV node dysfunction can be challenging. In patients with complex CHD and atrial arrhythmias, it is preferable to have rhythm control rather than just ventricular rate control. However, there does remain a potential role for rate control and preventing symptoms or to prevent the effect on ventricular function from rapid conduction of atrial arrhythmias. There is no single agent that would potentially be the best choice. β blockers and calcium channel blockers can be an effective first line of therapy in these patients. However, with the underlying sinus and AV node dysfunction, these drugs must be used with caution. Class I C drugs have the potential for an increased mortality in patients with ventricular scarring due to myocardial infarction or poor ventricular function. It has also been shown to be an increased risk of sudden death in patients with CHD.[1] Amiodarone is an effective agent at controlling atrial tachycardias and atrial arrhythmias. However, the toxicities of amiodarone limit its use. These toxicities include pulmonary and liver toxicity, corneal microdeposits, photosensitivity, thyroid dysfunction (hypo- or hyperthyroidism), and adverse cardiac effects (e.g., bradycardia, torsades de pointes). Amiodarone-induced thyrotoxicosis is especially common in women with CHD and cyanotic heart disease or univentricular hearts with Fontan palliation. Sotalol is a Class III antiarrhythmic that has shown efficacy in the treatment of atrial arrhythmias in adult patients with structural CHD.[2] Sotalol was initially developed as a β blocker and has a mild degree of β blocking effects in addition to its Class III activity. For this reason, sotalol should be used with caution and patients with sinus node dysfunction or underlying poor ventricular function. In addition, there is a proarrhythmic effect and it can promote the development of QT prolongation and torsades des pointes.

Dofetilide is a Class III antiarrhythmic that selectively inhibits the delayed rectifier potassium current. It is excreted by the kidneys and therefore should be used with caution in patients with renal dysfunction. Initiation of the medication should occur in the hospital and should not be administered if the corrected QT interval is greater than 440 in patients with a normal QRS duration and greater than 500 and patients with an underlying conduction disturbance. There is published experience with the use of dofetilide in patients with CHD with around a 5% incidence of significant side effects on initiation including torsades de pointes.[3] Caution must also be exercised as there is around 1% incidence of heart block with dofetilide.

Because of the potential for adverse effects with any of these medications, initiation as a hospital inpatient with continuous telemetry monitoring is warranted. In this manner, adverse proarrhythmic drug effects can be closely monitored and management decisions can be made based on the patient's response to a specific medication.

2. **Should he have been anticoagulated in 2007?**

Prevention of thromboembolism is of extreme importance in patients with structural CHD, particularly in the presence of atrial arrhythmias. An increased risk for thrombus formation in CHD patient is likely due to poor atrial synchrony from atrial scarring, the presence of dilated atria, associated hypercoagulable states, and both systolic as well as diastolic ventricular dysfunction. Decisions regarding anticoagulation must be made on an individual patient basis, but in general should use the CHA2DS2-VASC score as a guideline.[4] Using this guideline, most patients with CHD and atrial arrhythmias would qualify for anticoagulation. Guidelines for treating adults with CHD who have arrhythmias suggest treatment of intra-atrial reentrant tachycardia (IART) or atrial fibrillation with anticoagulant therapy.[5] This guideline can be reasonably extended to patients with frequent episodes of atrial ectopic tachycardia as well. Although the novel anticoagulants (NOACS) do hold some promise in the treatment of CHD, vitamin K antagonists (warfarin) have a relatively well-established safety and efficacy profile within the complex CHD population and are good choices for anticoagulation in this patient population.

This patient had two independent indications for anticoagulation. The first was his history of a TIA with his underlying cyanotic CHD. The second was his persistent atrial arrhythmias. A cerebrovascular insult can be devastating and have long-term consequences, so aggressive therapy to decrease the risk of a stroke is warranted when there are any significant risk factors.

3. **Was there any indication for PPM implantation prior to his syncopal episode?**

Sinus node dysfunction is a common problem in patients with CHD either due to the intrinsic nature of the CHD or to surgery that may disrupt the sinus node itself or the sinus node artery. In addition, AV nodal disease may also be seen in this patient population, particularly in patients with congenitally corrected transposition or heterotaxy. Guidelines for pacemaker implantation are generally based on the ACC/AHA/HRS 2008 Guidelines for device-based therapy of cardiac rhythm abnormalities.[6] However, these guidelines do not cover all patient situations and some degree of individual patient interpretation is required when applying the guidelines to complex ACHD patients. According to these guidelines, PPM implantation is definitely indicated for advanced second- or third-degree AV block associated with symptomatic bradycardia, ventricular dysfunction, or low cardiac output. PPM implantation is also indicated for sinus node dysfunction with correlation of symptoms during age-inappropriate bradycardia. PPM implantation is reasonable for patients with

CHD and sinus bradycardia (intrinsic or antiarrhythmic induced) for the prevention of recurrent episodes of IART. In addition, a pacemaker is reasonable for sinus bradycardia with complex CHD with a resting heart rate less than 40 bpm or pauses in ventricular rate longer than 3 s and in patients with CHD and impaired hemodynamics due to sinus bradycardia or loss of AV synchrony. In looking at these guidelines, a strong argument can be made for pacemaker placement in this patient. The pauses of 3.59 and 5.8 s (Fig. 15.5A and B) are concerning, especially considering that there is paroxysmal AV block in one tracing (Fig. 15.5B). In addition, there is evidence of infra-Hisian conduction disease with a rate-dependent bundle branch block (Fig. 15.3B). With the atrial arrhythmias, sinus node dysfunction, AV node dysfunction, and paroxysmal AV block with pauses up to 6 s, a very strong case can be made for implantation of a pacemaker even in the presence of only minor symptoms.

4. **Was the PPM definitely indicated at the time it was implanted?**

According to the 2008 ACC/AHA/HRS guidelines, PPM implantation is reasonable for unexplained syncope in the patient with prior congenital heart surgery complicated by transient complete heart block with residual fascicular block after a careful evaluation to exclude other causes of syncope. As a strong case can be made for pacemaker placement before his syncopal episode, this case is even stronger following his symptoms. Despite the major operation to place an epicardial system, PPM placement was definitely indicated at the time it was implanted. However, one has to exercise caution in attributing syncope to AV block as this patient is at risk for ventricular arrhythmias as well. A thorough evaluation is warranted to rule of the need for an implantable cardioverter-defibrillator (ICD) rather than just a pacemaker. This consideration is even stronger in a patient requiring an epicardial device as coil placement may need to be performed epicardially at the time of pacemaker lead implant.[7]

5. **What would be the preferred initial route for PPM implantation? And following the possible TIA?**

Transvenous leads incur a >twofold increased risk of systemic thromboembolism in patients with intracardiac shunts.[8] This is independent of documented right-to-left shunting, the presence of atrial or ventricular leads, ventricular function, and the number of leads. In addition, therapeutic anticoagulation may not be completely effective in preventing a cerebrovascular accident in the presence of transvenous leads. For this reason, the 2008 ACC/AHA guidelines for the management of adults with congenital heart disease state that epicardial pacemaker and device lead placement should be performed in all cyanotic patients with intracardiac shunts who require devices (Class I indication).[9] Although it is tempting to place a transvenous system in patients with complex CHD, the risk of a stroke makes an epicardial route the preferred route. Epicardial placement of a pacemaker or ICD can be challenging in complex adult patients who have had multiple previous surgeries. Careful planning to determine the least invasive approach that has the highest likelihood of obtaining good sensing and stimulation thresholds is important. For patients who have not had a previous left thoracotomy, this approach may provide access to both atrial and ventricular tissue for lead placement. A mini thoracotomy in the more anterior position or limited inferior sternotomy may also afford access for lead placement without performing a full sternotomy.

6. **Was there a role for a leadless device in this patient?**

For the reasons stated in the previous section, transvenous placement of any type of device is contraindicated in this patient. In addition, as leadless devices currently can only provide single chamber pacing, a leadless pacemaker would not be a good option in this patient. With both sinus node dysfunction and AV nodal disease, a dual chamber pacemaker is indicated. In addition, atrial pacing may be helpful in preventing atrial arrhythmias, particularly if the atrial tachycardia is related to tachy-brady syndrome. In adult patients with CHD, synchronous ventricular contraction is important for maintaining long-term ventricular function. Chronic ventricular pacing may have an adverse effect on ventricular function. In addition, with the potential difficulty in extracting leadless pacemakers, careful consideration of long-term consequences of leadless pacemakers should be undertaken prior to placing one of these devices.

7. **Should he undergo catheter ablation if he continues to experience atrial arrhythmia?**

Catheter ablation should be considered as a first line of therapy for adult congenital patients with atrial arrhythmias. Antiarrhythmic medications may be ineffective or have intolerable (or potentially life-threatening) side effects, making ablation an attractive alternative. There are some risks to performing an ablation as well, but the potential to eliminate the source of arrhythmias or make them easier to control may make these risks worthwhile. For patients with IART or atrial flutter, ablation is a very good choice to help control arrhythmias and has a relatively good success rate. However, with atrial tachycardia, the success rate may not be as high. The major limiting factor is having the arrhythmia actually occur in the electrophysiology laboratory in order to map and ablate it. Whereas IART or atrial flutter can frequently be induced by programmed stimulation, atrial ectopic tachycardia must occur spontaneously or be brought out by drugs such as isoproterenol in order to effectively map the source. Despite this fact, ablation should be strongly considered in patients in whom medications are not effective at controlling arrhythmias or in patients who have adverse medication effects or potential side effects. Ablation for atrial fibrillation is much more challenging in patients with CHD. It is technically possible in some patients with structural CHD to perform an atrial fibrillation ablation using the same basic principles as the procedure in adult patients with no structural heart disease, but the success rate is low and a large number of ablation lesions may be required in the ablation. However, in a significant number of patients, atrial fibrillation results from degeneration of another initial arrhythmia (IART or atrial tachycardia) and eliminating the initiating arrhythmia may help reduce the incidence of atrial fibrillation. It is difficult to determine which tachycardia is the predominant issue in this patient. Shows an organized tachycardia that may be amenable to ablation and this may be the initiating tachycardia for the atrial fibrillation. As there are many complicating factors in this patient, ablation in the hands of an experienced adult congenital electrophysiologist is worth an attempt to decrease the arrhythmia burden.

TAKE-HOME POINTS (EDITORS)

1. Brady- and tachyarrhythmias frequently coexist in complex ACHD patients. Management of one can complicate management of the other.
2. All ACHD patients with intracardiac shunts and/or sluggish blood flow (e.g., Fontan operation) should be anticoagulated even if asymptomatic. If, in addition, they have tachyarrhythmias, anticoagulation should be started regardless of symptoms.

3. In ACHD patients with intracardiac shunts, endocardial pacing (including the leadless pacemaker) should be avoided. The default method for pacing should be the epicardial approach.
4. Long-term amiodarone should be considered the last option for drug therapy.

REFERENCES

1. Fish FA, Gillette PC, Benson Jr DW. Proarrhythmia, cardiac arrest and death in young patients receiving encainide and flecainide. The Pediatric Electrophysiology Group. *J Am Coll Cardiol*. 1991;18:356–365.
2. Koyak Z, Kroon B, de Groot JR, et al. Efficacy of antiarrhythmic drugs in adults with congenital heart disease and supraventricular tachycardias. *Am J Cardiol*. 2013;112(9):1461–1467.
3. El-Assaad I, Al-Kindi SG, Abraham J, et al. Use of dofetilide in adult patients with atrial arrhythmias and congenital heart disease: a PACES collaborative study. *Heart Rhythm*. 2016;13(10):2034–2039.
4. Olesen JB, Torp-Pedersen C, Hansen ML, Lip GY. The value of the CHA2DS2-VASc score for refining stroke risk stratification in patients with atrial fibrillation with a CHADS2 score 0-1: a nationwide cohort study. *Thromb Haemost*. 2012;107(6):1172–1179.
5. Khairy P, Van Hare GF, Balaji S, et al. PACES/HRS expert consensus statement on the recognition and management of arrhythmias in adult congenital heart disease: developed in partnership between the Pediatric and Congenital Electrophysiology Society (PACES) and the Heart Rhythm Society (HRS). Endorsed by the governing bodies of PACES, HRS, the American College of Cardiology (ACC), the American Heart Association (AHA), the European Heart Rhythm Association (EHRA), the Canadian Heart Rhythm Society (CHRS), and the International Society for Adult Congenital Heart Disease (ISACHD). *Heart Rhythm*. 2014;11(10):e102–e165.
6. Epstein AE, Dimarco JP, Ellenbogen KA, et al. ACC/AHA/HRS 2008 guidelines for device-based therapy of cardiac rhythm abnormalities. *Heart Rhythm*. 2008;5(6):e1–62.
7. Schneider AE, Burkhart HM, Ackerman MJ, Dearani JA, Wackel P, Cannon BC. Minimally invasive epicardial implantable cardioverter-defibrillator placement for infants and children: an effective alternative to the transvenous approach. *Heart Rhythm*. 2016;13(9):1905–1912.
8. Khairy P, Landzberg MJ, Gatzoulis MA, et al. Transvenous pacing leads and systemic thromboemboli in patients with intracardiac shunts: a multicenter study. *Circulation*. 2006;113(20):2391–2397.
9. Warnes CA, Williams RG, Bashore TM, et al. ACC/AHA 2008 guidelines for the management of adults with congenital heart disease: a report of the American College of Cardiology/American Heart Association Task Force on practice guidelines (writing committee to develop guidelines on the management of adults with congenital heart disease). Developed in collaboration with the American Society of Echocardiography, Heart Rhythm Society, International Society for Adult Congenital Heart Disease, Society for Cardiovascular Angiography and Interventions, and Society of Thoracic Surgeons. *J Am Coll Cardiol*. 2008;52(23):e143–e263.

CHAPTER 16

Repaired Complete Atrioventricular Septal Defect Patient With Late Bradyarrhythmia

Case Presentation by Matthias Greutmann, MD, FESC

CASE SYNOPSIS

We report the case of a patient with repaired atrioventricular septal defect (AVSD) and trisomy 21. He underwent surgical repair at the age of 12 years by dual patch technique. Three years later he had a second repair operation for residual ventricular septal defect and severe regurgitation of both atrioventricular (AV) valves. At the age of 17 years he had an episode of intra-atrial reentrant tachycardia (IART) for which he underwent direct current cardioversion and was commenced on amiodarone.

The patient also had severe autism and was nonverbal. Since the age of 17 years he was living in a special care home, spending every second weekend with his parents. His caregiver and parents felt that his quality of life was fairly good and he seemed happy in his day-to-day life.

At the age of 18 years he had a convulsive syncope, which was attributed to a seizure disorder. No further investigations were undertaken at that time.

At the age of 19 years the patient was transferred to adult care and was subsequently followed at our center. Owing to his autism disorder with the inability to cooperate, physical examination and advanced investigations such as, Holter ECG monitoring and echocardiography were challenging. Echocardiography revealed significant residual left AV valve regurgitation, low-normal left ventricular ejection fraction, and mild pulmonary hypertension. The further course remained stable apart from hyperthyroidism at the age of 21 years, which normalized after cessation of amiodarone. The patient remained active and participated in social activities within the special care home and his family.

At the age of 30 years he had two episodes of "collapse" within 2 months. The nature of these collapses could not be further delineated and subsequent assessment by a neurologist did not clarify the cause of the collapse, although neither cerebral imaging nor electroencephalogram could be obtained due to lack of cooperation. Clinical findings, echocardiography, and electrocardiogram had remained unchanged compared with previous investigations. The electrocardiogram showed sinus rhythm with typical left axis deviation and complete right bundle branch block with normal PR intervals (Fig. 16.1, panel A).

While intermittent high-degree AV block was considered in a differential diagnosis of the "collapse," a decision was made against prophylactic pacemaker implantation at that time without ECG-symptom correlation. Three weeks later the patient was admitted to his local hospital with rapidly worsening exercise tolerance. At this time, he was found to be in complete AV block with slow ventricular escape rhythm at a rate of 25 beats per minute (Fig. 16.1, panel B).

The patient was transferred to our center and a temporary transvenous pacemaker was inserted. Transesophageal echocardiography demonstrated a persistent interatrial shunt with spontaneous right-to-left-shunting on bubble-contrast injection. Given the increased risk of paradoxical embolism with transvenous pacemaker leads in the setting of intracardiac shunts, it was decided to implant an epicardial dual-chamber pacemaker system (Fig. 16.2). The postoperative course was complicated by hemodynamic instability and the need for reintubation but the patient finally made a good recovery after a long hospital stay. In the initial period after pacemaker implantation he continued to have short "spells," manifesting as absences but never again fell or lost consciousness and his exercise capacity recovered to his usual level.

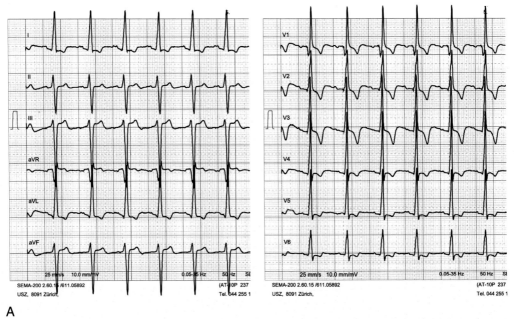

A

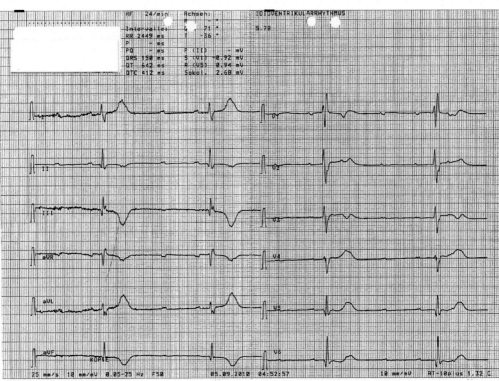

B

FIG. 16.1 *Panel A:* ECG at baseline, showing sinus rhythm at a ventricular rate of 78 beats per minute and normal PQ interval. The ECG shows typical left axis deviation, which is an almost universal finding in patients with atrioventricular septal defects. In addition, there is right bundle branch block with a QRS duration of 148 ms. *Panel B:* Complete heart block with low ventricular escape rhythm at 25 beats per minute.

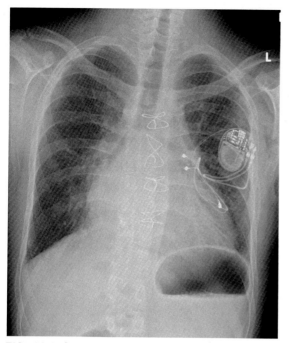

FIG. 16.2 Chest X-ray showing dual chamber epicardial pacemaker.

Given his autism, regular examinations including pacemaker interrogation remained challenging and, at times, impossible. Four years after pacemaker implantation the patient was referred for urgent assessment as he had shown unusual aggressive behavior and seemed to suffer from decreased exercise tolerance. An echocardiographic examination under general anesthesia was performed and revealed severe left AV valve regurgitation and moderately impaired left ventricular ejection fraction. More importantly, however, pacemaker interrogation surprisingly revealed unexpected loss of pacemaker battery voltage, only 5 months after the last pacemaker interrogation (Medtronic EnRhythm MRI). Owing to loss of battery voltage, the pacemaker had been automatically reprogrammed from DDD to VVI mode and hence loss of AV synchrony had occurred.

After extensive discussions with family and caregivers we opted for a stepwise approach with resolution of pacemaker issues first and then, AV valve repair, if needed. The patient underwent pacemaker box change with reprogramming to DDD mode, made a good recovery, and recovered rapidly to his normal exercise tolerance. Given the good quality of life thereafter, valve replacement was postponed and the patient remains under regular follow-up.

Questions

1. What other monitoring options are there for a nonverbal autistic patient with major life-threatening symptoms such as "collapse"?
2. Is there a role for catheter ablation for the tachyarrhythmia and would this have helped "prevent" the bradycardia?
3. What is the role of cardiac resynchronization therapy (CRT) in such a patient?

Consultant Opinion #1

JEFFREY J. KIM, MD • WILSON W. LAM, MD

ANSWERS

1. The 2017 ISHNE-HRS expert consensus statement on ambulatory ECG and external cardiac monitoring/telemetry is a useful resource when deliberating the various modalities for arrhythmia detection in unexplained syncope.[1] There are several options, with varying advantages and disadvantages, and the choice should be tailored to the individual case.

A 24- to 48-h Holter monitor is the traditional ambulatory electrocardiogram usually giving three leads of information using five electrodes. The yield in detecting arrhythmias for syncope is generally low (<10%–20%), but higher risk features such as prior heart disease, low ejection fraction, and older age seem to increase diagnostic yield with some studies suggesting male gender.[2,3] However, the device is bulky and limits activities such as showering, bathing, and swimming, as well as proximity to large magnets or high-voltage areas.[4] Additionally, in certain populations, such as in the described case, compliance related to "wearing" the device may be suboptimal. Newer models can extend to 30 days, allowing for longer periods of monitoring.[1]

Intermittent external loop recorders remain a staple for arrhythmia detection, and later models have automatic detection (rather than patient-triggered) for tachyarrhythmia and bradyarrhythmias, which would be necessary in patients with developmental delay or in those who are noncommunicative. These may be smaller than a standard Holter but are still bulkier than patch technology and should be worn continuously.[1] Patch technology was devised to alleviate the size of a recording device to improve compliance and allow for water exposure. From iRhythm Technologies, the ZIO Patch is a single-use, water-resistant 14-day continuous rhythm monitor and has data in adult and pediatric patients with very good patient compliance and excellent quality of recordings.[5,6] Mobile Cardiac Telemetry combines the benefits of Holter monitoring and loop recording and the Medtronic SEEQ remains a popular option, although temperature >80°F might be associated with discomfort and degraded performance.[7] In certain populations, where existing external recorders are considered too cumbersome, the smaller patches may be a reasonable alternative.

Finally, the implantable loop recorder is completely implanted and can be utilized for up to 3 years. It thus has the advantage of documenting events that are infrequent and difficult to capture, and once inserted, has minimal issues with patient compliance. Although more invasive, its longer duration of detection has been utilized to increase the diagnostic yield in atrial fibrillation.[8] The insertable/injectable loop recorder (Medtronic LINQ) might offer a minimally invasive approach requiring less sedation and shorter hospital times, particularly when concerned about incision healing.[9] High success with low complications has been demonstrated for advanced practice providers using this device.[10]

In this patient, we would consider starting with patch monitoring therapy (SEEQ or ZIO patch), and if index of suspicion remains high but no clear-cut indication for permanent pacing is detected, a LINQ injectable loop recorder would be considered. Given the patient's noncommunicative state and issues with compliance, as well as the relative infrequency of events, an implantable, durable monitor with automatic detection may be considered ideal.

2. Catheter ablation has become a mainstay of treatment for arrhythmias of all types over the past several years. The ultimate goal of these procedures is elimination of the mechanism for arrhythmias, and this holds true for IART. Functionally, however, the primary role for catheter ablation in IART is for treating patient symptoms, controlling the arrhythmia with a less intense antiarrhythmic regimen, or desire for a drug-free lifestyle. For all adult congenital heart disease (ACHD) patients, procedural success for these ablations is estimated to be ~75% with a 5-year recurrence rate between 30% and 50% (higher based on the complexity of the congenital heart disease).[11,12]

The tachy-brady syndrome is traditionally related to sinus node dysfunction, rather than progressive AV node dysfunction. In its most common descriptions, it is thought to result from progressive atrial fibrosis and apoptosis caused by atrial fibrillation. AV node dysfunction in congenital heart disease is more likely related to postoperative changes or intrinsic disease. Although rare, late development of postoperative AV block has been noted.[14] In recent years, genetic contributions to progressive AV block in congenital heart disease have been recognized, and there are reported murine models in congenital heart disease that exhibit progressive AV node dysfunction.[15,16] If the pathology is genetically predisposed or related to intrinsic disease or postoperative changes, it is unlikely that catheter ablation would alter the course toward advanced AV block requiring permanent pacing.

In the described patient, the potential role of catheter ablation of the tachyarrhythmia should be considered and discussed. As is typically the case, the risks of an invasive procedure should be weighed against the patient's quality of life, frequency of symptoms, and indication for anticoagulation. In hopes of staying off amiodarone, an antiarrhythmic with fewer side effects (e.g., sotalol, dronedarone, or dofetilide) might be offered. If tachycardia breaks through on antiarrhythmic therapy, or if the patient's family prefers an attempt at more definitive therapy, catheter ablation should be offered. It is likely that the procedural success rate would be relatively high considering the biventricular physiology, although the potential for recurrence would have to be addressed. Given the high association of Trisomy 21 with obstructive sleep apnea,[17] and the decreased success of catheter ablation for atrial arrhythmia in patients with untreated sleep apnea,[18,19] polysomnography might be considered as well. In any case, extensive discussions with the family and caregivers should play a large role in the decision.

3. In this case, the patient would meet the ACC/AHA/HRS class I indication for permanent pacing consideration due to symptomatic bradycardia and complete heart block.[20] The 2012 ACCF/AHA/HRS focused update on the guidelines highlights the role CRT might play in specific patient populations. In adults, when the left ventricular ejection fraction is <35% with NYHA II, III, or ambulatory IV symptoms and a left bundle branch block pattern with QRS duration >150 ms, there is significant likelihood of response with reduced hospitalizations and mortality.[21,22] In children, given the heterogeneity of disease, the results can be more varied.[23] With chronic epicardial ventricular pacing, a QRS duration wider than 150 ms would likely be expected as would an element of electromechanical dyssynchrony. Prophylactic multisite epicardial pacing has not, however, been the norm and there are no data to yet suggest a change in paradigm. Subsequent reoperation to place another lead would also be an invasive strategy with potential risk for morbidity given his prior difficulty with extubation and perioperative complications.

In this patient, the etiology of depressed left ventricular systolic function is likely multifactorial from volume load of mitral regurgitation, dyssynchrony of epicardial pacing, and underlying nonischemic cardiomyopathy exacerbated by prior interventions or possibly associated with sleep apnea. If he is already optimized on medical therapy, the most aggressive option would be to redo the left AV valve repair or replacement with addition of a second epicardial lead for cardiac resynchronization. A less invasive approach that does not involve repairing the valve and could be considered would be catheter-based closure of intracardiac shunts and placement of a transvenous biventricular pacing system. Cardiac resynchronization has been shown to benefit dilated cardiomyopathy with functional mitral regurgitation at high risk for surgical operation with roughly half improving their mitral regurgitation (grade improvement > or =1) and better survival in improvers than nonimprovers.[24] If the coronary sinus is not accessible for biventricular pacing, His bundle pacing has also been shown to be equivalent in outcomes with narrowing of the QRS duration.[25] If intracardiac shunts are not addressed, a transvenous system would pose a 1%–2%/year risk of stroke and an upgrade of the epicardial system will be preferred.[26,27]

Again, with regard to CRT, the risks, benefits, and alternatives of an invasive procedure should be weighed against the patient's desires and quality of life. The inability to reliably predict responders in the setting of congenital heart disease does have a tendency to make these discussions more difficult, although pacing-induced dyssynchrony is a subgroup that appears to be more likely to benefit.[23] Thus, it should, at minimum, be brought up in discussions. If the intracardiac shunts can be easily closed, cardiac resynchronization may be useful for restoring ejection fraction and reducing the volume load of mitral regurgitation.

REFERENCES

1. Steinberg JS, Varma N, Cygankiewicz I, et al. ISHNE-HRS expert consensus statement on ambulatory ECG and external cardiac monitoring/telemetry. *Heart Rhythm.* 2017;14(7):e55–e96.
2. Kühne M, Schaer B, Moulay N, Sticherling C, Osswald S. Holter monitoring for syncope: diagnostic yield in different patient groups and impact on device implantation. *QJM.* 2007;100(12):771–777.
3. Kühne M, Schaer B, Sticherling C, Osswald S. Holter monitoring in syncope: diagnostic yield in octogenarians. *J Am Geriatr Soc.* 2011;59(7):1293–1298.
4. http://www.heart.org/HEARTORG/Conditions/HeartAttack/DiagnosingaHeartAttack/Holter-Monitor_UCM_446437_Article.jsp#.WXYpJBRqlrU.
5. Tung CE, Su D, Turakhia MP, Lansberg MG. Diagnostic yield of extended cardiac patch monitoring in patients with stroke or TIA. *Front Neurol.* 2015;5:266.
6. Bolourchi M, Batra AS. Diagnostic yield of patch ambulatory electrocardiogram monitoring in children (from a national registry). *Am J Cardiol.* 2015;115(5):630–634.
7. Engel JM, Chakravarthy BL, Rothwell D, Chavan A. SEEQ™ MCT wearable sensor performance correlated to skin irritation and temperature. *Conf Proc IEEE Eng Med Biol Soc.* 2015;2015:2030–2033.
8. Mittal S, Rogers J, Sarkar S, et al. Real-world performance of an enhanced atrial fibrillation detection algorithm in an insertable cardiac monitor. *Heart Rhythm.* 2016;13(8):1624–1630.
9. Nguyen HH, Law IH, Rudokas MW, et al. Reveal LINQ versus reveal XT implantable loop recorders: intra- and post-procedural comparison. *J Pediatr.* 2017;187:290–294.
10. Kipp R, Young N, Barnett A, et al. Injectable loop recorder implantation in an ambulatory setting by advanced practice providers: analysis of outcomes. *Pacing Clin Electrophysiol.* 2017;40:982–985.

11. Khairy P, Van Hare GF, Balaji S, et al. PACES/HRS expert consensus statement on the recognition and management of arrhythmias in adult congenital heart disease: developed in partnership between the Pediatric and Congenital Electrophysiology Society (PACES) and the Heart Rhythm Society (HRS). *Heart Rhythm.* 2014; 11(10):e102–e165.

12. Philip Saul J, Kanter RJ, Writing Committee, et al. PACES/HRS expert consensus statement on the use of catheter ablation in children and patients with congenital heart disease: developed in partnership with the Pediatric and Congenital Electrophysiology Society (PACES) and the Heart Rhythm Society (HRS). *Heart Rhythm.* 2016;13(6): e251–e289.

13. Csepe TA, Kalyanasundaram A, Hansen BJ, Zhao J, Fedorov VV. Fibrosis: a structural modulator of sinoatrial node physiology and dysfunction. *Front Physiol.* 2015;6:37.

14. Lin A, Mahle WT, Frias PA, Fischbach PS, Kogon BE, Kirshbom PM. Early and delayed atrioventricular block after routine surgery for congenital heart disease. *J Thorac Cardiovasc Surg.* 2010;140(1):158–160.

15. Murray LE, Smith AH, Flack EC, Crum K, Owen J, Kannankeril PJ. Genotypic and phenotypic predictors of complete heart block and recovery of conduction after surgical repair of congenital heart disease. *Heart Rhythm.* 2017;14(3):402–408.

16. Chowdhury R, Ashraf H, Melanson M, et al. Mouse model of human congenital heart disease: progressive atrioventricular block induced by a heterozygous Nkx2-5 homeodomain missense mutation. *Circ Arrhythm Electrophysiol.* 2015;8(5):1255–1264.

17. Churchill SS, Kieckhefer GM, Landis CA, Ward TM. Sleep measurement and monitoring in children with Down syndrome: a review of the literature, 1960–2010. *Sleep Med Rev.* 2012;16(5):477–488.

18. Fein AS, Shvilkin A, Shah D, et al. Treatment of obstructive sleep apnea reduces the risk of atrial fibrillation recurrence after catheter ablation. *J Am Coll Cardiol.* 2013;62(4): 300–305.

19. Bazan V, Grau N, Valles E, et al. Obstructive sleep apnea in patients with typical atrial flutter: prevalence and impact on arrhythmia control outcome. *Chest.* 2013;143(5): 1277–1283.

20. Epstein AE, Dimarco JP, Ellenbogen KA, et al. ACC/AHA/HRS 2008 guidelines for device-based therapy of cardiac rhythm abnormalities: executive summary. *Heart Rhythm.* 2008;5(6):934–955.

21. Bristow MR, Saxon LA, Boehmer J, et al. Cardiac-resynchronization therapy with or without an implantable defibrillator in advanced chronic heart failure. *N Engl J Med.* 2004;350(21):2140–2150.

22. Cleland JG, Daubert JC, Erdmann E, et al. The effect of cardiac resynchronization on morbidity and mortality in heart failure. *N Engl J Med.* 2005;352(15):1539–1549.

23. Van der Hulst AE, Delgado V, Blom NA, et al. Cardiac resynchronization therapy in paediatric and congenital heart disease patients. *Eur Heart J.* 2011;32(18):2236–2246.

24. van Bommel RJ, Marsan NA, Delgado V, et al. Cardiac resynchronization therapy as a therapeutic option in patients with moderate-severe functional mitral regurgitation and high operative risk. *Circulation.* 2011;124(8):912–919.

25. Lustgarten DL, Crespo EM, Arkhipova-Jenkins I, et al. His-bundle pacing versus biventricular pacing in cardiac resynchronization therapy patients: a crossover design comparison. *Heart Rhythm.* 2015;12(7):1548–1557.

26. Khairy P, Landzberg MJ, Gatzoulis MA, et al. Transvenous pacing leads and systemic thromboemboli in patients with intracardiac shunts: a multicenter study. *Circulation.* 2006;113(20):2391–2397 [cited in original references].

27. DeSimone CV, Friedman PA, Noheria A, et al. Stroke or transient ischemic attack in patients with transvenous pacemaker or defibrillator and echocardiographically detected patent foramen ovale. *Circulation.* 2013; 128(13):1433–1441.

Consultant Opinion #2

PETER P. KARPAWICH, MsC, MD, FAAP, FACC, FAHA, FHRS

QUESTIONS

1. **What other monitoring options are there for a nonverbal autistic patient with major life-threatening symptoms such as "collapse"?**

Answer: Evaluation of syncope and/or collapse in any patient can be difficult. Typically, patient history just prior to the event often provides significant information to correctly define any particular etiology.

However, this obviously will be limited in a patient unable/unwilling to provide necessary facts pertaining to the event. In such instances, observations of any accompanying individuals can add useful information. Although autonomic tone issues are frequently causative in most individuals, among repaired congenital heart patients, transient brady- or tachyarrhythmias must always be included in the differential. These can include sudden and transient AV block, sometimes even years after surgical repair (Am Heart Journal 1987;114:654–656) as well ventricular arrhythmias. Currently, there are several ways to daily monitor heart rhythms among ambulatory patients. Although the traditional Holter monitors are useful, they are somewhat limited in their duration, typically for 24–48 h only. In that regard, they are not that useful for use among patients with infrequent arrhythmia episodes and are more effective to count ectopic complexes (e.g., premature ventricular contractions [PVC] burden). Ambulatory monitors have been available for decades and provide daily information over a longer period of time, often 1–2 months. Of these, both "loop"" and "nonloop" technologies are available. In the former, an external wearable device provides continuous heart rate information, comparable to the older Holter technology. This does require patient cooperation to wear the device. The "nonloop" devices are useful for less cooperative patients and are more of a handheld monitor in which the device is placed on the patient during an event. That requires the patient to communicate or an observer to identify when an event is occurring. Both devices use either telephone or satellite connections to transmit signals. In instances of a nonverbal and possibly noncooperative patient, small implantable monitoring devices are available for use (Am Heart J 2002;143:366–72). These require a minimally invasive surgical procedure with the device inserted subcutaneously, typically on the chest. These devices transmit heart rhythm information comparable to current pacemakers.

2. **Is there a role for catheter ablation for the tachyarrhythmia and would this have helped "prevent" the bradycardia?**

   Answer: Although surgical intervention of congenital heart defects can repair the problem, surgical incisions can be the nidus for later arrhythmias (Circ 2002;105(19):2318–2323). As such, electrophysiology studies with catheter ablation can be useful to localize and potentially modify or eradicate the abnormal rhythm. However, in instances of significant AV valve insufficiency causing altered hemodynamics, increased pressures, and resultant remodeling and thickening of cardiac musculature, correction of any abnormal hemodynamics should be performed first with ablation attempts reserved until normalization of hemodynamics. Ablation also, although effective for some arrhythmias, is never 100% guaranteed curative and can be associated with potential damage to the AV conduction system, depending on where ablation lesions are placed. Effective ablation of an atrial muscle reentrant arrhythmia would not be expected to prevent late-onset AV block caused by fibrotic changes in the proximal septal area as a result of AVSD repair.

3. **What is the role of cardiac resynchronization therapy in such a patient?**

   Answer: CRT can be an effective clinical intervention among some patients with repaired congenital heart disease and heart failure (J Am Coll Cardiol-EP 2017; 8:830–841). However, although among selected patients, CRT can improve quality of life with improvement in heart failure symptoms, it is not a panacea for cure as the underlying cardiac disease often progresses. In that regard, especially among repaired congenital heart disease patients, it can be viewed as a "bridge-to-transplant." Compared to standard dual chamber pacing, CRT requires two ventricular leads, one inserted in the venous (usually "right") ventricle and the other in the coronary sinus. Among patients in whom transvenous pacing is not recommended or feasible, two epicardial ventricular leads are required, usually implanted on opposite ventricular sides. Certain repaired congenital heart defects may require a "hybrid" combination of both transvenous and epicardial ventricular leads. However, efficacy of CRT to improve heart failure is dependent on the etiology of the myocardial dysfunction. In cases of heart failure caused by overcirculation, such as associated with AV valve insufficiency or septal defects, correction of the hemodynamic problem is required before consideration of CRT. In this patient, implant of the second ventricular lead would require an additional thoracotomy with associated potential morbidities. The particular pacemaker used (EnRhythm model) is known to have early battery depletion. As generator replacement with restoration of AV synchrony was associated with clinical improvement, CRT pacing would not be recommended at this time. If the patient does undergo eventual operative valve repair to improve the insufficiency, consideration for placement of a second ventricular lead can be made at that time.

TAKE-HOME POINTS (EDITORS)

1. Periodic (?annual) rhythm monitoring with Holter or other monitors should be considered part of the management regimen in patients with complex ACHD.
2. In patients with intellectual or psychiatric issues which confound management, placement of an implantable loop recorder can give long-term information about rhythm derangements.
3. Tachyarrhythmia therapy does not prevent the development of late bradyarrhythmias. Indeed, tachyarrhythmia therapy with medications can exacerbate bradyarrhythmia issues.
4. There is no role for "prophylactic" CRT in patients with biventricular hearts without systemic ventricular dysfunction. However, if such a patient undergoes placement of a ventricular or dual chamber pacemaker and subsequently develops ventricular dysfunction, dyssynchrony from pacing should be considered the likely cause of the ventricular dysfunction and upgrade to CRT device should be instituted.

REFERENCES

1. Ih S, Fukuda K, Okada R, Saitoh S. Histopathological correlation between the QRS axis and disposition of the atrioventricular conduction system in common atrioventricular orifice and in its related anomalies. *Jpn Circ J*. 1983; 47(12):1368–1376.
2. Blom NA, Ottenkamp J, Deruiter MC, Wenink AC, Gittenberger-de Groot AC. Development of the cardiac conduction system in atrioventricular septal defect in human trisomy 21. *Pediatr Res*. 2005;58(3):516–520.
3. St Louis JD, Jodhka U, Jacobs JP, et al. Contemporary outcomes of complete atrioventricular septal defect repair: analysis of the Society of thoracic surgeons congenital heart surgery database. *J Thorac Cardiovasc Surg*. 2014;148(6): 2526–2531.
4. Khairy P, Landzberg MJ, Gatzoulis MA, et al. Transvenous pacing leads and systemic thromboemboli in patients with intracardiac shunts: a multicenter study. *Circulation*. 2006;113(20):2391–2397.

CHAPTER 17

Postventricular Septal Defect Repair With Bradyarrhythmias and Sudden Death

Submitted by Berardo Sarubbi, MD, PhD

CASE SYNOPSIS

A.V., a 16-year-old male, was admitted to our cardiac tertiary center because of recurrent episodes of palpitations and recent episodes of "dizziness."

At the age of 1 year, he underwent a surgical repair of a perimembranous ventricular septal defect with a Gore-Tex patch, which was complicated by transient (4 days) complete heart block. His preoperative ECG was completely normal, without conduction disturbances.

Two years later, sporadic asymptomatic episodes of type 1 and type 2 second-degree atrioventricular (AV) blocks were diagnosed (Figs. 17.1 and 17.2).

At the age of 5 years, he was referred to our department for complete clinical and instrumental evaluation. A recent standard ECG showed asymptomatic episodes of 2:1 second-degree AV block associated with first-degree AV block (long PR interval 260 ms) and bifascicular block: complete right bundle branch block (QRS duration 160 ms) and left anterior hemi-block (frontal QRS axis—45 degrees) (Fig. 17.3).

Physical examination revealed an asymptomatic young boy of average build who was in no apparent distress and had stable vital signs. Cardiac examination was not significant.

His echocardiogram showed no residual shunt, with normal left ventricular dimensions and function.

ECG Holter confirmed the presence of episodes of type 1 and type 2 second-degree AV blocks with a mean heart rate of 54 b/min (range 40 b/min to 82 b/min) and no pauses >2 s or significant ST/T abnormalities.

A treadmill stress test was stopped at the beginning of the second stage of the Bruce protocol owing to the lack of compliance by the patient.

An electrophysiological study was performed and showed normal sinus node function; normal supra-His conduction time (AH interval 76 ms); a considerable infra-His conduction delay (HV interval 170 ms), essentially located in the main His bundle fascicle, given that its potential preceded the right bundle one by a 150-ms interval and the right bundle deflection was anterogradely activated (20 ms) (Fig. 17.4).

The validation of the His deflection was obtained both through atrial pacing and His bundle pacing. Spontaneous phases of infra-His type 1 second-degree AV block were found (Fig. 17.5).

A prophylactic pacemaker was prescribed. Due to the absence of any symptoms, the parents refused the pacemaker implant and opted instead for strict follow-up.

Aged 14 years, the patient experienced frequent episodes of presyncope, without loss of consciousness. No pauses were documented on Holter monitoring.

Aged 15 years, he started to have recurrent episodes of palpitation and recurrent episodes of "dizziness."

Aged 16 years, during hospitalization, telemetric electrocardiography monitoring showed repeated polymorphic ventricular tachycardia (VT) runs (Fig. 17.6).

Questions

1. Investigations in the patient with AV conduction disturbance
2. Time and indications for pacemaker implant in congenital heart disease
3. Indications for loop-recorded implantation and electrophysiological study
4. Use of antiarrhythmic drugs in patients with AV conduction disturbance

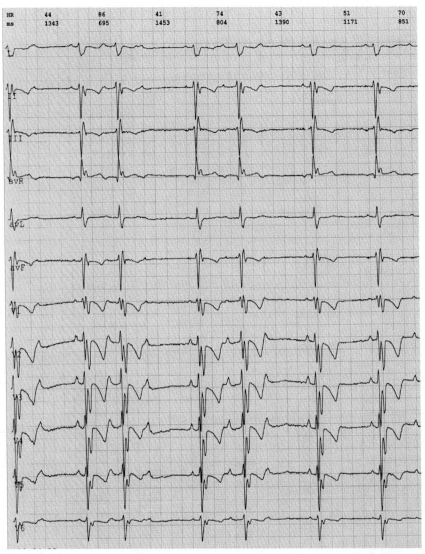

FIG. 17.1 Twelve-lead ECG: Wenckebach type 1 second-degree atrioventricular block. Note progressive prolongation of the PR interval in cycles preceding a dropped beat.

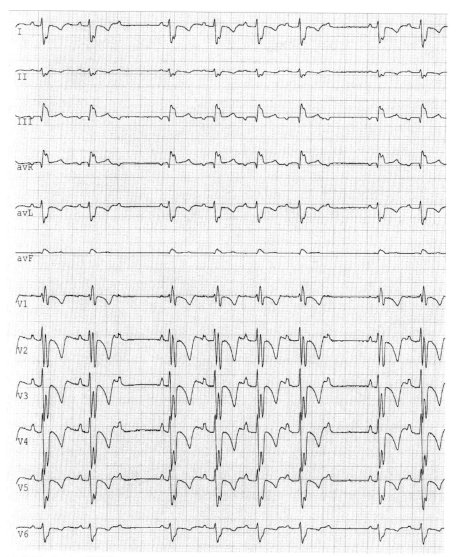

FIG. 17.2 Twelve-lead ECG: type 2 second-degree atrioventricular block. Note intermittent failure of atrial depolarizations to reach the ventricle.

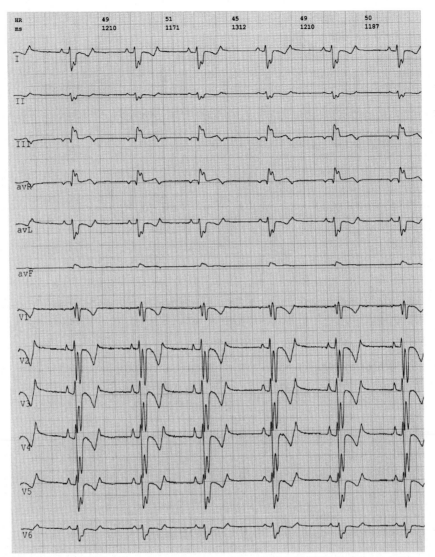

FIG. 17.3 Twelve-lead ECG: type 2 second-degree atrioventricular (AV) block with a 2:1 AV conduction associated with first-degree AV block (long PR interval 260 ms) and bifascicular block: complete right bundle branch block (QRS duration 160 ms) and left anterior hemiblock (frontal QRS axis—45 degrees).

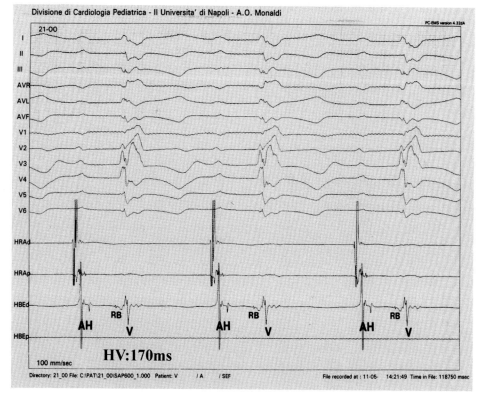

FIG. 17.4 Electrophysiological study: infra-His conduction delay (HV interval 170 ms). A, atrial electrogram; H, His bundle electrogram; RB, right bundle electrogram; V, ventricular electrogram.

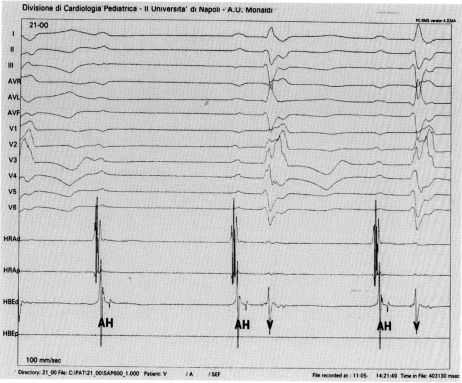

FIG. 17.5 Electrophysiological study: spontaneous episodes of infra-His type 1 second-degree atrioventricular block. A, atrial electrogram; H, His bundle electrogram; V, ventricular electrogram.

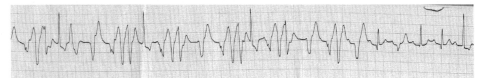

FIG. 17.6 ECG trace during telemetry monitoring: polymorphic ventricular tachycardia runs.

Consultant Opinion #1

AKASH R. PATEL, MD • RONN E. TANEL, MD

This patient illustrates the challenges with regard to the evaluation and management of acquired AV conduction disease after congenital heart surgery. Although the patient's heart block occurred after closure of a perimembranous ventricular septal defect, the discussion points below can be more generally applied to acquired postoperative AV conduction disease. In addition, rarely, tachyarrhythmias may arise in patients with postoperative AV block that occurs as a result of corrective congenital heart surgery (i.e., new scar), underlying anatomy, development of noncardiac diseases that may affect the AV conduction system, and bradyarrhythmias.

Currently, the overall incidence of postoperative heart block is between 1% and 3% for all congenital heart surgery.[1,2] The heart defects most commonly associated with the occurrence of acquired AV conduction disease include surgical repair of certain types of ventricular septal defects, aortic or AV valve surgery, septal myomectomy, and congenital defects with abnormal or displaced AV conduction tissues (i.e., congenitally corrected transposition of the great arteries, AV canal defects, and atrial isomerism).[1,2] This patient demonstrated no additional anatomic risk factors for early or late development of AV conduction disease based on anatomic considerations besides surgical repair of the perimembranous ventricular septal defect. In addition, the majority of postoperative AV block is transient with 43%–95% recovering in the first 7–10 days.[1,3–5] This patient initially had resolution of transient complete heart block within 4 days in the absence of residual conduction disease or symptoms (i.e., unexplained syncope), thus not necessitating the need for placement of pacemaker.

Over time, this patient demonstrated progressive conduction disease with the development of second-degree AV block and bifascicular block that would warrant pacing. This finding is not surprising as a small portion of patients (9%–16%), who develop transient postoperative heart block that resolves will go on to develop late-onset heart block.[3,5] AV node recovery can be seen late beyond 14 days which has been reported in up to 10%–32% of patients.[4,6–8] However, these patients whose early postoperative complete heart block lasts beyond 7 days are at highest risk of late-onset AV block.[5] The presence of early recovery still warrants careful follow-up evaluation including clinical and electrocardiographic monitoring.

The identification of significant and progressive AV conduction disease based on clinical electrocardiography over the course of this patient's postoperative history provided data to support the initiation of pacemaker therapy. In addition, the use of invasive testing was used to confirm clinical electrocardiographic concerns of pathologic AV conduction disease. The presence of untreated permanent postoperative complete heart block places patients at significant risk of symptoms and mortality (28%–100%).[3]

Finally, the presence of ventricular arrhythmias in the setting of complete heart block is a rare but known occurrence.[4,9] These life-threatening proarrhythmic events can be a result of several factors including consequences of surgery—ventricular scar or anatomic barriers due to surgical repair techniques—leading to reentrant VT, premature ventricular ectopy-induced ventricular arrhythmias, prolonged QT-dependent torsade de pointes, and pause-dependent ventricular arrhythmias. The lack of pacing makes management of proarrhythmia in this patient challenging and more importantly may be the primary modality for treatment.

Acquired AV conduction disease after congenital heart surgery resolves in the majority. However, this case illustrates the nontrivial aspect that even temporary AV nodal injury can have long-term implications including ongoing conduction and arrhythmia issues. This raises several important questions regarding optimal monitoring and evaluation, timing and indications for intervention, and appropriate treatment of unexpected arrhythmias.

1. **Investigations in the patient with atrioventricular conduction disturbance**

Clinical electrocardiography is the mainstay of investigating postoperative AV conduction disease. The resting electrocardiogram provides the initial evaluation of conduction disease. The preoperative ECG is important to determine underlying conduction disease that can be present including congenital complete heart block that should not be attributed to surgery and carries different implications. In this case, there was a normal preoperative electrocardiogram. The additional time points for monitoring include immediately postoperative to determine early-onset AV conduction disease, continuous telemetry monitoring after surgery, and during follow-up evaluations as AV conduction disease can be paroxysmal, progressive, or variable in recovery or development. Additionally, follow-up ECGs should be used during evaluation of symptoms such as unexplained syncope and during routine follow-up to identify significant asymptomatic conduction disease as was evident here. In particular, chronic bifascicular block carries a small risk of progressing to advanced second-degree AV or complete heart block.[10]

Ambulatory electrocardiographic monitoring provides additional information that resting electrocardiograms cannot, as AV conduction disease can be paroxysmal and asymptomatic. The choices of ambulatory monitoring technique vary based on modality of recording—event, continuous or autotriggered—and duration from <1 min for event monitors to >1 year for implantable loop recorders (ILRs). The choice of monitoring is dependent on symptoms and/or surveillance evaluation.[11] The monitor used here was a Holter monitor, which can be used for surveillance of pathologic AV block and should be considered as part of routine follow-up with postoperative AV block or chronic bifascicular block. The presence of first- and second-degree AV blocks should be evaluated to determine whether this is physiologic and associated with sleep or increased vagal tone or if it occurs during awake hours and/or faster heart rates which would raise

concern for underlying AV conduction disease. In addition, in younger children who are unable to perform exercise testing, ambulatory electrocardiographic monitoring may be used to demonstrate rate-related AV conduction disease that may result in impaired AV synchrony and chronotropic incompetence.

2. **Indications for loop-recorded implantation and electrophysiological study**

The particular role of an ILR in these patients is unclear. This patient already demonstrated significant AV conduction disease with noninvasive monitoring making the use of the ILR unnecessary. However, in patients with unexplained syncope with prior history of AV block and/or residual conduction disease (i.e., bifascicular block) the use of an ILR may be considered if other forms of ambulatory monitoring are unrevealing. In addition, the later development of palpitations and presyncope may have been identified earlier as due to polymorphic VT by using an ILR.

Exercise stress testing can be important for the evaluation of rate-related AV conduction disease. This should be considered in patients with symptoms or who are unable to achieve fast physiologic rates on Holter monitoring. The patient here was unable to comply with the exercise stress test.

The role of invasive evaluation of AV conduction disturbances with an electrophysiology study is limited in this case, as the clinical electrocardiographic findings have already demonstrated significant AV conduction abnormalities. However, electrophysiology study could be considered to assess level of conduction disease (intranodal vs. infra-Hisian) in situations that are unclear, such as 2:1 AV block or to exclude pseudo AV block due to premature, concealed junctional depolarizations suspected to cause a second- or third-degree AV block pattern.[12] This patient demonstrated significant infra-Hisian disease (HV > 100 ms) which, if untreated, has a poor prognosis, as patients with this finding progress to higher degrees of AV block and become symptomatic with syncope.[13]

3. **Time and indications for pacemaker implant in congenital heart disease**

The decision and timing for pacemaker implantation in congenital heart disease for postoperative AV conduction disease has been well established.[4] For postoperative advanced second- or third-degree AV block that is not expected to resolve or that persists at least 7 days after cardiac surgery, a permanent pacemaker is a Class I indication. This patient had recovery of AV node function at 4 days, thus deferring the need for pacemaker implantation unless there was transient postoperative third-degree AV block that reverted back to sinus rhythm with residual bifascicular block (Class IIB indication). However, the evidence for pacemaker therapy in this context is less clear. In the absence of transient AV block, postoperative bifascicular block with or without first-degree block does not warrant pacemaker therapy.

Once there is demonstration of higher degree AV block (Mobitz type II second-degree or higher) late after cardiac surgery, as was seen at 3 years of age, pacemaker therapy should be considered. The presence of asymptomatic Mobitz type II second-degree AV block with a narrow QRS complex would warrant pacemaker therapy (Class IIa) when not occurring during sleep or not thought to be vagally mediated. The presence of bifascicular block with a wide QRS, asymptomatic Mobitz type II second-degree AV block with a wide QRS, including isolated right bundle branch block, as seen at 5 years of age, would be a Class I indication for pacemaker therapy. The EP study provides further evidence for pacemaker implantation with asymptomatic second-degree AV block at intra- or infra-His levels IIA (HV > 100 ms) or if pacing-induced infra-Hisian block is seen (Class IIa).

Finally, The presence of advanced second-degree or third-degree AV blocks at any anatomic level that is associated with bradycardia and symptoms (including heart failure) or ventricular arrhythmias presumed to be due to AV block should warrant pacemaker therapy (Class I). At an age of 16 years, this patient developed episodes of symptomatic runs of polymorphic VT.

The indications for pacemaker therapy in the setting of postoperative AV conduction disturbances vary based on timing relative to surgery, symptoms, presence or absence of cardiac dysfunction or ventricular arrhythmias, and extent of conduction disease at the time a decision is undertaken. Additional factors to consider after the decision for pacemaker therapy is determined are the age and size of patient which have implications on type of device—single versus dual chamber and transvenous versus epicardial. The lack of symptoms had an impact on the parents' reluctance to proceed with pacemaker therapy but the long-term implications without therapy are clear, as demonstrated by the development of life-threatening polymorphic ventricular arrhythmias.

4. Use of antiarrhythmic drugs in patients with atrioventricular conduction disturbance

Ventricular arrhythmias in patients with postoperative AV conduction disease (advanced second-degree or third-degree AV block) after congenital heart surgery warrant immediate attention and initiation of pacemaker therapy as outlined above. The initiation of pacing can treat potential proarrhythmic factors such as bradycardia, pauses, ectopy suppression if paced at faster rates, and shortening and stability of the QT interval with uniform ventricular pacing. The use of antiarrhythmics in the setting of AV conduction disease is challenging and problematic and is thus not generally considered a first-line therapy. These agents may exacerbate AV conduction, slow the ventricular escape, induce or prolong pauses, and cause or exacerbate symptoms as a result of bradycardia, thus limiting their efficacy and potentially worsening the problem. Acutely, if temporary pacing cannot be initiated, isoproterenol can be used to increase the heart rate, minimize bradycardia, and pause-dependent events, and shorten the QT interval to reduce the risk of torsade de pointes. If after initiating pacemaker therapy, there continues to be tachyarrhythmias, identification of other substrates should be considered in postoperative congenital heart surgery patients, as medications and/or ablation may be required.

REFERENCES

1. Khairy P, et al. PACES/HRS expert consensus statement on the recognition and management of arrhythmias in adult congenital heart disease: developed in partnership between the Pediatric and Congenital Electrophysiology Society (PACES) and the Heart Rhythm Society (HRS). Endorsed by the governing bodies of PACES, HRS, the American College of Cardiology (ACC), the American Heart Association (AHA), the European Heart Rhythm Association (EHRA), the Canadian Heart Rhythm Society (CHRS), and the International Society for Adult Congenital Heart Disease (ISACHD). *Can J Cardiol.* 2014;30(10): e1−e63.

2. Anderson JB, et al. Postoperative heart block in children with common forms of congenital heart disease: results from the KID database. *J Cardiovasc Electrophysiol.* 2012; 23(12):1349−1354.

3. Gross GJ, et al. Natural history of postoperative heart block in congenital heart disease: implications for pacing intervention. *Heart Rhythm.* 2006;3(5):601−604.

4. Epstein AE, et al. ACC/AHA/HRS 2008 guidelines for device-based therapy of cardiac rhythm abnormalities: a report of the American College of Cardiology/American Heart Association Task Force on Practice Guidelines (writing committee to revise the ACC/AHA/NASPE 2002 guideline update for implantation of cardiac pacemakers and antiarrhythmia devices): developed in collaboration with the American Association for Thoracic Surgery and Society of Thoracic Surgeons. *Circulation.* 2008;117(21): e350−e408.

5. Weindling SN, et al. Duration of complete atrioventricular block after congenital heart disease surgery. *Am J Cardiol.* 1998;82(4):525–527.

6. Batra AS, et al. Late recovery of atrioventricular conduction after pacemaker implantation for complete heart block associated with surgery for congenital heart disease. *J Thorac Cardiovasc Surg.* 2003;125(6):1291–1293.

7. Bruckheimer E, et al. Late recovery of surgically-induced atrioventricular block in patients with congenital heart disease. *J Interv Card Electrophysiol.* 2002;6(2):191–195.

8. Siehr SL, et al. Incidence and risk factors of complete atrioventricular block after operative ventricular septal defect repair. *Congenit Heart Dis.* 2014;9(3):211–215.

9. Kearney, K., et al., From bradycardia to tachycardia: complete heart block. Am J Med. 128(7): p. 702–706.

10. McAnulty JH, et al. Natural history of "high-risk" bundle-branch block: final report of a prospective study. *N Engl J Med.* 1982;307(3):137–143.

11. Steinberg JS, et al. 2017 ISHNE-HRS expert consensus statement on ambulatory ECG and external cardiac monitoring/telemetry. *Heart Rhythm.* 2017;14(7): e55–e96.

12. Zipes DP, et al. Guidelines for clinical intracardiac electrophysiological and catheter ablation procedures. A report of the American College of Cardiology/American Heart Association Task Force on Practice Guidelines (Committee on Clinical Intracardiac Electrophysiologic and Catheter Ablation Procedures), developed in collaboration with the North American Society of Pacing and Electrophysiology. *J Am Coll Cardiol.* 1995;26(2): 555–573.

13. Dhingra RC, et al. The significance of second degree atrioventricular block and bundle branch block. Observations regarding site and type of block. *Circulation.* 1974;49(4): 638–646.

Consultant Opinion #2

ANDREA LEE, MD, FRCPC •
SANTABHANU CHAKRABARTI, MBBS, MD, FRCPC, FRCP (EDIN), FRCPCH, FACC, FHRS

This 15-year-old young man initially had AV node block post VSD surgery which resolved after 4 days. In follow-up, he had evidence of progressive Hisian and infra-Hisian conduction system. Postsurgical complete AV block is attributed to inflammation, hemorrhage, ischemia, necrosis, and direct disruption of AV nodal tissue. This complication is usually associated after mitral and aortic valve surgery along with VSD, Tetralogy of Fallot, and LTGA surgical procedures. Approximately, 30% of patients with postoperative AV block requires permanent pacemaker implantation.

1. **Investigations in the patient with atrioventricular conduction disturbance**

   Isolated AV conduction disturbance is rare in the pediatric population but should be suspected in certain clinical settings, as syncope and presyncope in the background of structural heart disease. Apart from congenital complete heart block and postcardiac surgery heart block, other causes include undiagnosed causes of congenital heart disease as LTGA. Acquired causes include Lyme disease, infectious mononucleosis, myocarditis, endocarditis, toxins, electrolyte disturbances, and sarcoidosis. Genetic disorders such as mitochondrial cytopathies and muscular dystrophies can also cause AV conduction delay.

   Accurate definition of AV conduction usually requires more than a standard 12-lead ECG. Sometimes a long rhythm strip with carotid sinus massage is useful, otherwise a 24–48 h Holter record or even a 7–14 days external loop recorder should be considered. For intermittent symptoms, ILR should be considered. Invasive electrophysiology (EP) study to assess the sinus and AV node and infra-Hisian conduction parameters may also be useful if there is relative urgency to establish diagnosis, especially if the presenting symptoms are profound. Once the electrophysiological diagnosis is established, further testing to the possible etiology is important

2. **Time and indications for pacemaker implant in congenital heart disease**

   The development of syncope or presyncope, heart failure or chronotropic incompetence limiting the level of physical activity justifies the implantation of a PM.[1] Therefore, focused history and examination in these patients should be taken at regular follow-up. Objective assessment with ambulatory Holter recording and exercise stress test for chronotropic incompetence is reasonable.

The risk of AV blocks is greatest for the surgical repair of ventricular septal defects and mitral/aortic valve surgery. Spontaneous resolution of complete AV block in the early postoperative period can occur, usually within 7–10 days after the operation with good prognosis for patients who develop normal conduction on ECG.[2,3]

However, residual bifascicular block persisting after the disappearance of transient postsurgical complete heart block has been associated with a high incidence of late recurrence of AV block or even sudden death.[4]

In selective patients, postoperative HV interval determination may help to assess the risk of late-onset AV block in patients with residual conduction disorder. Indications of pacing in AV block in patients with congenital heart disease are shown in Table 17.1.[1]

3. **Indications for loop-recorded implantation and electrophysiological study**

In suspected conduction system disorder in the pediatric age group, conventional diagnostic investigations may be unable to establish a diagnosis, making it difficult to determine patient risk. The ILR device is a useful tool to help unmask arrhythmias as a cause of unexplained syncope in children.[5] Data suggest that the diagnostic yield of the ILR device in unmasking the cause for symptoms in a pediatric population is approximately 64% with manually activated events accounting for 71% of all documented episodes and 68% of the cases involving hemodynamically important arrhythmias or transient rhythm changes. No long-term adverse event was associated with placement of ILR in children.[6,7]

The ILR in congenital heart disease is a useful adjunct to other diagnostic studies. Patient selection is critical as the conventional ILR should not be utilized for malignant arrhythmias but recent devices with automatic transmission capabilities (Reveal LINQ) may be considered for early notification. A firm diagnosis is expected to be available in the majority of symptomatic patients with bradyarrhythmias.[8]

Invasive EP study helps in further risk stratification in suspected conduction disorders in children allowing accurate anatomic diagnosis of conduction delay.

EP testing is rarely necessary in bradycardic patients as other modalities as event recorders, Holters and exercise testing often suffice. Differentiation of supra- or infra-Hisian conduction block with EP study has potential prognostic implication because

TABLE 17.1
Pacing Indication in Patients With Congenital Heart Disease

Recommendations	Class of Evidence	Level of Evidence
Congenital AV block: Pacemaker implantation indicated in symptomatic patients and asymptomatic patients with high risk: • Ventricular dysfunction • Long QTc • Complex ventricular ectopy • Wide QRS escape rhythm • V rate <50 bpm • V pause >three times the cycle length of underlying sinus rate	I	C
Congenital AV block: pacemaker implantation may be considered in patients without high-risk characteristics	IIB	C
Postoperative AV block: pacemaker implantation indicated in high-grade AV block or complete AV block persisting more than 10 days	I	B
Postoperative AV block: pacemaker implantation should be considered in persistent, asymptomatic bifascicular block associated with transient complete AV block	IIA	C

infra-Hisian block more often progresses to complete block and needs to be treated more aggressively. Rarely, sinus node function tests may be required with autonomic blockade in selected patients.[9] In current practice, ole of EP studies is usually to exclude a potentially treatable cause when the presenting event has been profound to allow continued monitoring in high-risk patients with other monitoring (e.g., with ILR).

4. **Use of antiarrhythmic drugs in patients with atrioventricular conduction disturbance**

Antiarrhythmic drugs should be used with utmost caution in patients with known or suspected AV conduction disturbance. These agents work by changing the conduction velocity, suppression of automaticity or alteration, the excitability of cardiac cells by alteration of the membrane ion channel conductance properties.

The AV nodal cells depend on the inward calcium ions to depolarize, hence calcium channel blockers reduce AV nodal conduction. On the other hand, β1-adrenergic blocking agents work indirectly by affecting the potassium and calcium conductance, hence should be used with utmost caution in suspected AV node conduction disorders. Sodium blockers (e.g., flecainide, propafenone) affect the infra-Hisian conduction tissues more than AV node physiology. However, muscarinic receptors such as atropine may be used to reduce vagus activity–related conduction slowness in the AV node.

Potassium blockers—Class III agents in the Vaughan-Williams-Singh classification scheme (amiodarone, dronedarone, sotalol, ibutilide, bretylium, and dofetilide) bind to and block the potassium channels that are responsible for phase III repolarization and delays repolarization. This leads to an increase in action potential duration and also increase the effective refractory period of the cell, which reflects as a QT interval prolongation on ECG.

While amiodarone and dronedarone have Class I (sodium channel blocking), II (β blocking), III and IV (calcium channel blocking) action, sotalol has only Class II and III actions.

Dofetilide is a very selective potassium blocker but ibutilide also has Class IV action, both can cause life-threatening ventricular arrhythmias.

Class IV agents block L type calcium channels especially at sino atrial and AV node and have to be used with caution with preexistent SA/AV node dysfunction. Class I agents have the potential to produce second- or third-degree AV conduction block. Quinidine, ajmaline,

disopyramide, and lidocaine induce more high-grade AV conduction block than mexiletine or procainamide. On the other hand, procainamide has more infra-Hisian conduction suppression than other Class I agents.

Digoxin results in increase of intracellular calcium, shortening of the action potential and hence increased and abnormal automaticity of all cardiac cells, potentiated by other electrolyte disturbances, especially hypokalemia. Due to the narrow therapeutic index, its propensity to produce clinical arrhythmia is relatively high and unpredictable. Unifocal or multifocal atrial and/or ventricular ectopy resulting in sustained arrhythmias may occur. Bidirectional ventricular arrhythmia can occur. On the other hand, AV nodal block can also occur.

Therefore, all antiarrhythmic agents should be used with utmost caution and judgment in patients with congenital heart disease under the supervision of appropriate specialist. Investigations to find out reversible factors and determine the etiology and location of conduction delay/block are crucial in successful management of these patients.

MANAGEMENT OF POLYMORPHIC VENTRICULAR TACHYCARDIA

This depends on the etiology of the polymorphic VT. Usual considerations include ischemia, hypoxia, electrolyte and temperature disturbance, drug toxicities, and inflammation (e.g., myocarditis). Management involves initial stabilization of the patient using ACLS protocol and administration of amiodarone for torsades des pointes, intravenous magnesium should be strongly considered while electrolyte disturbance and hypoxia are corrected. An assessment of the LV and RV ejection fractions should be made and optimized as priority.

The index patient has a relative pattern to his ventricular ectopy, which may be sometimes observed in ectopy from Purkinje fibers and is reported to have good response to hydroxyquinidine.[10]

TAKE-HOME POINTS (EDITORS)

1. Progressive or late-occurring bradyarrhythmias are an important cause of problems in ACHD.
2. "Symptoms" due to bradycardia can be vague and atypical.
3. All "symptomatic" bradycardia patients should be considered for pacemaker implantation.

REFERENCES

1. European Society of Cardiology (ESC), European Heart Rhythm Association (EHRA), Brignole M, et al. 2013 ESC guidelines on cardiac pacing and cardiac resynchronization therapy: the task force on cardiac pacing and resynchronization therapy of the European Society of Cardiology (ESC). Developed in collaboration with the European Heart Rhythm Association (EHRA). *Europace.* 2013; 15(8):1070–1118.
2. Gross GJ, Chiu CC, Hamilton RM, Kirsh JA, Stephenson EA. Natural history of postoperative heart block in congenital heart disease: implications for pacing intervention. *Heart Rhythm.* 2006;3(5):601–604.
3. Weindling SN, Saul JP, Gamble WJ, Mayer JE, Wessel D, Walsh EP. Duration of complete atrioventricular block after congenital heart disease surgery. *Am J Cardiol.* 1998; 82(4):525–527.
4. Krongrad E. Prognosis for patients with congenital heart disease and postoperative intraventricular conduction defects. *Circulation.* 1978;57(5):867–870.
5. Frangini PA, Cecchin F, Jordao L, et al. How revealing are insertable loop recorders in pediatrics? *Pacing Clin Electrophysiol.* 2008;31(3):338–343.
6. Al Dhahri KN, Potts JE, Chiu CC, Hamilton RM, Sanatani S. Are implantable loop recorders useful in detecting arrhythmias in children with unexplained syncope? *Pacing Clin Electrophysiol.* 2009;32(11): 1422–1427.
7. Kenny D, Chakrabarti S, Ranasinghe A, Chambers A, Martin R, Stuart G. Single-centre use of implantable loop recorders in patients with congenital heart disease. *Europace.* 2009;11(3):303–307.
8. Atallah J, Erickson CC, Cecchin F, et al. A multi-institutional study of implantable defibrillator lead performance in children and young adults: results of the Pediatric Lead Extractability and Survival Evaluation (PLEASE) study. *Circulation.* 2013;127(24):2393.
9. Balaji S. Indications for electrophysiology study in children. *Indian Pacing Electrophysiol J.* 2008;8(suppl 1): S32–S35.
10. Laurent G, Saal S, Amarouch MY, et al. Multifocal ectopic Purkinje-related premature contractions: a new SCN5A-related cardiac channelopathy. *J Am Coll Cardiol.* 2012; 60(2):144–156.

CHAPTER 18

Atrial Fibrillation and Thrombus in a Patient With a Fontan Circulation

Submitted by Lara Curran, MBBS, BSc, Konstantinos Dimopoulos, MD, MSc, PhD, FESC and Rafael Alonso-Gonzalez, MD, MSc, FESC

CASE SYNOPSIS

A 38-year-old gentleman presented to a routine clinic appointment describing a 4-month history of daily episodes of palpitations lasting between 10 and 20 min and declining exercise tolerance. Although he was continuing to work full time as a support worker in a care home, the severity of his symptoms meant that he was struggling to complete daily activities of living without becoming limited by breathlessness.

His background was that of situs solitus, tricuspid atresia with a rudimentary right ventricle, severe pulmonary stenosis, and normally related great vessels. When the patient was 2 months old, a right Blalock-Taussig shunt was performed, and he subsequently underwent a classic atriopulmonary Fontan at 10 years of age. During his childhood, the patient suffered from severe kyphoscoliosis, for which he underwent a spinal fusion procedure at the age of 18 years.

The patient was under regular follow-up at a specialist adult congenital heart disease (ACHD) institution and had enjoyed a long preceding period of clinical stability. During his previous clinical review, he had described symptoms consistent with New York Heart Association Class II—III. At that point, a cardiac MRI had showed reduced left ventricular function (LVEF 42%), long-standing severe right atrial dilatation, and patent Fontan pathways, without evidence of intracardiac thrombus. His regular medications included enalapril 2.5 mg twice daily and warfarin, with a target INR range between 2 and 3.

At presentation, he was found to be slightly hypotensive (95/57 mmHg) and tachycardic (120 bpm), with normal oxygen saturations (97%) measured on room air. Auscultation of his chest revealed that he was in an irregular cardiac rhythm, with a single second heart sound present and no additional murmurs audible. He had normal vesicular breath sounds and no hepatosplenomegaly or ascites were detected. There was no sign of peripheral edema and peripheral pulses were easily palpated.

An electrocardiogram performed on admission showed atrial fibrillation (AF) with fast ventricular response (120 bpm), normal axis, and a normal QRS interval (Fig. 18.1). His previous resting electrocardiogram had showed sinus rhythm with stable first-degree atrioventricular block, normal QRS interval, and signs of right atrial dilatation. In addition, a recent 48-h Holter monitor, requested prior to his clinic attendance, had not revealed any significant arrhythmias.

The patient was admitted to hospital for further evaluation, including blood pathology and imaging. His laboratory data revealed a significantly elevated BNP and a mild rise in CRP, with normal renal and liver functions (Table 18.1). A chest radiograph showed clear lung fields, with cardiomegaly due to a prominent bulging at the right heart border relating to the grossly enlarged atrium (Fig. 18.2).

Transthoracic echocardiography demonstrated a nondilated single left ventricle with moderately to severely impaired systolic function (LVEF 36%). A small rudimentary right ventricle was present, with a nonrestrictive VSD. The mitral valve was of normal function. The aortic valve was trileaflet, with no sign of significant stenosis or regurgitation. The Fontan connections were patent with low velocity, phasic flow. Of particular note, a large thrombus was detected within the severely dilated right atrium, extending from the mouth of the inferior vena cava (IVC) up to the right atrium (RA) connection (7.9 × 3.3 cm, area: 24.6 cm^2).

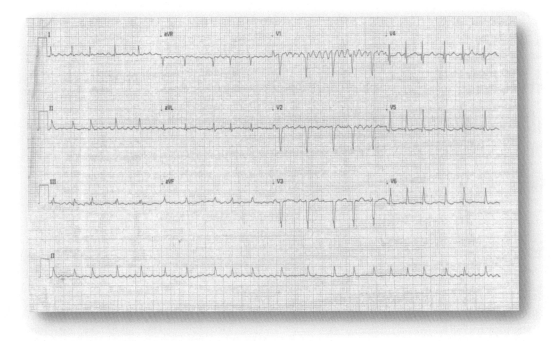

FIG. 18.1 Electrocardiogram at presentation.

TABLE 18.1
Laboratory Data Collected at Point of Admission

	Value	Normal Range
Hemoglobin (g/L)	144	[134–166]
Hematocrit (%)	45	[40–49]
MCV (fL)	88	[84–98]
MCH (pg)	28	[28.3–33.3]
Platelets (10^9/L)	205	[136–343]
WBC total (10^9/L)	6.9	[4.4–10.1]
Neutrophils (10^9/L)	4.8	[2.1–6.7]
Lymphocytes (10^9/L)	1.5	[1.3–3.7]
INR	2.5	[2–3]
Sodium (mmol/L)	134	[133–146]
Potassium (mmol/L)	4.6	[3.5–5.3]
Creatinine (μmol/L)	60	[60–120]
Bilirubin (μmol/L)	20	[<20]
ALP (U/L)	122	[30–130]
ALT (IU/L)	37	[8–40]
Total protein (g/L)	80	[60–80]
Albumin (g/L)	43	[35–50]
BNP (ng/L)	563	[<20]
CRP (mg/L)	14	[<10]

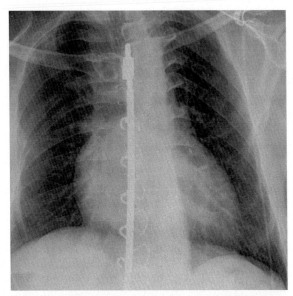

FIG. 18.2 Chest radiograph showing a spinal fixation bar in situ with slight residual thoracic scoliosis, concave to the right. There is prominence of the right heart border relating to the grossly enlarged right atrium. The lung fields are clear.

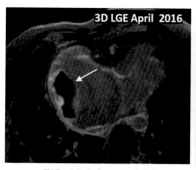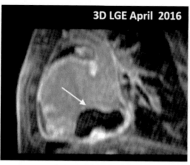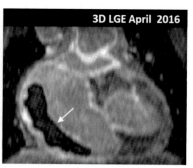

FIG. 18.3 Late gadolinium-enhanced cardiac magnetic resonance imaging showing (left to right) transverse, sagittal, and coronal views of a large thrombus (9.1 × 2.3 cm) inferiorly and anteriorly from IVC-RA connection.

A cardiac magnetic resonance (CMR) examination confirmed the presence of a large thrombus (9.1 × 2.3 cm) situated inferiorly and anteriorly from the IVC-RA connection (Fig. 18.3). The left ventricular ejection fraction was significantly reduced at 36%, a clear deterioration from the preceding CMR study (LVEF 43%). There was unobstructed flow within the Fontan connections.

Questions

1. Should an attempt be made to restore sinus rhythm in this symptomatic patient?
2. Assuming that electric cardioversion is deemed too risky, what are the pros and cons of chemical cardioversion?
3. Should one go with a rate control strategy?
4. What drugs do you recommend for rate control?
5. What anticoagulation strategy would you recommend for this clot?
6. Is he a candidate for surgery to remove the clot + convert to a newer style Fontan with a biatrial Maze?
7. If the thrombus can be made to get smaller and denser-appearing on imaging, can he be considered for cardioversion? Electric cardioversion? Or is that still too risky? What about chemical cardioversion?
8. If the thrombus can be resolved with anticoagulation, can he be considered for ablation?
9. If ablation is not an option, what would be the drug of choice for antiarrhythmic management?

Consultant Opinion #1

MADHUKAR S. KOLLENGODE, MD • DUY T. NGUYEN, MD

Since the introduction of a surgical technique to separate the systemic and pulmonary circulations in 1971 by Dr. Fontan and associates, single ventricle palliation has undergone numerous modifications.[1] The initial atriopulmonary (AP) approaches incorporated contractile right atrial tissue into the systemic venous circulation, resulting in marked RA dilation and a high burden of atrial arrhythmias. Although these approaches have been largely abandoned in favor of lateral tunnel or extracardiac conduits, the aging population of patients who underwent AP Fontan palliation means that many adult patients may have a surgical history of this type of Fontan. The ACHD specialist should be familiar with management decisions unique to these patients. This particular case presents a complex set of circumstances not infrequently seen in this population and is an important therapeutic challenge to highlight and discuss.

Thromboembolism is an important cause of late mortality in Fontan patients.[2,3] The RA dilation seen in AP Fontan patients often results in hemodynamic derangement with atrial stasis with a predisposition to thrombus development.[4] Right-sided thrombus in the setting of AF is associated with an increased risk of pulmonary embolism.[5-7] In 38% of noncongenital patients with an intracardiac thrombus, a manifest pulmonary embolism has been found.[6] Prior studies in Fontan patients have demonstrated a prevalence of 9%—33% of RA thrombus and up to 16% of asymptomatic pulmonary embolism.[6,8-10] Pulmonary embolism results in ventilation-perfusion mismatch and an elevation in pulmonary vascular resistance, both of which are deleterious to Fontan hemodynamics.[11] Thrombus within the Fontan pathway and AF are independent predictors of thromboembolic death.[2]

The first consideration in this patient with AF associated with hypotension and worsening ventricular systolic function is whether or not restoration of sinus rhythm should be attempted. AF with rapid ventricular response is poorly tolerated in patients with the Fontan circulation, where pulmonary blood flow is highly dependent on low filling pressures and diastolic filling. Therapeutic options include rate control or restoration of sinus rhythm (via pharmacologic or electric cardioversion or catheter ablation). Unfortunately, management is confounded by the presence of newly discovered RA thrombus, as restoration of sinus rhythm may result in embolization. Although electric cardioversion is more efficacious than pharmacologic cardioversion, both carry an equivalent risk of embolization and postconversion atrial stunning.[12] Regardless, isolated cardioversion without use of concurrent antiarrhythmic medications in Fontan patients is unlikely to be effective.[13] Catheter ablation of AF in Fontan patients is challenging,[4,14] and, in this case, carries additive risk of thrombus dislodgement. Thus, we do not advocate initial rhythm control strategy in this situation. We would favor temporizing with a rate control strategy with the intent to improve hemodynamics and allow recovery of systolic function, which has likely deteriorated due to tachycardia-induced cardiomyopathy. β-Blockade should be initially utilized, although dose tolerance may be limited secondary to depressed systolic function and hypotension. Alternative rate control options include digoxin or short-term low dose amiodarone (while an antiarrhythmic, the low dose of

amiodarone will have low likelihood of pharmacologic cardioversion, the risks of which are offset by its rate control properties and relative tolerance in those with severe systolic dysfunction). Calcium channel blockers are likely to be poorly tolerated.

Because this patient developed a thrombus while ostensibly on therapeutic warfarin, a review of anticoagulation strategy is warranted. Thromboprophylaxis with both aspirin and warfarin has been shown to reduce the incidence of thromboembolism in Fontan patients,[15] but there is ongoing uncertainty about which strategy is best suited for long-term therapy. In a recent single-center retrospective review of Fontan patients with atrial arrhythmias, treatment with warfarin rather than aspirin was associated with lower rates of thromboembolism.[10] We agree with the utilization of warfarin over antiplatelet therapy with aspirin in this patient. Lack of adequate intensity of anticoagulation is the primary reason for thrombosis while on therapeutic anticoagulation.[16,17] To prevent clot propagation, we recommend the utilization of high-intensity warfarin therapy (goal INR 2.5—3.5). Alternative considerations include the addition of aspirin or transition to an alternative regimen such as low-molecular-weight heparins. Although non—vitamin K oral anticoagulants (NOACs) have not been studied extensively in patients with congenital heart disease, early reports are encouraging. NOACs may have an increasing role in this population in the future.[18] There is no role for thrombolytic therapy in the absence of hemodynamic instability.

It is unlikely that the thrombus will resolve with 4—6 weeks of increased intensity of anticoagulation. **If thrombus is resolved, rhythm control with antiarrhythmic therapy and/or catheter ablation is an option.** Antiarrhythmic medications can be considered as an initial option, concurrently with electric or pharmacologic cardioversion. Vaughan Williams Class III agents are good first options. Dofetilide may be a more appealing choice than sotalol if ventricular function remains depressed, to avoid excessive negative inotropy and allow for the addition of guideline-directed medical therapy of ventricular systolic dysfunction. Amiodarone is an efficacious short-term agent, but should be avoided long-term due to toxicity. Given his impaired NYHA functional classification, ventricular dysfunction, and arrhythmias consistent with Fontan failure, dronedarone should ideally be avoided. Vaughan Williams Class Ic agents are probably best avoided in this patient with structural heart disease and poor ventricular function. Catheter ablation can also be considered. Although catheter ablation of atrial arrhythmias in Fontan patients is challenging, a focused ablative approach targeting mechanisms of AF initiation and maintenance can provide durable results.[4,19,20]

Fontan conversion with thrombus evacuation and arrhythmia surgery or cardiac transplantation should be considered in this patient with a failing Fontan as evidenced by poor functional status, depressed ventricular function, atrial arrhythmias, and poor flow dynamics. However, he has multiple risk factors for early mortality following Fontan conversion, including gender, age, abnormal hemodynamics, and presence of an intratrial thrombus.[3] Ideally, hemodynamic evaluation with heart catheterization to evaluate and optimize filling pressures would be undertaken prior to consideration of both surgical options. Attempts at rate control and medical therapy for ventricular dysfunction should be utilized and, if unsuccessful or not tolerated, then Fontan conversion with thrombus evacuation and arrhythmia surgery should be attempted.

SUMMARY

AF is associated with ventricular dysfunction, and functional deterioration in Fontan patients should be managed aggressively. Ideally, if no intracardiac thrombus is present, initial management strategies should incorporate prompt cardioversion and initiation of antiarrhythmic therapy as well as anticoagulation. Catheter ablation, either as isolated or adjunctive therapy, can be considered. The presence of an intracardiac thrombus is an important finding that precludes initial rhythm control strategies due to risk of embolism. Attempts to intensify anticoagulation for a period of 4–6 weeks, or as long as patient is stable and improving hemodynamically, and thereafter assess for thrombus resolution are reasonable; however, efforts should be made in the interim to optimize rate control and encourage ventricular functional recovery. Fontan conversion or cardiac transplantation should be considered if medical management is not tolerated or unsuccessful to allow time for thrombus resolution.

REFERENCES

1. Fontan F, Baudet E. Surgical repair of tricuspid atresia. *Thorax.* 1971;26(3):240–248. https://doi.org/10.1136/thx.26.3.240.

2. Khairy P, Fernandes SM, Mayer JE, et al. Long-term survival, modes of death, and predictors of mortality in patients with Fontan surgery. *Circulation.* 2008;117(1):85–92. https://doi.org/10.1161/CIRCULATIONAHA.107.738559.

3. Said SM, Burkhart HM, Schaff HV, et al. Fontan conversion: identifying the high-risk patient. *Ann Thorac Surg.* 2014;97(6):2115–2122. https://doi.org/10.1016/j.athoracsur.2014.01.083.

4. Deal BJ, Mavroudis C, Backer CL. Arrhythmia management in the Fontan patient. *Pediatr Cardiol.* 2007;28(6):448–456. https://doi.org/10.1007/s00246-007-9005-2.

5. Gallagher MM, Hennessy BJ, Edvardsson N, et al. Embolic complications of direct current cardioversion of atrial arrhythmias: association with low intensity of anticoagulation at the time of cardioversion. *J Am Coll Cardiol.* 2002;40(5):926–933. https://doi.org/10.1016/S0735-1097(02)02052-1.

6. Ogren M, Bergqvist D, Eriksson H, Lindblad B, Sternby NH. Prevalence and risk of pulmonary embolism in patients with intracardiac thrombosis: a population-based study of 23,796 consecutive autopsies. *Eur Heart J.* 2005;26(11):1108–1114. https://doi.org/10.1093/eurheartj/ehi130.

7. Lafuente-Lafuente C, Mouly S, Long?s-Tejero MA, et al. Antiarrhythmic drugs for maintaining sinus rhythm after cardioversion of atrial fibrillation. *Arch Intern Med.* 2006;166(7):719. https://doi.org/10.1001/archinte.166.7.719.

8. Varma C, Warr MR, Hendler AL, Paul NS, Webb GD, Therrien J. Prevalence of "silent" pulmonary emboli in adults after the Fontan operation. *J Am Coll Cardiol.* 2003;41(12):2252–2258. https://doi.org/10.1016/S0735-1097(03)00490-X.

9. Balling G, Vogt M, Kaemmerer H, Eicken A, Meisner H, Hess J. Intracardiac thrombus formation after the Fontan operation. *J Thorac Cardiovasc Surg.* 2000;119(4 Pt 1):745–752. https://doi.org/10.1067/mtc.2000.104866.

10. Egbe AC, Connolly HM, McLeod CJ, et al. Thrombotic and embolic complications associated with atrial arrhythmia after Fontan operation: role of prophylactic therapy. *J Am Coll Cardiol.* 2016;68(12):1312–1319. https://doi.org/10.1016/j.jacc.2016.06.056.

11. Balling G. Fontan anticoagulation: a never-ending debate? *J Am Coll Cardiol.* 2016;68(12):1320–1322. https://doi.org/10.1016/j.jacc.2016.06.050.

12. Van Gelder IC, Tuinenburg AE, Schoonderwoerd BS, Tieleman RG, Crijns HJG. Pharmacologic versus direct-current electrical cardioversion of atrial flutter and fibrillation. *Am J Cardiol.* 1999;84(9):147–151. https://doi.org/10.1016/S0002-9149(99)00715-8.

13. Egbe AC, Connolly HM, Niaz T, McLeod CJ. Outcome of direct current cardioversion for atrial arrhythmia in adult Fontan patients. *Int J Cardiol.* 2016;2016(208):115–119. https://doi.org/10.1016/j.ijcard.2016.01.209.

14. Deal BJ, Jacobs ML. Education in Heart. Management of the failing Fontan circulation. *Heart.* 2012;98:1098–1104. https://doi.org/10.1136/heartjnl-2011-301133.

15. Viswanathan S. Thromboembolism and anticoagulation after Fontan surgery. *Ann Pediatr Cardiol.* 2016;9(3): 236−240. https://doi.org/10.4103/0974-2069.189109.
16. Kyrle PA. How I treat recurrent deep-vein thrombosis. *Blood.* 2017;127(6):696−703. https://doi.org/10.1182/blood-2015-09-671297.modi.
17. McCrindle BW, Manlhiot C, Cochrane A, et al. Factors associated with thrombotic complications after the Fontan procedure: a secondary analysis of a multicenter, randomized trial of primary thromboprophylaxis for 2 years after the Fontan procedure. *J Am Coll Cardiol.* 2013;61(3): 346−353. https://doi.org/10.1016/j.jacc.2012.08.1023.
18. Pujol C, Niesert A-C, Engelhardt A, et al. Usefulness of direct oral anticoagulants in adult congenital heart disease. *Am J Cardiol.* 2016;117(3):450−455. https://doi.org/10.1016/j.amjcard.2015.10.062.
19. Ruckdeschel ES, Kay J, Sauer WH, Nguyen DT. Atrial fibrillation ablation without pulmonary vein isolation in a patient with Fontan palliation. *Card Electrophysiol Clin.* 2016;8(1):161−164. https://doi.org/10.1016/j.ccep.2015.10.018.
20. Szili-Torok T, Kornyei L, Jordaens LJ. Transcatheter ablation of arrhythmias associated with congenital heart disease. *J Interv Card Electrophysiol.* 2008;22(2):161−166. https://doi.org/10.1007/s10840-007-9198-6.

Consultant Opinion #2

SRUTI RAO, MD • PETER F. AZIZ, MD

DIAGNOSIS

The patient is in AF with rapid ventricular response that is causing hemodynamic instability as evidenced by new-onset hypotension and tachycardia.

Risk factors for development of atrial arrhythmia:

Risk factors for atrial tachyarrhythmia in this patient include severe, long-standing right atrial dilation, decreased left ventricular function (LVEF 42%), and the presence of a classic atriopulmonary Fontan.

Other potential risk factors for the development of atrial tachyarrhythmias in a Fontan include preoperative bradycardia, sinus node dysfunction, older age at Fontan, longer postoperative interval, greater than mild atrioventricular valve regurgitation, and heterotaxy syndrome.[1]

INCIDENCE AND PREVALENCE OF ATRIAL ARRHYTHMIAS

The incidence of atrial arrhythmias is 60% in an atriopulmonary Fontan and 12% in an extracardiac Fontan. Atrial reentrant tachycardias compose 75% of all the supraventricular tachycardias with focal tachycardias seen in up to 15% of the patients. The most common mechanism of the tachyarrhythmia is a macroreentrant circuit in the atria, also known as atrial flutter/intraatrial reentrant tachycardia.[1]

MEDICAL MANAGEMENT OF ARRHYTHMIA

AF is not well tolerated in the Fontan circulation and all measures must be taken to restore sinus rhythm due to the risk of sudden hemodynamic compromise of the lone systemic ventricle. The presence of a large atrial thrombus with right to left shunting at the atrial level increases the risk of a cerebrovascular accidents from embolic phenomena. Hence rhythm control and cardioversion are not attractive options. Preventing rapid ventricular response by rate control can be achieved by AV node blocking agents.[2] Drugs that increase the AV nodal refractoriness include β-blockers, non−dihydropyridine calcium channel blockers, and digoxin. From the results of the AFFIRM study, β-blockers were more successful than calcium channel blockers in achieving rate control when used alone or in combination with digoxin.[3] β-Blockers can be additionally helpful in those with coronary artery disease and congestive heart failure, in combination with digoxin.[4] However, prospective studies comparing the relative efficacy of a calcium channel blocker and a β-blocker in achieving rate control in ED patients with rapid ventricular rate from AF found diltiazem to be more effective than metoprolol.[5] Limitations of the study include the fact that this study was underpowered.

Class IC agents (flecainide) or Class III agents (ibutilide and dofetilide) have also been used but are not very effective as rate control agents. There has been some hesitation to implement flecainide because of the results of the CAST I trial in patients with reduced ejection fraction.[6] The study concluded that premature ventricular complex suppression in the immediate post-MI period was associated with a higher mortality rate when compared with the placebo group. However, the results were inappropriately extrapolated to patients in more chronic settings such as nonischemic cardiomyopathy and supraventricular tachycardias that have led to physician reluctance to use this medication. As Class Ic agents can lead to higher ventricular rates by converting AF to atrial flutter and subsequently slowing the flutter rate to allow for 1:1 AV conduction, these agents are often given in combination with AV nodal slowing agents such as β-blockers. Intravenous amiodarone used as a slow infusion can achieve rate control in critically ill patients when used in the acute setting. Dofetilide is another Class III antiarrhythmic agent that has been widely used in the adult population with persistent AF/atrial flutter. The Pediatric and Congenital Electrophysiology Society/Heart Rhythm society (PACES/HRS) expert consensus statement on atrial arrhythmia in ACHD recommends its use as a first line alternative to amiodarone.[6] It is also used as a second-line antiarrhythmic agent in individuals with severe ventricular dysfunction and hence can be used in our patient as long as it is administered in a closely supervised setting provided meticulous monitoring of electrolytes, including renal function is performed to prevent adverse effects such as torsades de pointes and ventricular arrhythmias.[7–9] A recent PACES collaborative study by El-Assaad et al. showed that out of a total of 64 patients with congenital heart disease with AF/Afib, 49% remained on dofetilide with adequate or partial rhythm control.[10]

MANAGING A LARGE INTRAATRIAL THROMBUS

After achieving rate control, management of the intraatrial thrombus must be undertaken. Because the thrombus is large, surgical removal of the thrombus/thrombectomy is favored. In the study by Tsang et al., 68% of patients had tricuspid atresia who underwent surgical thrombectomy.[11] In this study, patients who were hemodynamically stable at the time of surgery had a lower mortality rate when compared with the hemodynamically unstable group. Our patient was hemodynamically stable at presentation. Hence he would have better outcomes with an elective rather than emergent thrombectomy.

THE CONCEPT OF "FONTAN CONVERSION"

The development of late arrhythmias in the Fontan is not only due to a rhythm problem but more of an electromechanical problem. Hence early Fontan conversion rather than isolated treatment of the arrhythmia with medication and/or ablation is warranted to prevent deterioration to the point of listing for cardiac transplantation.[12] The Fontan conversion consists of revision to an extracardiac total cavopulmonary connection, right atrial reduction, and performance of a biatrial maze. Factors such as the presence of a right atrial thrombus at the time of surgery and older age at Fontan conversion increase the risk for failure. Fontan conversions have better success rates when performed in nonemergent conditions after achieving hemodynamic stability.

The right atrial maze procedure as part of the Fontan conversion is done to eliminate the possibility of a right atrial macroreentrant tachycardia (atrial flutter) in the future. The presence of AF warrants an additional left atrial Cox Maze III, which consists of pulmonary vein isolation by an encircling lesion, left atrial appendage excision, and placing a cryoablation lesion connecting the base of the resected appendage to the encircling pulmonary vein lesion.[1] Despite long-term predictors for Maze failure such as arrhythmia duration prior to the procedure and increased size of the left or single atrium (atrial size >6 cm) as seen in our patient,[13–15] we would advocate for a left atrial Maze, as numerous studies have shown improvement in NYHA functional classification post-Fontan conversion, with reduction in the recurrence of atrial arrhythmias.[1,16–18] An 80% freedom from recurrence was observed at 5-year follow-up among patients undergoing Fontan.[1]

There is also an increased prevalence of atrioventricular block, either due to intrinsic conduction abnormalities or damage to the conduction system for which we could consider implantation of an epicardial pacemaker system at the time of Fontan conversion to avoid the morbidity associated with a repeat sternotomy, difficult venous access to the atrium, and the risk of endocardial lead thrombosis.[19,20]

Tsao et al. described the success of dual chamber antitachycardia pacemaker with bipolar steroid eluting epicardial leads and excellent device longevity in Fontan patients at the time of Fontan conversion based on an experience with 120 cases[1]. Hence the pacemaker system can also be used to treat commonly encountered rhythm issues such as sinus node dysfunction, provide antitachycardia pacing, and prevent bradycardia-induced tachycardia syndromes.

CONCLUSION

Management of atrial tachyarrhythmias in Fontan patients provides a unique challenge to the pediatric and adult congenital electrophysiologist.

Acute stabilization of this patient consisting of rate control, heart failure management, and anticoagulation takes precedence before attempting surgical thrombectomy and Fontan conversion.

TAKE-HOME POINTS (EDITORS)

1. All patients with ACHD and AF, atrial flutter, or intraatrial reentrant tachycardia should undergo transthoracic and transesophageal echocardiography to rule out a thrombus prior to cardioversion.
2. In patients with Fontan operation presenting with AF, flutter, or IART, the search for an intracardiac thrombus should be performed regardless of the duration of the arrhythmia and prior anticoagulant therapy.
3. Fontan patients with a large intracardiac thrombus should be considered for surgical removal of the thrombus. Conversion to a newer style Fontan can be combined with the thrombectomy operation.

REFERENCES

1. Deal BJ, Jacobs ML. Management of the failing Fontan circulation. *Heart.* 2012;98:1098–1104.
2. Heist EK, Mansour M, Ruskin JN. Rate control in atrial fibrillation: targets, methods, resynchronization considerations. *Circulation.* 2011;124:2746–2755.
3. Olshansky B, Rosenfeld LE, Warner AL, et al. The Atrial Fibrillation Follow-up Investigation of Rhythm Management (AFFIRM) study: approaches to control rate in atrial fibrillation. *J Am Coll Cardiol.* 2004;43:1201–1208.
4. Khand AU, Rankin AC, Martin W, Taylor J, Gemmell I, Cleland JG. Carvedilol alone or in combination with digoxin for the management of atrial fibrillation in patients with heart failure? *J Am Coll Cardiol.* 2003;42: 1944–1951.
5. Demircan C, Cikriklar HI, Engindeniz Z, et al. Comparison of the effectiveness of intravenous diltiazem and metoprolol in the management of rapid ventricular rate in atrial fibrillation. *Emerg Med J.* 2005;22:411–414.
6. Echt DS, Liebson PR, Mitchell LB, et al. Mortality and morbidity in patients receiving encainide, flecainide, or placebo. *New Engl J Med.* 1991;324:781–788.
7. Khairy P, Van Hare GF, Balaji S, et al. PACES/HRS expert consensus statement on the recognition and management of arrhythmias in adult congenital heart disease: developed in partnership between the Pediatric and Congenital Electrophysiology Society (PACES) and the Heart Rhythm Society (HRS). Endorsed by the governing bodies of PACES, HRS, the American College of Cardiology (ACC), the American Heart Association (AHA), the European Heart Rhythm Association (EHRA), the Canadian Heart Rhythm Society (CHRS), and the International Society for Adult Congenital Heart Disease (ISACHD). *Can J Cardiol.* 2014;30: e1–e63.
8. Singh S, Zoble RG, Yellen L, et al. Efficacy and safety of oral dofetilide in converting to and maintaining sinus rhythm in patients with chronic atrial fibrillation or atrial flutter: the symptomatic atrial fibrillation investigative research on dofetilide (SAFIRE-D) study. *Circulation.* 2000;102: 2385–2390.
9. Norgaard BL, Wachtell K, Christensen PD, et al. Efficacy and safety of intravenously administered dofetilide in acute termination of atrial fibrillation and flutter: a multicenter, randomized, double-blind, placebo-controlled trial. Danish Dofetilide in Atrial Fibrillation and Flutter Study Group. *Am Heart J.* 1999;137: 1062–1069.
10. El-Assaad I, Al-Kindi SG, Abraham J, et al. Use of dofetilide in adult patients with atrial arrhythmias and congenital heart disease: a PACES collaborative study. *Heart Rhythm.* 2016;13:2034–2039.
11. Tsang W, Johansson B, Salehian O, et al. Intracardiac thrombus in adults with the Fontan circulation. *Cardiol Young.* 2007;17:646–651.
12. Deal BJ, Mavroudis C, Backer CL. Arrhythmia management in the Fontan patient. *Pediatr Cardiol.* 2007;28:448–456.
13. Gaynor SL, Schuessler RB, Bailey MS, et al. Surgical treatment of atrial fibrillation: predictors of late recurrence. *J Thorac Cardiovasc Surg.* 2005;129:104–111.
14. Gillinov AM, Sirak J, Blackstone EH, et al. The Cox maze procedure in mitral valve disease: predictors of recurrent atrial fibrillation. *J Thorac Cardiovasc Surg.* 2005;130: 1653–1660.
15. Kawaguchi AT, Kosakai Y, Isobe F, et al. Factors affecting rhythm after the maze procedure for atrial fibrillation. *Circulation.* 1996;94:Ii139–i142.
16. Mavroudis C, Deal BJ, Backer CL, Johnsrude CL. The favorable impact of arrhythmia surgery on total cavopulmonary artery Fontan conversion. *Semin Thorac Cardiovasc Surg Pediatr Card Surg Annu.* 1999;2:143–156.

17. Mavroudis C, Deal BJ, Backer CL. The beneficial effects of total cavopulmonary conversion and arrhythmia surgery for the failed Fontan. *Semin Thorac Cardiovasc Surg Pediatr Card Surg Annu.* 2002;5:12—24.

18. Hiramatsu T, Iwata Y, Matsumura G, Konuma T, Yamazaki K. Impact of Fontan conversion with arrhythmia surgery and pacemaker therapy. *Eur J Cardiothorac Surg.* 2011;40:1007—1010.

19. Figa FH, McCrindle BW, Bigras JL, Hamilton RM, Gow RM. Risk factors for venous obstruction in children with transvenous pacing leads. *Pacing Clin Electrophysiol.* 1997;20:1902—1909.

20. Gillette PC, Zeigler V, Bradham GB, Kinsella P. Pediatric transvenous pacing: a concern for venous thrombosis? *Pacing Clin Electrophysiol.* 1988;11:1935—1939.

Index

Note: Page numbers followed by "f" indicate figures, "t" indicate tables.

Printed in the United States
By Bookmasters